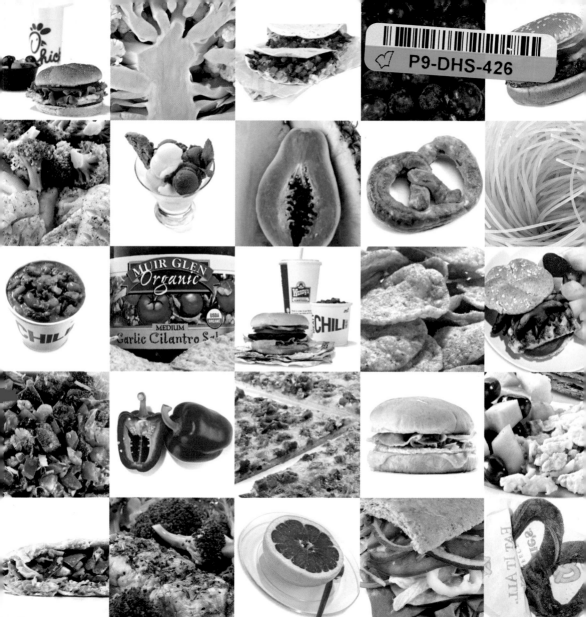

EAT THIS NOT THAT!

The Best (& Worst!) Foods in America!

BY DAVID ZINCZENKO
WITH MATT GOULDING

RODALE

Eat This, Not That! is a registered trademark of Rodale Inc.
© 2009 by Rodale Inc.

All rights reserved. No part of this publication may be reproduced or transmitted in any form
or by any means, electronic or mechanical, including photocopying, recording, or any other information storage
and retrieval system, without the written permission of the publisher.

Rodale books may be purchased for business or promotional use or for special sales. For information, please write to:
Special Markets Department, Rodale Inc., 733 Third Avenue, New York, NY 10017

Printed in the United States of America

Rodale Inc. makes every effort to use acid-free ♾, recycled paper ♻.

Book design by George Karabotsos

Cover photographs by Jeff Harris. Food styling by Susan Sugarman. Hand model: Ashly Covington.
All interior photos by Mitch Mandel and Thomas MacDonald/Rodale Images,
with the exception of the following: pages 37 through 61: Kevin Cooley; pages 256 through 259: Jeff Harris; page 316:
© Brett Danton/StockFood Munich (celeriac); page 318: © Williams/StockFood UK (açai berries), © Image 100
(alligator), © Image Source (fenugreek); page 320: © Ellert/StockFood Munich (kamut), © Peter Rees/StockFood
Munich (goldenberries), © Spathis Miller/Foodpix (jicama); page 322: © Image Source (mung beans), © Elizabeth Watt/
Foodpix (sardines), © Dorling Kindersley/Getty Images (sunchokes); page 324: © Dorling Kindersley/Getty Images
(sweet-potato leaves), © Anthony Masterson/Digital Vision (watercress); page 325: © Renee Comet Photography/
StockFood (pork chop), © Dorling Kindersley/Getty Images (iceberg lettuce), © Digital Vision/Getty Images
(mushrooms/Swiss cheese), © Corbis/Jupiter Images (vinegar), © Photos.com/Jupiter Images (red-pepper flakes)

Library of Congress Cataloging-in-Publication Data is on file with the publisher.
ISBN-10 1-60529-461-6 paperback
ISBN-13 978-1-60529-461-2 paperback

Distributed to the trade by Macmillan
2 4 6 8 10 9 7 5 3 1 paperback

RODALE
LIVE YOUR WHOLE LIFE™

ACKNOWLEDGMENTS

This book is the product of thousands of meals, hundreds of conversations with nutritionists and industry experts, and the collective smarts, dedication, and raw talent of dozens of individuals. Our undying thanks to all of you who have inspired this project in any way. In particular:

Steve Murphy, who captains the ship called Rodale Inc. with grace, courage, and remarkable vision. Thanks for continuing to make this the best publishing company on the planet.

The Rodale family, whose dedication to improving the lives and well-being of their readers is apparent in every book and magazine they put their name on.

George Karabotsos, whose vision and design savvy has once again turned a jumble of words and numbers into something that's impossible to put down.

Stephen Perrine, with whom we've conferred over many a fast-food lunch and who never met an exclamation point he didn't like.

Clint Carter, whose heroic efforts help make sense out of a daunting database of numbers, ingredients, and bogus label claims.

Allison Falkenberry, whose tremendous talent and dedication has helped spread the *Eat This, Not That!* message to millions of people.

The entire *Men's Health* editorial staff: a smarter, more inspiring group of writers, editors, researchers, designers, and photo directors does not exist, in the magazine world or beyond.

To the Rodale book team: Karen Rinaldi, Chris Krogermeier, Nancy Bailey, Sara Cox, Tara Long, Mitch Mandel, Tom MacDonald, Troy Schnyder, Melissa Reiss, Nikki Webber, Jennifer Giandomenico, Wendy Gable, Keith Biery, Liz Krenos, Brooke Myers, Marc Sirinsky, Sean Sabo, and Caroline McCall. Your extraordinary sacrifices of time and sanity brought another project to reality in record time.

Special thanks to: Carolyn Kylstra, Anna Maltby, Sophie Fitzgerald, Brett LeVecchio, Mark Michaelson, Laura White, and Adam Campbell. You guys make these books possible.

And to the people who matter most to us in this world: Sorry for all the talk about calorie counts.

—Dave and Matt

CONTENTS

Meet the Good Guys

Batman and the Joker.
Obi-Wan Kenobi and Darth Vader.
Harry Potter and Lord Voldemort.

Whether your tale takes place in a modern city, a distant galaxy, or a castle straight out of medieval England, great stories all share one simple element: good guys versus bad guys. The world's stage is filled with bit players and middle-of-the-road characters, but it's the heroes and the villains that make an adventure come to life.

Well, in these pages, you're going to meet lots and lots of villains. But only one character has the chance to be the hero: you.

That's because the book that you hold in your hands is something different from a traditional diet book. It's not a book designed for reading; it's a book designed for *using*. It's a book you can use in the aisles of your local supermarket, behind the wheel at your regular drive-thru window, or even at the tables of your favorite chain restaurant. If you're going to be the hero of your own personal weight loss story, you don't need a book. You need a secret weapon, an insider's advantage, a magic decoder ring for your daily meals.

Well, this *is* your secret weapon. You can use it to strip away belly fat; build lean, firm muscle; and look and feel fitter and healthier than you have in years.

And you can achieve all of that without putting yourself on a diet!

(and the Bad Guys)

The Secret to Eating Well

The first thing you need to know is that smart eating is much easier than it seems. See, most of the foods you eat during the day are relatively good for you. (Indeed, as you'll see in these pages, even a lot of what's offered at places like McDonald's, Burger King, and KFC fits in just fine with a sensible eating plan.) But some foods are so bad for you—so laden with fat, calories, sodium, and other nutritional land mines—that letting them slip into your diet can completely destroy your weight loss goals.

The result? Your weight begins to climb, so you swear off the foods you love, spend hours slogging along on the treadmill or stair climber, and start wondering whether you're actually going to live longer—or if your life is just going to seem longer!

But no matter how hard you work or how much you deny yourself, the fact is you don't have control. All you have to do is unwittingly eat one or two of these bad guys and guess what? Up goes your weight again like a balloon at the Macy's Thanksgiving Day Parade.

Well, it's time to stop the cycle. We've used the latest nutritional research and countless hours scouring the menus and nutrition labels of American restaurants and supermarkets to identify the really bad guys on the nutritional landscape—those trouble-packing toughs who make every trip to the supermarket or the local eatery a perilous adventure. Indeed, given how nutritionally damaging some of today's food can be, it seems easier to fight your way through the bar scene in the original *Star Wars* than to tackle the dangerous, devious, and downright damnable deceptions that can be found on today's food labels and dinner menus.

INTRODUCTION

Does that sound a little extreme? Maybe, but so are the food hazards awaiting you and your family at the drive-thru, along the supermarket aisles, or at your favorite sit-down restaurant chain. It sometimes seems as though today's food manufacturers are on a mission to fill your body with as many cheap, empty calories as possible, and they'll use any trick in the book to make that happen—supersizing your belly and damaging your health in the process. Consider this:

- You try to start your day right, so you pour a bowl of Quaker 100% Natural Granola Oats, Honey & Raisins. But that good-for-you-sounding cereal actually packs more sugar than a bowl of Cocoa Pebbles—and as many calories as eight chicken wings.

- You want a smart lunch, so at Blimpie you order the Veggie Supreme sandwich. (Sounds healthy, right?) You've just snarfed down a very unhealthy 1,106 calories—more calories than two Big Macs!

- Maybe a seemingly good-for-you frozen dinner would be better, but no: A Healthy Choice Complete Meals Sweet & Sour Chicken dinner will give you a "healthy" dose . . . of sugar. It's got more sugar than two scoops of Breyers All Natural Chocolate Crackle ice cream.

- What about dessert? Romano's Macaroni Grill Dessert Ravioli has as many calories—1,630—as four Quarter Pounders and more than half a day's allotment of sodium!

These crimes against nutritional sanity are exactly why we've written this book. Because you shouldn't have to worry about picking your way through your favorite restaurant or supermarket, concerned that all your attempts at eating smartly and healthfully might be undermined by a single sandwich that contains more than half of a day's calories, or a granola cereal with more sugar than a bowl of Cocoa Pebbles, or a kid's meal that could feed an entire third-grade classroom.

Now you don't have to.

Join the Food Revolution!

What you have in your hands here is a proven weapon against the fat-, salt-, and calorie-laden foodstuffs lurking in today's marketplace. Since the publication of the original *Eat This, Not That!* in 2007, more than 2 million people have bought copies of our books. More than 40 million people have explored our Web site (EatThis.com). And more than 600,000 have signed up to receive our free weekly newsletter.

The response from America's consumers? Terrific. Tens of thousands of e-mails and posts on our Web site testify to how *Eat This, Not That!* has made food shopping and restaurant ordering easier than ever and how simple it's been for people just like you to shed 10, 20, 30 pounds or more—without ever dieting again.

And the response from America's food marketers? Well, um . . . they haven't been amused. The companies that manufacture and sell the majority of supermarket and restaurant foods spend billions of dollars a year researching ways to trick your taste buds into craving more of their products. And they spend $30 billion more on advertisements designed to make you and your children think you can't be happy/cool/emotionally fulfilled unless you're cramming as much of their stuff into your face as possible. So when we launched the *Eat This, Not That!* movement to call them out on it? Let's just say our e-mail and voice mail were pretty jammed with angry, sometimes threatening messages.

But then a funny thing started to happen: As more and more people began demanding nutritional information from their favorite restaurants and started looking for alternatives to the most nutritionally unsound foods lurking in the supermarket aisles, a lot of America's food manufacturers and marketers started to change their ways. For example:

● Shortly after we named the Baskin-Robbins Heath Shake the Unhealthiest Drink in America—a title it earned by packing in 2,310 calories and an elephantine 108 grams of fat—the company quietly removed that nutritional disaster from its menu.

- Chili's removed the Awesome Blossom from their menu, after we argued it should be called the Awful Blossom thanks to the terrifying 2,710 calories and more than 6,000 milligrams of sodium it contained. (That's about three times as much sodium as you should be getting a day! And that was an appetizer!)

- After we bestowed upon Jamba Juice's Chocolate Moo'd Smoothie the dubious distinction of being one of the worst drinks in America, they retracted the 900-calorie glorified milk shake from their menu and went about adding a handful of healthier, legitimate smoothies.

- Romano's Macaroni Grill used to serve a 1,210-calorie portion of Double Macaroni 'n' Cheese as a kids' meal. We took them to task on it over the years and they finally downsized to a single mac with a more reasonable (but still unsettling) 670 calories.

Indeed, since we published our original list of the 20 Worst Foods in America, 10 of them—fully half!—have been substantially altered or discontinued entirely. And many more restaurants—including Red Lobster, Olive Garden, and Quiznos—have begun posting nutritional information on their Web sites, something many restaurants refused to do, until we called them out.

Become a Weight Loss Superhero

Sure, we've made an impact on the nutritional landscape, pushing aside some really terrible foods and empowering people to eat better than ever. But that doesn't mean our job is done. No, not by a long shot. Because even while supermarkets, restaurant chains, and other food purveyors have seen what happens when educated eaters vote with their wallets, they've been heading back to the food labs—cooking up new recipes, tinkering with existing formulas, and using every trick in the book to find new ways to fool our taste buds into making fattening and unhealthy choices.

And remember: They don't necessarily care about your family, your health, or your waistline. They care most about your wallet. It's no wonder, then, that:

- Two-thirds of US adults are now overweight. In fact, the obesity rate has increased by almost 50 percent since 1960. A lot of that damage is due to the "Worst" foods you'll find in the coming pages. And a lot of it can be undone simply by choosing the "Best."

- Traditional foods that our parents ate have now been supersized—calories and all! A bag of potato chips and a soda now pack 142 more calories than they did when your parents were dating. Eat that on a daily basis and after 1 year, you'd weigh 15 pounds more than Mom or Dad did when they were eating the same food!

- The health condition most directly tied to obesity—diabetes—now eats up one in five dollars Americans spend on health care. (Indeed, several years ago doctors eliminated the term adult-onset diabetes, because for the first time, our children are coming down with the disease!)

- A study from the University of North Carolina found that we consume 222 additional calories a day from beverages than we did 37 years ago. That's enough to add an extra 23 pounds a year onto our frames!

- In an effort to produce cheaper, tastier, longer-lasting foods, marketers are adding new types of preservatives, fats, sugars, and other foodlike substances to our daily meals. There are more than 3,000 substances on the FDA's list of "safe" food additives, and any one (or 20) could be in your next meal.

But now you have the power to fight back. Now you can eat smart, eat healthy, and eat well and still lose all the weight you want. You don't have to diet, or spend hours at the gym, or limit your food choices to wilted lettuce and cottage cheese. All you need is the ability to avoid the bad guys and make the smart choices in any eating situation.

You have the power to be the hero of your own weight loss story. And the power is right here in your hands. Why not turn the page?

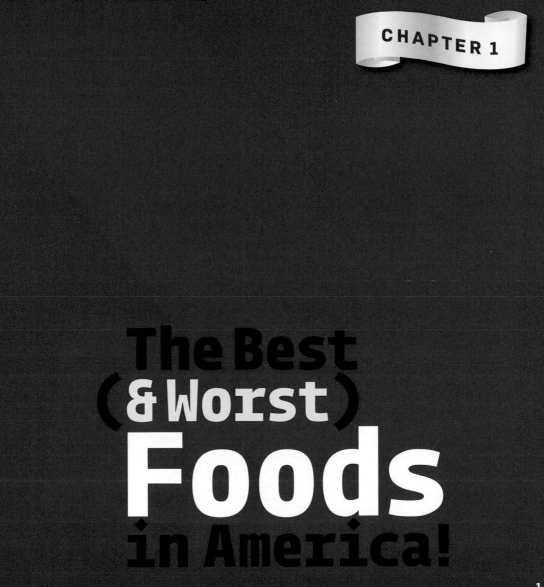

CHAPTER 1

The Best (& Worst) Foods in America!

Eat This

Ruby Tuesday Peppercorn Mushroom Sirloin

with Premium Baby Green Beans

468 calories
21 g fat
18 g carbohydrates

Save more than 1,700 calories!
Strip away half a pound of fat from your diet by simply switching steaks.

Save 71 g fat!
That's 5 Snickers bars' worth of the bad stuff.

Not That!

Chili's Fajita Quesadillas Beef

with Rice and Beans, 4 flour tortillas, and condiments

2,240 calories
92 g fat
(43.5g saturated)
6,390 mg sodium
253 g carbs

A bona fide condiment catastrophe. The tortillas and toppings add 690 calories to your fajita platter.

Think sizzling meat and vegetables make for a decent dinner? Think again. These Tex-Mex fat-traps contain a full day's worth of calories and 277 percent of your recommended daily intake of sodium.

3

It doesn't matter how religiously you diet.

It doesn't matter how intensely you exercise.

It doesn't matter if you try to make the smartest choices, pick the healthiest foods, and watch what you eat at every meal.

It doesn't matter, because in America's restaurants, fast-food joints, and grocery aisles, all it takes to sabotage your weight loss goals is one simple mistake.

Today's food marketers have loaded many of their offerings with so much fat, sugar, and sodium that any single food in this chapter can destroy all your hard work and best intentions. Welcome any one of these nutritional neutron bombs into your diet just once a month—let me repeat that, just once a month!— and you could add nearly 7 pounds of flab to your frame in the coming year.

Sure, some of them may seem obvious:

Anything that goes by the name Double Trouble Brownie Sundae at least earns points for giving consumers fair warning. But the terrible, troublesome tour-de-fats in this chapter mostly sound like wholesome fare— the kind you might make for your family, the kind your mom made for hers. Banana pancakes, veggie sandwiches, tuna melts, heck, even a salad! How bad could they be?

The truth is enough to make your jaw drop. And then to make you want to close your jaw back up quickly and swear to never, ever let any of these foods past your lips again.

Meet the Terrible 20

When we first launched *Eat This, Not That!*, we knew we'd encounter some pretty horrific crimes against America's waistlines. But we had no idea we'd be confronted with an appetizer—let me say that again, an appetizer! —that carries the caloric

2,580 calories
Outback Steakhouse Baby Back Ribs

Here's a typical scenario at Outback: Split the Aussie Cheese Fries to start; nosh on free bread and a house salad next; order the ribs with a sweet potato; finish by spliting a slice of cheesecake. The damage? 5,525 calories. Ouch.

equivalent of 13 Krispy Kreme original glazed doughnuts. The 2,710-calorie Awesome Blossom was one of the center-pieces of Chili's national chain restaurant menu. But when we revealed how insanely bad for you this giant, fat-fried onion really was, Chili's did the right thing: They banished the blossom from their restaurants.

Indeed, from our original list of Unhealthiest Foods in America, fully half have either been shown the kitchen door entirely or been substantially altered to be more in line with reasonable edible expectations. But the more things change, the more they stay the same: Food marketers are back with plenty more ways to wallop your waistline.

And we're back to give you the tools to protect yourself and your family —and lose the weight you want without giving up your favorite foods!

WORST KIDS' MEAL
20 Chili's Pepper Pals Little Chicken Crispers
with Ranch Dressing and Homestyle Fries

- *1,110 calories*
- *82 g fat (15 g saturated)*
- *1,980 mg sodium*
- *56 g carbohydrates*

Most kids, if given the choice, would live on chicken fingers for the duration of their adolescent lives. If those chicken fingers happened to come from Chili's, it might be a pretty short life. A moderately active 8-year-old boy should eat around 1,600 calories a day. This single meal plows through 75 percent of that allotment. So unless he plans to eat carrots and celery sticks for the rest of the day (and we know he doesn't), find a healthier chicken alternative.

Eat This Instead!
Pepper Pals Grilled Chicken Platter with Cinnamon Apples
- *340 calories • 8 g fat (2.5 g saturated)*
- *755 mg sodium • 38 g carbohydrates*

WORST SUPERMARKET MEAL
19 Stouffer's White Meat Chicken Pot Pie (large)

- *1,160 calories*
- *66 g fat (26 g saturated)*
- *1,780 mg sodium*

Whether ordered in restaurants or eaten straight from the microwave, potpies are seriously problematic. Why? The flaky, oil-strewn crust and the viscous, cream-based filling, to start with. Stouffer's creation suffers because of its size, packing within its carbo-walls as much saturated fat as you'll find in 6 scoops of Breyers All Natural Butter Almond ice cream.

Eat This Instead!
Stouffer's Grilled Herb Chicken
- *250 calories • 6 g fat (1 g saturated)*
- *740 mg sodium*

WORST "HEALTHY" SANDWICH
18 Blimpie Special Vegetarian (12")

- *1,186 calories*
- *60 g fat (19 g saturated)*
- *3,532 mg sodium*
- *131 g carbohydrates*

Sure, a Special Vegetarian sandwich sounds healthy, but

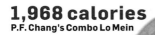

1,968 calories
P.F. Chang's Combo Lo Mein

Traditional ordering strategy dictates that each customer order his or her own entrée, but if you follow that strategy at Chang's, you'll float away on a tide of excess calories and sodium. Instead, order a starter and plan on one entrée per two people.

Research shows that starting your day off with refined carbs will lead to higher consumption levels throughout the rest of the day. Just imagine, then, how many calories you'll knock back with 198 grams of low-quality carbs in your belly.

1,543 calories
Bob Evans Stacked & Stuffed Pancakes

this foot-long comes with 3 different kinds of cheese and a thick slick of oil. Hard to believe you'd be better off with 2 Big Macs.

Eat This Instead!
Mediterranean Ciabatta
· *447 calories* · *8 g fat (2 g saturated)*
· *1,635 mg sodium* · *65 g carbohydrates*

WORST STEAK
17 Outback Steakhouse Rib Eye Steak

· *1,190 calories*

Start with a 14-ounce hunk of beef and you're already skating on thin nutritional ice. To make matters worse, rib eye is one of the most heavily marbled cuts of beef on the cow. Factor in the whole meal—including bread, salad, baked potato, and seasonal veggies—and you're looking at a 2,195-calorie steak dinner! Cut that number in thirds by sticking to leaner cuts of beef—sirloins and fillets—slicing the serving size in half, and passing on the bread.

Eat This Instead!
Prime Minister's Prime Rib (8 ounces)
· *350 calories*

WORST FAST-FOOD BREAKFAST
16 McDonald's Deluxe Breakfast (large-size biscuit) with syrup and margarine

· *1,370 calories*
· *64.5 g fat (21.5 g saturated)*
· *2,340 mg sodium*
· *161 g carbohydrates*

This breakfast comes with the works—scrambled eggs, sausage, biscuit, hash browns, you name it. Problem is, it also comes with more than half your day's allotment of calories and an entire day's worth of sodium. It's the caloric equivalent of 4 McDonald's cheeseburgers —can you imagine starting your day off like that? Embrace the McMuffin, but just steer clear of sausage.

Eat This Instead!
Egg McMuffin
· *300 calories* · *12 g fat (5 g saturated)*
· *820 mg sodium* · *30 g carbohydrates*

WORST BREAKFAST
15 Bob Evans Stacked & Stuffed Caramel Banana Pecan Hotcakes

· *1,543 calories*
· *77 g fat*
  (26 g saturated, 9 g trans)

· *2,259 mg sodium*
· *109 g sugars*

It's not a good sign when it takes you nearly 5 seconds to spit out the name of your breakfast. This bad boy packs in more than 75 percent of your calories for the day, along with more sugar and fat than 8 glazed Dunkin' Donuts and nearly as much sodium as 5 Bloody Marys. That's why it's back on our list of the 20 Worst Foods in America again this year.

Eat This Instead!
3 Scrambled Egg Lites with 2 slices of bacon and fresh fruit
· *502 calories* · *19 g fat (7 g saturated)*
· *832 mg sodium* · *19 g sugars*

WORST ICE CREAM DESSERT
14 Così Double Trouble Brownie Sundae

· *1,594 calories*
· *95 g fat*
· *1,039 mg sodium*
· *163 g carbohydrates*

This dessert is dubbed Double Trouble for a reason. Così doesn't provide sugar content, but the 163 grams of carbohydrates suggests that this sundae racks up at least

100 grams of the sweet stuff, easily. That's the sugar equivalent of 10 Krispy Kreme original glazed donuts. And there could be even more. Add to that enough calories to fill you up for almost an entire day (not to mention a disturbingly high level of sodium) and this dessert is sure to absolutely trash your diet.

Eat This Instead!
S'Mores
- *361 calories • 10 g fat • 234 mg sodium*
- *61 g carbohydrates*

WORST CHICKEN ENTRÉE
13 **Dairy Queen 6-Piece Chicken Strip Basket with Country Gravy**

- *1,640 calories*
- *74 g fat*
  (12 g saturated, 1 g trans)
- *3,690 mg sodium*
- *121 g carbohydrates*

It's amazing how many calories DQ can pack into 6 strips of fatty fried chicken. Don't blame the trans-fatty gravy alone—it adds only about 400 extra calories. This disastrous basket will send your blood pressure soaring with the sodium equivalent of 112 saltine crackers, and it'll drag you down for the rest of the day with its carbohydrate overload.

Eat This Instead!
Grilled Flamethrower Chicken Sandwich

- *590 calories • 36 g fat (9 g saturated)*
- *1,480 mg sodium • 34 g carbohydrates*

WORST SALAD
12 **On the Border Grande Taco Salad with Taco Beef and Chipotle Honey Mustard Dressing**

- *1,700 calories*
- *124 g fat (37.5 g saturated)*
- *2,620 mg sodium*
- *86 g carbohydrates*

Greasy ground beef, shredded cheese, and a massive tortilla bowl lend this taco "salad" the caloric heft of 8½ Taco Bell beef tacos! The only way to escape unscathed at On the Border is to use the Create Your Own Combo option on the

The Best and Worst Vocabulary Guide

Restaurant language is littered with ambiguities, embellishments, and euphemisms. Use this dictionary to decode the jargon and save yourself time, money, and a whole lot of empty calories.

Blackened
Covered in a piquant blend of spices such as paprika, onion powder, cumin, and cayenne pepper and then grilled or pan seared in a cast-iron skillet. It's a healthier way to enjoy big flavor without adding excessive calories.

Complimentary
Usually attached to one of the following words: chips, bread, desserts, refills. In any case, the act of giving away low-cost foods and beverages is a common tactic restaurants use to add value to the "customer experience." It might seem like a treat, but these empty calories add up quickly.

Create your own
The safest or most dangerous phrase you'll find on a menu, depending on how you play it. Mexican menus feature this prominently, and if you choose wisely (crunchy tacos, enchiladas), it could be your safest strategy. But free-wheeling pizza and pasta creations require restraint.

menu; this salad-taco plate is the best meal you could hope to have—just be sure to skip the rice and beans.

Eat This Instead!
Mexican Chopped Salad and a Crispy Chicken Taco
- 450 calories • 25 g fat (7 g saturated)
- 1,120 mg sodium • 40 g carbohydrates

WORST SANDWICH
11 Quiznos Tuna Melt (large)
- 1,760 calories
- 133 g fat
  (25 g saturated, 1.5 g trans)
- 2,120 mg sodium
- 92 g carbohydrates

When we first launched *Eat This, Not That!,* we singled out this troublesome tuna sandwich for its massive caloric load. In response, Quiznos claims to have shaved a good 300 calories from between the bread. But incredibly enough, it's still the most atrocious sandwich we found in our latest round of menu-scouring. Blame the gobs of calorie- and fat-packed mayo, the endless inches of carb-heavy bread, and the full day's worth of sodium.

Eat This Instead!
Small Honey Bourbon Chicken on Wheat Bread
- 320 calories • 4.5 g fat (0.5 g saturated)
- 920 mg sodium
- 920 mg carbohydrates

WORST ITALIAN ENTRÉE
10 Romano's Macaroni Grill Spaghetti and Meatballs with Meat Sauce
- 1,810 calories
- 118 g fat (54 g saturated)
- 4,900 mg sodium
- 109 g carbohydrates

With nearly three times your recommended daily intake of saturated fat and 2 days' worth of salt, these ain't your mama's meatballs (at least we hope not). This dish debuted on last year's list, but there's still no other pasta that delivers this bad a blow.

Eat This Instead!
Capellini Tre Pomodoro
- 640 calories • 25 g fat (3 g saturated)
- 990 mg sodium • 96 g carbohydrates

Crispy
The restaurant industry's euphemism of choice for breaded and deep-fried fare. Expect it to carry a massive load of fat and excess calories.

Italian cold cuts
An umbrella term used by delis and sub shops to denote any mix of the following cured meats: ham, salami, capicola, prosciutto, bologna, mortadella, and sopressata. High in fat and sodium, Italian-style sandwiches are always among the worst you'll find in a deli.

Lightly breaded
The phrase most restaurants use to distract diners from the fact the food they're about to eat has been rolled in flour, egg, and bread crumbs before taking a dip in a vat of hot oil. Doesn't matter how light the breading is; it's the oil part that will get you.

Pan pizza
Synonymous with "deep dish," meaning your pizza is too large and topping-laden to be cooked in the traditional manner and instead requires the use of a cast-iron baking pan to cook properly. Expect slices of pan pizza to be up to 50 percent more caloric than their regular-size counterparts.

The Worst Foods in America

WORST CHINESE ENTRÉE
9 P.F. Chang's Combo Lo Mein

- *1,968 calories*
- *96 g fat (12 g saturated)*
- *5,860 mg sodium*

Lo mein is normally looked at as a side dish, a harmless pile of noodles to pad your plate of orange chicken or broccoli beef. This heaping portion (to be fair, Chang's does suggest diners share an order) comes spiked with chicken, shrimp, beef, and pork, not to mention an Exxon *Valdez*–size slick of oil. The damage? A day's worth of calories, 1½ days' worth of fat, and 2½ days' worth of sodium. No meat-based dish beats out the strip.

Eat This Instead!
Asian Marinated New York Strip

- *558 calories • 30 g fat (12 g saturated)*
- *864 mg sodium*

WORST BURGER
8 Ruby Tuesday Colossal Burger

- *2,014 calories*
- *141 g fat*
- *95 g carbohydrates*

Ordering this burger would be a Colossal mistake. In between 2 buns is the number of calories you should consume over the course of an entire day. And though Ruby Tuesday doesn't provide saturated fat content, we're willing to guess it's not a pretty number. Ruby Tuesday offers only 5 burgers that ring in at less than 1,000 calories apiece—and not a single one that offers less than 800 calories. If you must go the burger route at this restaurant, forget side dishes, appetizers, or sugary drinks to keep your meal within the realm of reasonability. Better yet, remember what Mick Jagger said: "Good-bye, Ruby Tuesday."

Eat This Instead!
Blackened Fish Burger

- *861 calories • 53 g fat*
- *44 g carbohydrates*

The Best and Worst Vocabulary Guide—*Continued*

Prime
A term doled out by the USDA that means a piece of beef is sufficiently marbled, i.e., strewn with intramuscular fat. Only 3 percent of beef processed in the US receives this rating, and most goes to restaurants. If your steak is prime, count on it packing 50 percent more calories.

Roasted
A fancy way of saying "baked." Oven-cooking generally requires the use of less oil and butter than sautéing (and certainly less than pan-frying), making it one of the healthiest ways to have your vegetables, meat, and fish prepared.

Secret sauce
In the vast majority of cases, this refers to a spread of about 80 percent mayonnaise and 20 percent ketchup. It might also have a smattering of relish mixed in, making it nearly identical to Thousand Island dressing. Expect it to add an extra 120 calories to your sandwich.

Supersize
Term once used by McDonald's to indicate an increase in the size of French fries and soda that come with a combo meal. Other establishments have since adopted other terms—Upsize, Biggie Size, King Size—to denote the same. Regardless of the moniker used, research shows

7 Romano's Macaroni Grill Parmesan-Crusted Sole

- *2,190 calories*
- *141 g fat (58 g saturated)*
- *2,980 mg sodium*
- *145 g carbohydrates*

Fish is normally a safe bet, but this entrée proves that it's all in the preparation. If you fry said fish in a shell of cheese, be prepared to pay the consequences. Here that means meeting your daily calorie, fat, saturated fat, and sodium intake in one sitting.

Eat This Instead!
Simple Salmon
- *590 calories · 32 g fat (6 g saturated)*
- *1,800 mg sodium · 15 g carbohydrates*

6 Chili's Fajita Quesadillas Beef with Rice and Beans, 4 flour tortillas, and condiments

- *2,240 calories*
- *92 g fat (43.5 g saturated)*
- *6,390 mg sodium*
- *253 g carbohydrates*

Since when has it ever been a smart idea to combine 2 already calorie- and sodium-packed dishes into one monstrous meal? This confounding creation delivers nearly a dozen Krispy Kreme original glazed donuts' worth of calories, the sodium equivalent of 194 saltine crackers, and the saturated fat equivalent of 44 strips of bacon. Check please.

Eat This Instead!
Guiltless Carne Asada Steak
- *371 calories · 10 g fat (7.5 saturated)*
- *1,436 mg sodium · 11 g carbohydrates*

5 Uno Chicago Grill Chicago Classic Deep Dish Pizza

- *2,310 calories*
- *165 g fat (54 g saturated)*
- *4,920 mg sodium*
- *120 g carbohydrates*

A horrific 254 percent of your daily allowance of fat and 295 percent of your daily sodium intake. It also wipes out your whole day's caloric allotment. It may be a Chicago classic, but so was Al Capone.

that, on average, an extra 17 percent more money will buy customers 55 percent more calories, making upsizing a sound investment in flab. Here's a novel idea: If chains offer supersize possibilities, why not also offer a downsize option to customers?

Tempura
The Japanese version of battering and deep-frying. And just like the American version, it smothers vegetables and seafood alike under a fat-loaded armor of crispy flour.

Vinaigrette
A vinaigrette is technically a dressing made from 3 parts oil and 1 part vinegar. While generally better for you than the viscous white dressings (ranch, Caesar, blue cheese), many restaurant vinaigrettes pack up to 300 calories per serving, so keep it on the side and use sparingly.

Wrap
A "healthy" alternative to a sandwich. The problem is the typical tortilla packs up to 300 calories and provides ample surface for a surplus of cheese and dressing. All told, the average chicken wrap weighs in at 600 calories—about 50 percent more than the average grilled chicken sandwich.

The Worst Foods in America

Eat This Instead!
Cheese and Tomato Flatbread Pizza (half) and a house side salad

- *515 calories • 22 g fat (8 g saturated)*
- *1,355 mg sodium*

WORST STARTER
4 Uno Chicago Grill Pizza Skins (full order)

- *2,400 calories*
- *155 g fat (45 g saturated)*
- *3,600 mg sodium*

This appetizer is like eating a Large Domino's Hand-Tossed Sausage Pizza all by yourself. Split among 4 people, it's still a full dinner's worth of calories. Order the Thai Vegetable Pot Stickers —the only starter with fewer than 800 calories.

Eat This Instead!
Thai Vegetable Pot Stickers

- *400 calories • 20 g fat (2 g saturated)*
- *1,080 mg sodium • 46 g carbohydrates*

WORST MEXICAN ENTRÉE
3 On the Border Dos XX Fish Tacos with Chipotle Sauce and Refried Beans and Rice

- *2,550 calories*
- *151 g fat (31 g saturated)*
- *4,790 mg sodium*

This dish is an astonishing example of a restaurant defying all preconceived notions about so-called healthy food. No food is safe, not even fish, at least not when it's breaded, fried, and slapped on a plate with more calories than you'd get in three sticks of butter. Is nothing sacred?

Eat This Instead!
Pico Shrimp Tacos

- *490 calories • 5 g fat (1 g saturated)*
- *1,650 mg sodium*

WORST ENTRÉE
2 Outback Steakhouse Baby Back Ribs (full rack)

- *2,580 calories**

Let's be honest: Ribs are rarely served alone on a plate. When you add a sweet potato and Outback's Classic Wedge salad, this meal is a 3,460-calorie blowout. (Consider that it takes only 3,500 calories to add a pound of fat to your body. Better plan for a very, very long "walkabout" when this meal is over!)

Eat This Instead!
Prime Rib (8 ounces) with Fresh Seasonal Veggies

- *500 calories**

*Outback refuses to disclose complete nutritional data for their dishes.

THE WORST FOOD IN AMERICA
1 Baskin-Robbins Chocolate Oreo Shake (large)

- *2,600 calories*
- *135 g fat (59 g saturated, 2.5 g trans)*
- *263 g sugars*
- *1,700 mg sodium*

We didn't think anything could be worse than Baskin-Robbins' 2008 bombshell, the Heath Bar Shake. After all, it had more sugar (266 grams) than 20 bowls of Froot Loops, more calories (2,310) than 11 actual Heath Bars, and more ingredients (73) than you'll find in most chemistry sets. Yet the folks at Baskin-Robbins have shown that when it comes to making America fat, they're always up to the challenge. The large Chocolate Oreo Shake is soiled with more than a day's worth of calories and 3 days' worth of saturated fat. Worst of all, it takes less than 10 minutes to sip through a straw.

Drink This Instead!
Peach Passion Fruit Blast (small)

- *270 calories • 0 g fat • 65 g sugars*
- *10 mg sodium*

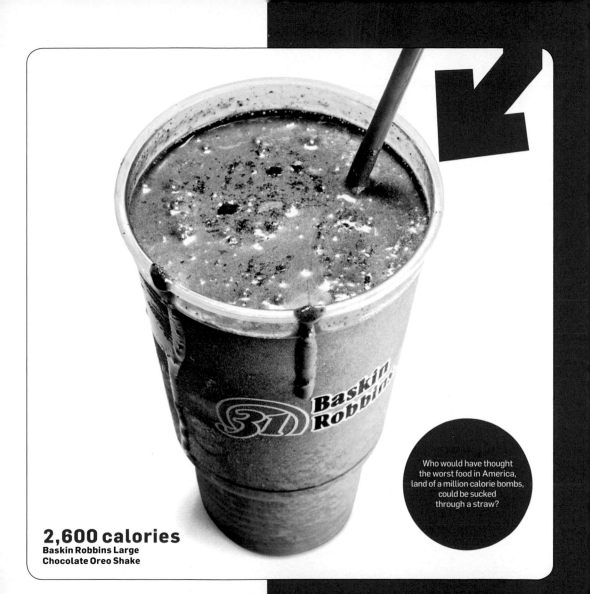

2,600 calories
Baskin Robbins Large
Chocolate Oreo Shake

Who would have thought
the worst food in America,
land of a million calorie bombs,
could be sucked
through a straw?

The Best Foods in Ame

THE FINEST CHOICES FOUND UP AND DOWN THE FOOD CHAIN

BEST APPETIZER
Outback Seared Ahi Tuna (small)

· 360 calories

In the first *Eat This, Not That!* book, we named Outback's infamous Aussie Cheese Fries the Worst Food in America, so it's nice to see they have the good side of the caloric spectrum covered, too. This one couldn't be simpler: hunks of lean tuna pan seared and served with a wasabi vinaigrette. Tons of protein and healthy omega-3 fats for minimal calories. In fact, with dozens of land mines lurking in the entrée department, it would be a smart move to make this your main course for the night.

BEST BREAKFAST
McDonald's Egg McMuffin

· 300 calories
· 12 g fat (5 g saturated)
· 820 mg sodium

Surprised that the maligned McMuffin is actually a model of solid morning eating? Don't be. For just 300 calories, you get a big dose of protein, plus some healthy fat from the eggs to boot.

BEST FISH ENTRÉE
Uno Chicago Grill Grilled Mahi Mahi with **Mango Salsa**

· 240 calories
· 2 g fat (0 g saturated)
· 980 mg sodium

Nearly every calorie comes from protein. The fat-free mango salsa wins the award for condiment of the year.

BEST STEAK
Ruby Tuesday Peppercorn Mushroom Sirloin with Premium Baby Green Beans

· 468 calories
· 21 g fat
· 18 g carbohydrates

Ruby Tuesday may make some of the planet's most fattening burgers, but their line of sirloins is surprisingly lean and reliable. Flank this one with a pile of baby green beans to soak up the sauce and you have yourself a pretty serious—and seriously nutritious—meal.

BEST BURGER
Wendy's ¼-Pound Single

· 430 calories
· 20 g fat (7 g saturated)
· 870 mg sodium
· 25 g protein

Sure, you can find hamburgers with fewer calories, but they'll most likely be paltry hockey pucks incapable of satisfying the average 8-year-old's appetite. This Wendy's classic, though, packs plenty of substance—4 ounces of beef, 25 grams of belly-filling produce—for a very respectable 430 calories.

rica

360 calories
Outback Seared Ahi Tuna

BEST SANDWICH

Subway 6" Double Roast Beef with all the fixings on 9 Grain Wheat

- 360 calories
- 7 g fat (3.5 g saturated)
- 1,300 mg sodium

Why double the meat? Because for an extra 50 calories, you get nearly twice as much metabolism-spiking protein, which helps build muscle and burn fat. Plus doubling up on a 6-inch sub will save you 220 calories over the other alternative for hungry sandwich hounds: the dreaded footlong. Get your money's worth by loading up on the free veggies: peppers, olives, onions, tomatoes, and spinach.

BEST DESSERT

Breyers All Natural Vanilla and Chocolate Ice Cream (½ cup)

- 130 calories
- 7 g fat (4.5 g saturated)
- 15 g sugars

Truth is, most restaurant desserts are treacherous; they have the potential to derail an otherwise healthy meal with just a few seemingly innocent spoonfuls. Save the calories and the cash and wait until you get home to serve yourself a scoop from our favorite line of ice cream. Everything in Breyers All Natural portfolio is great, but we love the simple yin-yang satisfaction of the chocolate-vanilla combo.

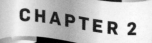
The Best
(& Worst)
"Healthy"
Foods
in America

Eat This

Chili's Cedar Plank Tilapia

with Kettle Black Beans and Seasonal Veggies

369 calories
9 g fat
(3 g saturated)
1,519 mg sodium
17 g carbohydrates

Like most of Chili's creations, this dish is high in sodium, but it offers a counterbalancing punch of potassium, plus 14 grams of fiber.

Save 132 g fat!
That's more than you'd find in 26 Hostess Cup Cakes!

Save more than 1,800 calories!
Make this swap once a week and you'll save 26 pounds in a year.

Not That!

Romano's Macaroni Grill Parmesan-Crusted Sole

2,190 calories
141 g fat
(58 g saturated)
2,980 mg sodium
145 g carbohydrates

Don't flounder with this tortured sole: You could eat 2 whole sticks of butter and still save 500 calories.

Leave it up to Macaroni Grill to take one of the leanest proteins on the planet and transform it into a dish that packs more calories than 4 Big Macs and as much saturated fat as you should consume in 3 days.

If you want a good idea of how food marketers like to sell their products, all you need to do is go onto Google and type in "properties for sale" in your neighborhood.

Now take a look at the brilliant use of hot-button adjectives in those real estate ads. All the views are "breathtaking." The yards are almost always "expansive." But once you see the property, those adjectives begin to take on different meanings. Maybe the joint with the "cozy" living room has space for a TV or a couch—but not both.

They're not outright lies, per se, because one person's "claustrophobic" is another person's "cozy." And so it is with the hot-button words on food labels. "Reduced-fat" products usually have less fat and "all-natural" foods often do come from ingredients actually found in nature. But not all health-related words on food packaging are defined by the Food and Drug Administration, leaving certain gray areas for manufacturers to exploit. So while those phrases, and others like them, would seem to indicate that the products inside the packages are somehow "healthy," the reality is often something very different. As likely as not, "reduced fat" means "increased sugar." As for products that are "all natural"? Well, so are hurricanes and tidal waves.

And the most deceptive word of all? That might be the word "healthy." Because there is no way to really define it, the FDA has no way to regulate it. And just about anything out there can be healthy—or unhealthy—in the right amounts. In this chapter, we dig deep, below the surface labels, and expose the real truth behind some of the food industry's most specious health claims.

20 grams of sugar
Dole Tropical Mixed Fruit in Passion Fruit Nectar

When will food manufacturers learn that fruit, teeming with concentrated natural sugars, needs no additional sweeteners to taste delicious? Make it a policy to keep fruit products with added sugar out of your pantry.

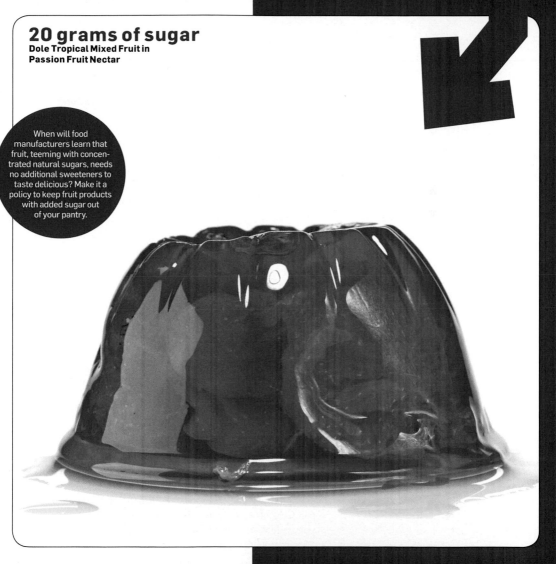

The Worst "Healthy" Foods in America

15 **Dole Tropical Mixed Fruit in Passion Fruit Nectar** (½ cup)

- *90 calories*
- *0 g fat*
- *20 g sugars*

If there's one thing we love about fruit, it's that nature prepackages it with the perfect amount of sugar. That's why fruit packed in syrup bothers us so much. Apparently the folks who can these fruits don't trust nature's recipe, so they augment it with a gob of extra sugar, which downgrades nature's wonder food into canned candy. Stick with nature's recipe instead and buy only fruits packed in 100 percent juice.

Eat This Instead!
Del Monte 100% Juice Tropical Fruit Salad (½ cup)
- *60 calories • 0 g fat • 14 g sugars*

WORST DIP

14 **Dean's Guacamole Flavored Dip** (2 Tbsp)

- *90 calories*
- *9 g fat (2.5 g saturated)*
- *170 mg sodium*

This "guacamole" dip is comprised of less than 2 percent avocado; the rest of the green goo is a cluster of fillers and chemicals, including modified food starch, soybean oils, locust bean gum, and food coloring. Dean's isn't alone in this guacamole fake-out; most guacs with the word "dip" don't deliver on the avocado.

Eat This Instead!
Wholly Guacamole Classic (2 Tbsp)
- *50 calories • 4 g fat (0.5 g saturated)*
- *75 mg sodium*

WORST YOGURT

13 **Yoplait 99% Fat Free Cherry Orchard**

- *170 calories*
- *1.5 g fat (1 g saturated)*
- *27 g sugars*
- *5 g protein*

Think those 27 grams of sugar come from the cherries? Think again: After milk, sugar's the first ingredient on this list. And there's as much of it in here as there is in a Kit Kat candy bar. Choose Fage Greek-style yogurt instead; the megadose of protein makes it a great postworkout meal, and it's sweetened with more fruit than sugar.

Eat This Instead!
Fage 2% Strawberry
- *130 calories • 2.5 g fat (1.5 g saturated)*
- *17 g sugars • 17 g protein*

WORST "HEALTHY" CEREAL

12 **Quaker 100% Natural Granola, Oats & Honey & Raisins** (1 cup)

- *420 calories*
- *12 g fat (7 g saturated)*
- *6 g fiber*
- *30 g sugars*

Granola, despite its earthy reputation, is usually weighed down by a deluge of added sugars. For the caloric investment, you could eat 8 chicken wings; for the same amount of sugar, you could have a bowl of Cocoa Pebbles more than twice the size. Even scarier is the fact that if you did switch to Cocoa Pebbles, you'd get more fiber and save about 60 calories in fat.

Eat This Instead!
Kashi GoLean (1 cup)
- *140 calories • 1 g fat • 10 g fiber*
- *6 g sugars*

11 Au Bon Pain Homestyle Lemonade (large)

- *460 calories*
- *0 g fat*
- *104 g sugars*
- *120 g carbohydrates*

Lemons are naturally tart, which is why you'll never find a legitimate lemonade that isn't loaded with sugar. That being said, this drink is just absurd, even by lemonade standards. It's basically a full meal's worth of calories, but because nearly every single calorie comes from sugar, it will have absolutely zero impact on your hunger. If you plan on having a drink at Au Bon Pain, make it a small. Otherwise, you'll have to skip your meal to make up for the extra calories.

Drink This Instead!
Orange Juice (small)
- *110 calories • 0 g fat • 26 g sugars*
- *26 g carbohydrates*

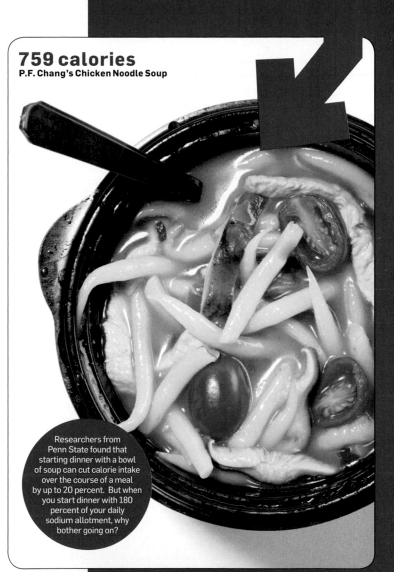

759 calories
P.F. Chang's Chicken Noodle Soup

Researchers from Penn State found that starting dinner with a bowl of soup can cut calorie intake over the course of a meal by up to 20 percent. But when you start dinner with 180 percent of your daily sodium allotment, why bother going on?

The Worst "Healthy" Foods in America

WORST "REDUCED-CALORIE" SMOOTHIE

10 Dunkin' Donuts Reduced-Calorie Berry Smoothie (32 ounces)

- *490 calories*
- *4 g fat (2.5 g saturated fat)*
- *83 g sugars*
- *97 g carbohydrates*

Sure, this blend may not completely derail your diet, but it's a perfect example of how the restaurant industry fools health-conscious consumers with labels like "reduced calorie." The truth is it has more calories than a Quarter Pounder from McDonald's, and it's not alone: Every medium fruit-and-yogurt smoothie on the menu packs at least 60 grams of sugar. That's more than four times as much as one of Dunkin's own Chocolate-Frosted Cake Doughnuts.

Drink This Instead!
Peach Flavored Iced Tea (32 ounces)
- *30 calories • 0 g fat • 6 g carbohydrates*

WORST "HEALTHY" BREAKFAST

9 Atlanta Bread Company Banana Nut Muffin

- *610 calories*
- *36 g fat (5 g saturated)*
- *38 g sugars*

Here's what you don't want for a breakfast: 610 calories based on sugar and refined carbs glued together with half your day's fat. Start your morning with a recipe like that and you'll need a pot of coffee just to fight off the impending sugar crash. Instead, what you want is a breakfast that will provide long-lasting energy, one with more protein and fewer carbs. Breakfast sandwiches, so long as they're not covered with sausage and bacon, are great—and if you order them on whole wheat English muffins, they're even better.

Eat This Instead!
Egg and Cheese Sandwich
- *440 calories • 17 g fat (6 g saturated)*
- *790 mg sodium*

WORST "LOW-FAT" SANDWICH

8 Subway Footlong Sweet Onion Chicken Teriyaki

- *770 calories*
- *9 g fat (2.5 g saturated)*
- *34 g sugars*
- *2,290 mg sodium*

It's a wonder that this sandwich ever made it onto Subway's healthy subs menu. Sure, a foot-long sub is a lot of food, but that doesn't explain the teriyaki sauce that covers this chicken like a blanket of briny syrup, simultaneously providing a day's worth of sodium and 4 Peanut Butter Twix bars' worth of sugar. Plus, like all posted calorie counts at Subway, this doesn't include cheese or any other condiments, so if you like to load up your sandwich, expect to see this number inch toward 1,000 calories.

Eat This Instead!
Oven-Roasted Chicken Breast (6")
- *320 calories • 5 g fat (1.5 g saturated)*
- *7 g sugars • 880 mg sodium*

The "Health" Food Decoder

As many health-food impostors as there are lurking on restaurant menus across America, you'll find even more tangled up in the aisles of your local supermarket. You know the ones—products emblazoned with those bold, purposefully ambiguous claims that may or may not actually mean anything to your well-being. Don't waste another dime (or calorie) on reduced-fat(!) fake-outs and all-natural(!) nutritional nightmares. Consider this your lie detector, a secret cheat sheet that will teach you how to sniff out a faux health food from the parking lot.

THE CEREAL CONUNDRUM

Kellogg's Smart Start Cereal

The Claim: "Lightly sweetened"
The Truth: Unregulated by the USDA, the word "lightly" gets tossed around like a Frisbee in the food-packaging world. Always take it with a grain of salt; in many instances, "light" is the first sign of trouble. With this healthy-sounding cereal, "lightly" means 14 grams of sugar from 5 different sources, all of which adds up to a cereal with more added sugars per serving than Froot Loops, Frosted Flakes, or Apple Jacks.
What you really want: A cereal with less than 10 grams of sugar per serving (and ideally less than 5), with at least 3 grams of fiber. Look at cereal as a sugar-to-fiber ratio; you want a ratio no higher than 2 to 1.

THE FAT FAKE-OUT

Smucker's Reduced Fat Creamy Peanut Butter

The Claim: "25 percent less fat than regular natural peanut butter"
The Truth: Smucker's has indeed removed some of the fat from the peanut butter, but they've replaced it with maltodextrin, a carbohydrate used as a cheap filler in many processed foods. This means you're trading the healthy fat from peanuts for empty carbs, double the sugar, and a savings of a meager 10 calories.
What you really want: The real stuff: no oils, fillers, or added sugars. Just peanuts and salt. Smucker's Natural fits the bill, as do many other peanut butters out there.

THE UNNATURAL FRUIT

Nutri-Grain Strawberry Cereal Bar

The Claim: "Naturally and artificially flavored"
The Truth: While the FDA requires manufacturers to disclose the use of artificial flavoring on the front of the box, the requirements for what is considered "natural" and "real" are not strict: Even trace amounts of the essence or extract of fruit counts as natural. So yes, there is fruit in this bar, but it falls 3rd in the ingredients list, behind high-fructose corn syrup and corn syrup.
What you really want: An honest snack with nothing to hide. Lärabars, one of our favorite snacks in the aisle, are made with nothing more than dried fruit and nuts.

THE "HEALTH FOOD" THAT ISN'T

Healthy Choice Sweet & Sour Chicken

The Claim: "Healthy Choice"
The Truth: A company can call itself whatever it wants, but that doesn't give credence to the name. With 29 grams of sugar from 6 different forms of sweeteners, this meal has as much in common with a Snickers bar as it does a truly great dinner. Many Healthy Choice selections are reliably nutritious; this is not one of them.
What you really want: Dinner that doesn't taste like a bowl of ice cream. While fat and calories are important considerations in everything you eat, be sure to read the fine print. Companies with healthy label claims often pull the bait and switch, going low in fat but then elevating the sugar or sodium to up the flavor quotient.

Learn to translate the special language of food labels and you'll know how to stock your pantry to perfection.

The Worst "Healthy" Foods in America

WORST "HEALTHY" SOUP
7 P.F. Chang's Chicken Noodle Soup

- *759 calories*
- *24 g fat (4 g saturated)*
- *4,135 mg sodium*
- *92 g carbohydrates*

It's the best part about getting sick: the promise of chicken noodle soup to come. Studies have shown it works, too, but no study could have planned on the torrent of sodium that swirls among Chang's noodles. Experts recommend capping your daily sodium intake at 2,400 milligrams. Any more than that can put you at an increased risk for heart disease, not to mention swell you up with retained water. Unfortunately, all Chang's soups suffer a similar fate. Your only choice is to swap out your bowl for a smaller cup.

Eat This Instead!
Egg Drop Soup (cup)

- *61 calories • 2 g fat • 1,122 mg sodium*

WORST TURKEY BURGER
6 T.G.I. Friday's California Turkey Burger

- *950 calories**

There was a time when turkey was a reliably lean substitution for ground beef, but then eager-to-please restaurants started "beefing" up the turkey by slathering it with oil, increasing the portions, and sticking it between 2 buns dripping with butter. Pastoral as this burger may sound, it can't escape the fact that it delivers more calories than a Wendy's Baconator. Unfortunately, T.G.I. Friday's doesn't offer anything decent in the burger department, so if you want something meaty to nibble on, you'd better go with a half rack of ribs.

Eat This Instead!
Half Rack of Ribs

- *500 calories**

*T.G.I. Friday's refuses to disclose full nutritional information for the food they're serving you.

WORST VEGGIE BURGER
5 Ruby Tuesday Veggie Burger

- *952 calories*
- *53 g fat*
- *95 g carbohydrates*

This inauspicious burger might be made of veggies, but those veggies still manage to pack this burger with as many calories as you'll find in 4 Butterfinger candy bars. Always remember, it's not about the headliner, it's about the supporting cast; in this case, a huge bun and a cluster of lackluster condiments drag down something that should be a reliable health-food staple. Unfortunately, there's no good substitution on the burger menu; everything Ruby jams into a bun comes out as a massive wad of fat. For a truly healthy vegetarian choice, choose the Signature House Salad. Just take it easy with the dressing, okay?

Eat This Instead!
Signature House Salad

- *391 calories • 30 g fat*
- *19 g carbohydrates*

4 Denny's Grilled Chicken Sandwich
with Honey Mustard Dressing

- *970 calories*
- *58 g fat (10 g saturated)*
- *2,070 mg sodium*
- *69 g carbohydrates*

Here's a distinction you should familiarize yourself with: honey mustard versus honey mustard *dressing*. If you're like most people, you probably assume they're 2 terms for the same thing, and that's exactly what Denny's is banking on. The truth is honey mustard dressing, unlike honey mustard, is calorically more akin to ranch or mayonnaise than it is to mustard. Don't waste the calories; instead look for items labeled Fit Fare— they represent the best Denny has to offer.

Eat This Instead!
Fit Fare Chicken Sandwich with Applesauce
- *490 calories • 7 g fat (1.5 g saturated)*
- *1,460 mg sodium • 67 g carbohydrates*

770 calories
Subway Footlong Sweet Onion Chicken Teriyaki

Not pictured: 12 bags of Lay's Classic Potato Chips and 7 Chewy Chips Ahoy! cookies. Those contain the same amounts of sodium and sugar, respectively, as you'll find in this sandwich.

The Worst "Healthy" Foods in America

WORST VEGGIE SANDWICH
3 Blimpie Special Vegetarian (12")

- *1,186 calories*
- *60 g fat (19 g saturated)*
- *3,532 mg sodium*
- *131 g carbohydrates*

Let's clear something up: Just because a meal is vegetarian doesn't mean it's healthy. And if this sandwich doesn't prove that point, then we don't know what will. This off-menu item (you have to "special" request it) consists of diced vegetables resting on a bed of crumbled Doritos held together with a wad of melted American cheese and covered in a sugar-loaded chutney. Sure, it's cool to know about the secret menu, but if you care about your health, you'll stick with the not-so-special regular menu.

Eat This Instead!
Mediterranean Ciabatta
- *447 calories • 8 g fat (2 g saturated)*
- *1,635 mg sodium*

WORST WRAP
2 Applebee's Chicken Fajita Rollup

- *1,450 calories*

For some curious reason, wraps have come to be viewed as a healthy upgrade from sandwiches, as if those massive tortillas can be filled with nothing but anticalories. But that couldn't be further from the truth. The problem with wraps is that they function as holding tanks for fluids, so hurried fry-cooks can squirt in as much sauce as they want without making it look messy. With Applebee's rollup, the offending sauce is a Mexi-ranch sauce, which looks suspiciously more like ranch than anything eaten in Mexico. But here's the final insult: This "healthy" meal is served with fries. Eat them and you tack on 400 extra calories.

Eat This Instead!
Garlic Herb Chicken
- *370 calories*

WORST "HEALTHY" FOOD IN AMERICA
1 Romano's Macaroni Grill Parmesan-Crusted Sole

- *2,190 calories*
- *141 g fat (58 g saturated)*
- *2,980 mg sodium*
- *145 g carbohydrates*

Lean sole served with capers and spinach-strewn orzo sounds like the safest bet on the Mac Grill menu, but it turns out to be not just one of the worst dishes in this restaurant, but one of the worst entrées we've found in any restaurant in America. From a nutritional standpoint, "Parmesan crusting" is akin to coating one of the healthiest proteins in the world with a blanket of fried cheese. Fish should make for healthy eating, but restaurants like Macaroni Grill are doing their best to challenge that age-old adage.

Eat This Instead!
Simple Salmon
- *590 calories • 34 g fat (6 g saturated)*
- *1,980 mg sodium*

Wraps have a great PR manager. Over the years, they've won the undeserving reputation as a nutritionally superior sandwich, but the stats just don't support it. Exhibit A: a chicken wrap with more calories than a 20-ounce T-bone steak.

1,450 calories
Applebee's Chicken Fajita Rollup

The Best Healthy Foods

THESE SNACKS, SOUPS, AND ENTRÉES ARE EVERY BIT AS GOOD FOR YOU

BEST FISH ENTRÉE

Red Lobster Full Portion Wood-Grilled Cod
with Broccoli

- 305 calories
- 3.5 g fat
  (0.5 g saturated)
- 340 mg sodium

Exactly what a lean fillet of fish with vegetables is supposed to be—one of the healthiest meals in the world. Red Lobster will grill nearly any fish in the sea, but make cod one of your go-to fish. It's one of the leanest on the menu, it offers a dependable dose of omega-3 fats, and it's absolutely loaded with selenium, an antioxidant that protects your blood vessels and promotes a healthy thyroid.

BEST SANDWICH

Così Fire-Roasted Veggie Sandwich

- 328 calories
- 8 g fat
- 259 mg sodium

Così's sandwich keeps the calories down by using flatbread in place of an oversized bun, but it's what's inside the flatbread that makes this sandwich great: red and yellow peppers, eggplant, artichoke hearts, zucchini, squash, red onions, and romaine lettuce. Wow, sounds like the nutritional Garden of Eden.

BEST DRIVE-THRU

Taco Bell Fresco Grilled Steak Soft Tacos

- 160 calories
- 4.5 g fat
  (1.5 g saturated)
- 550 mg sodium

Hopefully, one day every fast-food chain in America will offer some variation of Taco Bell's Fresco Menu, but for now, you'll have to settle for this. And here's what it does for you: Opt to have your Steak Taco served Fresco style and you cut 100 calories of pure fat. Fast-food choices don't get any easier than that.

BEST SALAD

Panera Bread Full Asian Sesame Chicken Salad

- 410 calories
- 19 g fat
  (3.5 g saturated)
- 900 mg sodium

Here's a salad that does something unusual in today's supersize culture: It lives up to the potential of a salad. In fact, it has a near-perfect balance of protein, fat, and fiber, thanks to an all-star list of ingredients that includes romaine lettuce, almonds, and lean chicken. But here's what really sets this salad above the rest: It's topped with a reduced-sugar vinaigrette instead of a viscous blanket of ranch or Thousand Island.

in America

AS THEY SOUND. DIG IN

BEST PACKAGED SNACK
Reduced-Fat Triscuits
(7 crackers)

- *120 calories*
- *3 g fat (0.5 g saturated)*
- *160 mg sodium*

Most snack foods that make the leap to "reduced fat" do so by packing in extra servings of sugar, salt, and empty carbohydrates, but not Triscuits. To scale back the fat in this cracker, Nabisco did the obvious thing—they used less oil. That's why, just as with regular Triscuits, the reduced-fat crackers have only 3 ingredients: whole wheat, soybean oil, and salt.

BEST SOUP
Amy's Light in Sodium Organic Split Pea Soup
(1 cup)

- *100 calories*
- *0 g fat*
- *280 mg sodium*

Scan the ingredient list on Amy's soup and you'll notice something odd: You've used every one of these ingredients in your own kitchen. There's nothing in this can besides vegetables, herbs, and split peas, which is why the entire can carries only 200 calories and close to a third of your day's fiber. If only every soup were so good.

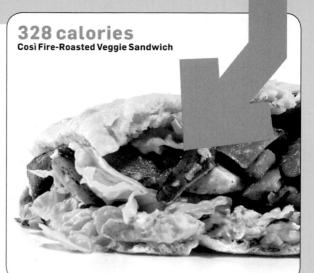

328 calories
Così Fire-Roasted Veggie Sandwich

460 calories
Baja Fresh Grilled Mahi Mahi Fish Tacos (2)

In a perfect nutritional world, fish tacos would be reliably healthy eats. Too bad many restaurants bombard them with batter, cheese, and fatty condiments. But these handheld Mahi bites offer a heap of heart-healthy fats for just 230 calories a pop.

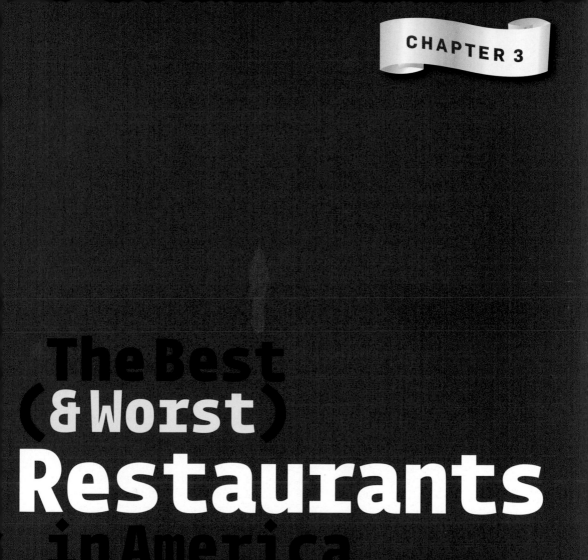

CHAPTER 3

The Best (& Worst) Restaurants in America

Control.

It's the word you hear all the time when people talk about managing their weight. "Portion control," they urge. "Control your cravings," they say. But what's the first thing you give up the minute you decide to go out to eat? Control.

Once you hop into the car and head to your local eatery, you're giving up control over what's in your food and forking that control over to a handful of folks who have a lot less invested in your health and well-being than you do. Sure, you can special order, you can parse through the menu, and you can quiz the waitress about your meal's ingredients (although in many cases, the waitstaff knows as much about what they're serving as they know about quantum physics).

But you don't really know what's happening back there behind the kitchen doors, where that sizzling sound could be caused by fresh vegetables being sautéed in virgin olive oil—or by frozen nuggets hitting the deep fryer.

So once you and your family have solved the major questions about eating out—Sit-down or drive-thru? Burgers or pizza? Plastic sporks or silverware?—you still have some important choices to make. Which restaurant you choose,

and what you order off the menu, will determine whether or not you feel confident showing up at the pool without a cover-up. Indeed, deciding which burger joint to haunt isn't just a choice between scary clown Ronald McDonald and that creepy Burger King. Making the right decision—the healthy decision—could spell a difference of hundreds of calories in a meal, more than 20 unnecessary pounds over the course of a year, and countless health woes over the course of

Drive-thru debacle

USDA scientists found that people consume 500 calories more on the days they eat fast food than on the days they don't.

a lifetime. That's why *Eat This, Not That!* put 65 major chain restaurants under the nutritional microscope—for both your benefit and that of your family.

To separate the commendable from the deplorable, we calculated the total number of calories per entrée. This gave us a snapshot of how each restaurant compared in average serving size—a key indicator of unhealthy portion distortion. Then we rewarded establishments that offer fruit and vegetable side-dish choices, as well as whole wheat bread. Finally, we penalized places for excessive amounts of trans fat and menus laden with gut-busting desserts. We call our report the Restaurant Report Card.

Did your favorite restaurant make the grade?

RESTAURANT REPORT CARD

APPLEBEE'S

F We've tried repeatedly to get Applebee's to cough up the nutritional info on their menu items, but they won't deliver. Without full disclosure, we have no choice but to give them a flunking grade. (And while Applebee's takes its sweet time coming clean, we took advantage of New York legislation requiring chain restaurants to publish calorie counts to find out what they're hiding.)

SURVIVAL STRATEGY
The saving grace here is the handful of items created in partnership with Weight Watchers, the only items for which the restaurant offers any nutritional information at all. That doesn't leave you much to choose from, but unless you want to play nutritional Russian roulette, you're better off sticking to this menu.

Best
Garlic Herb Chicken
· *370 calories*

Worst
Oriental Chicken Rollup
· *1,550 calories*

ARBY'S

C+ Too bad Arby's didn't toss out their oversize breads when they removed the trans fat from the frying oil in 2006. If they had, you wouldn't have to worry about the extra 360 calories in the honey wheat sandwich bread. In fact, Arby's might be just a little too proud of its trans fat—free frying oil; the restaurant doesn't offer a single side that hasn't had a hot oil bath, and any added oil means added calories.

SURVIVAL STRATEGY
Don't think you're doing yourself any favors by ordering off the Market Fresh menu. You're far better off with a regular roast beef or Melt Sandwich, which will save you an average of nearly 300 calories over a Market Fresh sandwich or wrap.

Best
Ham & Swiss Melt · *268 calories · 8 g fat (3 g saturated) · 1,042 mg sodium*

Worst
Roast Turkey Ranch & Bacon Market Fresh Sandwich
· *769 calories · 39 g fat (10 g saturated) · 1,380 mg sodium*
· *92 g carbohydrates*

ATLANTA BREAD COMPANY

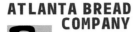 **B-**

The bad news is the breakfast menu is riddled with unnecessary fats and refined carbohydrates, and most of the sandwiches are a little too high calorie for comfort. The good news is that there's also a robust selection of healthy soups and salads to offset these problems, so focus your appetite there and you'll escape relatively unscathed.

SURVIVAL STRATEGY

Atlanta Bread Company lets you order a half sandwich with a half salad or a cup of soup, which are perfect compromises for those who prefer a handheld lunch. Hold the mayo on your sandwich and this is a pretty safe bet. Oh, and avoid the pizzas, pastas, and calzones at all costs.

Best
Chopstix Chicken Salad with Asian Sesame Dressing
· 360 calories · 20 g fat (3 g saturated)
· 850 mg sodium · 29 g carbohydrates

Worst
Turkey Bacon Rustica Sandwich · 960 calories · 56 g fat
(19 g saturated) · 2,480 mg sodium
· 62 g carbohydrates

AU BON PAIN

A-

There are plenty of ways you could go wrong here, but Au Bon Pain couples an extensive inventory of healthy items with an unrivaled standard of nutritional transparency. Each store has an on-site nutritional kiosk to help customers find a meal to meet their expectations, and the variety of ordering options provides dozens of paths to a sensible meal.

SURVIVAL STRATEGY

Most of the café sandwiches are in the 650-calorie range, so make a lean meal instead by combining soup with one of the many low-calorie options on the Portions menu. And if you're in the mood to indulge, pass up the baked goods in favor of a cup of fruit and yogurt or a serving of chocolate-covered almonds.

Best
Jamaican Black Bean Soup (large) · 330 calories · 2 g fat
(0 g saturated) · 590 mg sodium

Worst
Turkey Melt · 780 calories
· 32 g fat (13 g saturated)
· 2,350 mg sodium

AUNTIE ANNE'S

C+

Is there anything redeeming on Auntie Anne's menu? Not really. The average pretzel is about 360 calories of refined carbohydrates, and they supplement the twisted-bread menu with a long list of sweetened beverages and smoothies. But you can find far worse indulgences on just about any dessert menu in the country, so go here in search of relatively healthy indulgences, not genuinely nutritious food.

SURVIVAL STRATEGY

Cut most of the fat and half of the sodium by skipping the butter and salt that go on most pretzels, relying instead on a healthier dipping sauce such as marinara or sweet mustard for big flavor.

Best
Jalapeño Pretzel (no butter or salt) with Marinara Sauce
· 320 calories · 1.5 g fat (0 g saturated)
· 810 mg sodium · 68 g carbohydrates

Worst
Jumbo Pretzel Dog with Hot Salsa Cheese
· 720 calories · 37 g fat
(16.5 g saturated, 1 g trans)
· 1,150 mg sodium · 71g carbohydrates

BAJA FRESH

D⁻ It's a surprise that Baja Fresh's menu has not yet collapsed under the weight of its own fatty fare. About a third of the items on the menu have more than 1,000 calories, and most are spiked with enough sodium to melt a polar ice cap. Order the Steak Fajitas, for instance, and you're looking at 3,440 milligrams of sodium—nearly 2 days' worth in one sitting!

SURVIVAL STRATEGY

Unless you're comfortable stuffing 110 grams of fat into your arteries, avoid the nachos at all costs. In fact, avoid almost everything on this menu. The only safe options are the Baja tacos or a salad topped with salsa verde and served without the elephantine tortilla bowl.

Best
Baja Chicken Tacos (2)
· 420 calories · 10 g fat (2 g saturated)
· 460 mg sodium · 56 g carbohydrates

Worst
Charbroiled Steak Nachos
· 2,120 calories · 118 g fat
  (44 g saturated, 4.5 g trans)
· 2,990 mg sodium
· 163 g carbohydrates

BASKIN-ROBBINS

D⁺ Baskin-Robbins could earn a D on the atrocity of its line of Premium Sundaes and Shakes alone. But the reality is that it would take more than just a little pruning to really clean up this menu; its soft serve is among the most caloric in the country, the smoothies contain more sugar than fruit, and anything that Baskin sticks into a cup winds up with more fat than a steakhouse buffet.

SURVIVAL STRATEGY

With frozen yogurt, sherbet, and no-sugar-added ice cream, Baskin's lighter menu is the one bright spot. Just be sure to ask for it in a sugar or cake cone—the waffle cone will swaddle your treat in an extra 160 calories.

Best
Premium Churned Reduced Fat No Sugar Added Caramel Turtle Truffle (2 scoops)
· 200 calories · 5 g fat (4 g saturated)
· 46 g carbohydrates · 8 g sugars

Worst
Fudge Brownie 31 Below (large) · 1,900 calories
· 85 g fat (36 g saturated, 1.5 g trans)
· 265 g carbohydrates · 233 g sugars

BEN AND JERRY'S

C What sets B&J's apart from the competition amounts to more than just an affinity for jam bands and green pastures. The shop also adheres to a lofty commitment to the quality and source of its ingredients. All dairy is free from rBGH (growth hormones) and the chocolate, vanilla, and coffee ingredients are all Fair Trade Certified. From a strict nutritional standpoint, though, it's still just an ice cream shop.

SURVIVAL STRATEGY

With half of the calories of the ice cream, sorbet makes the healthiest choice on the menu. If you demand dairy, the frozen yogurt can still save you up to 100 calories per scoop.

Best
Half Baked Frozen Yogurt (1 scoop) · 160 calories · 2.5 g fat
  (1 g saturated) · 20 g sugars

Worst
Coconut Seven Layer Bar Ice Cream (1 scoop) · 276 calories
· 17 g fat (11 g saturated, 0.5 g trans)
· 20 g sugars

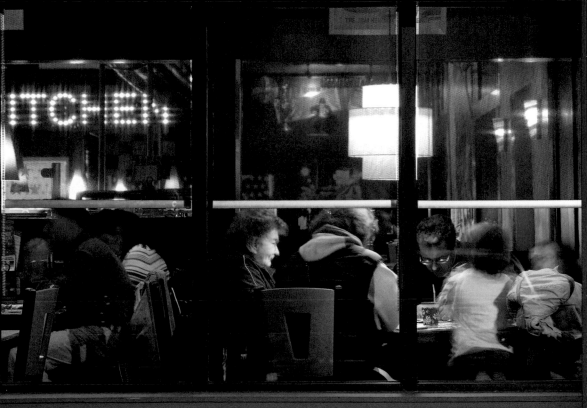

Sit down for this
Our research shows that the average entrée at a sit-down restaurant contains 345 more calories than an entrée from a fast-food establishment.

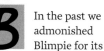

BLIMPIE

B In the past we admonished Blimpie for its love of trans fat. Since then, the chain has quietly removed all the dangerous oils from its menu and earned itself a worthy spot in our good book. But that doesn't mean the menu is free from danger. Blimpie likes to splash oil on just about everything with deli meat, and there are a handful of subs that top the 1,000-calorie mark.

SURVIVAL STRATEGY

A ham Bluffin makes a decent breakfast, and the Grilled Chicken Teriyaki Sandwich is one of the best in the sandwich business. But skip the wraps and most of the hot sandwiches. And no matter which sandwich you choose, swap out mayo and oil for mustard or light dressing.

Best
Club Sandwich (6")

· *363 calories · 11 g fat (5 g saturated)*
· *1,003 mg sodium*

Worst
Super Stacked BLT Sandwich (12")
· *1,265 calories*
· *82 g fat (18 g saturated)*
· *2,870 mg sodium · 84 g carbohydrates*

BOB EVANS

C- Sure there are plenty of healthy entrée and side options on the menu, but too much of Bob's food suffers from an overdose of dangerous trans fat. The Stacked & Stuffed Pancakes, for instance, have between 6 and 9 grams per serving, and the Slow Roasted Chicken Pot Pie has a near heart-stopping 13 grams.

SURVIVAL STRATEGY

If it sounds unhealthy (chicken fried steak, potpie, stuffed hotcakes), it is. Breakfast should be staples like oatmeal, eggs, fruit, and yogurt; for lunch and dinner, stick with grilled chicken or fish paired with one of the fruit and vegetable sides that avoid the fry treatment.

Best
Fit from the Farm Breakfast with Oatmeal · *364 calories*
· *13 g fat (3 g saturated)*
· *815 mg sodium · 37 g carbohydrates*
· *24 g sugars*

Worst
Stacked & Stuffed Caramel Banana Pecan Hotcakes
· *1,543 calories · 77 g fat*
  (29 g saturated, 9 g trans)
· *2,259 mg sodium*
· *198 g carbohydrates · 109 g sugars*

BOSTON MARKET

B+ Boston Market's menu has plenty of land mines— including nutritional disasters disguised as comfort food, such as potpies and creamed spinach. But those items are offset by a host of lean, roasted meats and steamed vegetables, which are among the healthiest contributions from the kitchens of the Deep South.

SURVIVAL STRATEGY

Pair roasted turkey, ham, white-meat chicken, or even sirloin with a vegetable side or two and you've got a solid dinner. But avoid calorie-laden dark-meat chicken, meat loaf, potpie, or hot Carver Sandwiches.

Best
¼ White Rotisserie Chicken (no skin) with Green Beans and Garlic Dill New Potatoes
· *440 calories · 10.5 g fat*
  (3.5 g saturated) · 1,190 mg sodium
· *32 g carbohydrates· 55 g protein*

Worst
Crispy Country Chicken Carver · *1,020 calories · 42 g fat*
  (7 g saturated) · 2,210 mg sodium
· *114 g carbohydrates · 45 g protein*

BURGER KING

C We got word from Burger King in October 2008 that they were finally removing the trans fat from their deep fryer. Excellent news, but don't think that means BK's menu is completely sans trans fat. The burgers and Whoppers are still sullied with the dangerous oils. Plus BK likes to smear 160 calories' worth of mayonnaise on just about everything, so you'd better get used to asking for your sandwich without. The unhealthiest of the Big Three burger joints.

SURVIVAL STRATEGY

For breakfast, pick the Ham Omelet Sandwich. For lunch, match the regular hamburger, the Whopper Jr., or the Tendergrill Sandwich with Apple Fries and water and you'll escape for less than 500 calories.

Best

Tendergrill Chicken Sandwich without Mayo · *380 calories · 9 g fat (2 g saturated) · 1,130 mg sodium*

Worst

Triple Whopper Sandwich with Cheese · *1,250 calories*
· *84 g fat (32 g saturated, 3.5 g trans)*
· *1,600 mg sodium*

CARL'S JR.

D+ Congrats to Carl's for finally getting with the times and removing the trans-fatty frying oil. Unfortunately, this West Coast staple is still swimming against the nutritional current, trying to lure the last of a dying breed of customers free of health concerns. The breakfast menu doesn't have a single entrée under 500 calories, the burgers are as bad as any in the country, and there's not a side on the menu that hasn't been dipped in oil.

SURVIVAL STRATEGY

Settle on either the Charbroiled Chicken Salad with Low-Fat Balsamic or the Charbroiled Chicken Sandwich, the only sandwich with less than 400 calories.

Best

Charbroiled BBQ Chicken Sandwich · *380 calories · 7 g fat (1.5 g saturated) · 1,010 mg sodium*

Worst

The Guacamole Bacon Six Dollar Burger · *1,040 calories*
· *70 g fat (25 g saturated)*
· *2,240 mg sodium*

CHEVYS

D Don't let the made-fresh-daily shtick distract you from the massive portions that push many of Chevys' meals beyond the 1,000-calorie threshold. Beyond the dangerous amount of fat found in most dishes (the average salad has 67 grams), you'll be hard-pressed to find an entrée with less than 2,000 milligrams of sodium.

SURVIVAL STRATEGY

The best items on the menu are the Homemade Tortilla Soup and the Santa Fe Chopped Salad. If you can't resist an entrée, order it without all the fixin's—tamalito, rice, sour cream, and cheese. That should knock more than 300 calories off your meal.

Best

Santa Fe Chopped Salad (no cheese) · *471 calories · 23 g fat (6 g saturated) · 1,067 mg sodium*
· *29 g carbohydrates*

Worst

Juicy Shrimp Fajitas
· *1,592 calories · 74 g fat (32 g saturated)*
· *4,993 mg sodium*
· *164 g carbohydrates*

CHICK-FIL-A

 Between the breakfast and lunch menus, there are only 3 entrées that break the 500-calorie barrier (the sausage biscuit, its bacon-strewn cohort, and the Chick-n-Strips Salad with ranch). And unlike the typical fast-food chain, Chick-fil-A offers a list of sides that goes beyond breaded and fried potatoes and onions. That's why we dub the Atlanta-based chicken shack one of our all-time favorite fast-food restaurants. Now, if they could just cut back on the salt.

SURVIVAL STRATEGY
Instead of nuggets or strips, look to the Chargrilled Chicken Sandwiches, which average only 315 calories apiece. And sub in a healthy side—fruit, carrot salad—for the standard fried fare.

Best
Chargrilled Chicken Sandwich
· 270 calories · 3 g fat (1 g saturated)
· 1,270 mg sodium

Worst
Chick-n-Strips Salad with Buttermilk Ranch Dressing
· 610 calories · 39 g fat (8.5 g saturated)
· 1,440 mg sodium

CHILI'S

 From burgers to baby back ribs, Chili's serves up some of the saltiest and fattiest fare in the country. In fact, 73 percent of its starters and entrées have more than 1,000 milligrams of sodium. The Guiltless Grill menu is Chili's admirable attempt to offer healthier options, but even there the average entrée carries 1,320 milligrams of sodium.

SURVIVAL STRATEGY
There's not too much to choose from after you cut out the ribs, burgers, fajitas, chicken, and salads. You're better off with a Classic Sirloin and steamed vegetables or broccoli. Another solid option is the Fajita Pita Chicken with Black Beans and Pico de Gallo.

Best
Fajita Pita Chicken · 455 calories
· 13 g fat (2 g saturated)
· 1,401 mg sodium · 52 g carbohydrates

Worst
Crispy Honey-Chipotle Chicken Crispers · 1,960 calories
· 108 g fat (17 g saturated)
· 4,780 mg sodium · 187 g carbohydrates

CHIPOTLE

There are only a few bad items on Chipotle's menu: the 290-calorie flour tortillas, the 130-calorie servings of white rice, and the 570-calorie chips. Unfortunately, these are the backbones of most meals. Without realizing it, the careless customer can easily construct a 1,000-calorie burrito. Still, Chipotle gets bonus points for using responsible, sustainable purveyors like Niman Ranch.

SURVIVAL STRATEGY
Chipotle assures us that they'll make anything a customer wants—except a smaller burrito—as long as they have the ingredients. With fresh salsa, beans, lettuce, and grilled vegetables, you can do plenty of good, like our protein favorite below.

Best
Crispy Tacos (3) with Carnitas, Black Beans, Lettuce, and Salsa
· 515 calories · 15 g fat (4 g saturated)
· 1,340 mg sodium

Worst
Carnitas Fajita Burrito with Rice, Beans, Corn Salsa, Cheese, Sour Cream, and Guacamole
· 1,205 calories · 55 g fat
  (20 g saturated) · 2,720 mg sodium

Free for all,
good for none

The restaurant industry is essentially
a lawless society, nutrition-wise: Aside
from regulations in specific places
(like Manhattan), no rule exists that says
restaurants must publish their nutritional
information. Some do it anyway
(God bless 'em), but at least 10 major
national chains keep those numbers
under suspicious lock and key.

CHUCK E. CHEESE'S

 While the average impact of a regular slice at Chuck E.'s stacks up well with most other pie places, it's the other areas of the menu that don't make the grade. Combine the oversize sandwiches with the no-thin-crust policy and you see what we mean. The distraction of video games may be the best thing Chuck E. Cheese has going for itself.

SURVIVAL STRATEGY

The safest bet is the salad bar, but good luck getting the kids to eat anything but pizza. Otherwise, stick to the Canadian bacon and vegetable toppings and cap the munching at 2 slices. That should keep the damage below 500 calories.

Best
Small Veggie Combo pizza
(2 slices) · 270 calories · 10 g fat
(4 g saturated) · 638 mg sodium
· 40 g carbohydrates

Worst
Italian Sub Oven-Baked
Sandwich · 790 calories · 39 g fat
(12 g saturated) · 2,374 mg sodium
· 78 g carbohydrates

CICI'S PIZZA

Cici's began in Texas in 1985 and now boasts more than 600 locations, proving definitively that Americans love a good buffet. The good news for our waistlines is that the crust is moderately sized and the pizza comes in varieties beyond simple sausage and pepperoni. But if you check your willpower at the door, you're probably better off skipping the pizza buffet entirely.

SURVIVAL STRATEGY

It takes 20 minutes for your brain to tell your body it's full, so start with a salad and then proceed slowly to the pizza. Limit yourself to the healthier slices like the Zesty Veggie, Alfredo, and the Olé, which is a Mexican-inspired pie with only 108 calories per slice.

Best
Olé Pizza (1 slice, buffet pizza)
· 110 calories · 3 g fat (1 g saturated)
· 290 mg sodium · 20 g carbohydrates

Worst
Bar-B-Que Pizza (1 slice, to-go
pizza) · 240 calories · 6 g fat
(3 g saturated) · 710 mg sodium
· 36 g carbohydrates

COLD STONE CREAMERY

"Overindulge" is the not-so-silent mantra emanating from Cold Stone's menu board. Their largest-size ice cream bears the dubious name Gotta Have It; small milk shakes weigh in at 1,000 calories; and even a modest scoop of ice cream can be spoiled with an extra 190 calories' worth of Reese's. On the other hand, Cold Stone does offer a nice variety of sorbet, frozen yogurt, and fat-free ice cream.

SURVIVAL STRATEGY

Go low by filling a Like It—size cup with a Sinless scoop and with fresh fruit strewn on top. Or opt for one of the creamery's 16-ounce real-fruit smoothies, which average 290 calories apiece.

Best
Sinless Sans Fat Sweet
Cream with Blackberries (Like It)
· 150 calories · 0 g fat (0 g saturated)
· 11 g sugars

Worst
Nutter Butter Ice Cream
with Reese's Peanut Butter Cups
(Gotta Have It) · 1,130 calories
· 70 g fat (34 g saturated, 1 g trans)
· 101 g sugars

COSÌ

 Answering the call for healthier options, Così recently unveiled the new Lighten Up! Menu, which relies on light dressings, low-fat mayo, and modest cheese servings to turn some of the more egregious menu items into some fairly decent nosh. That's a step in the right direction, to be sure, but it does little to rein back the breakfast menu's oversize muffins or bagel-sandwich belt busters, and every sandwich flanked by Così's Etruscan Whole Grain Bread is still saddled with an extra 470 calories from the oversize bread.

SURVIVAL STRATEGY

Get cozy with Così's Lighten Up! Menu. Only 2 items top the 500-calorie mark: the Light Cobb Salad and the Light Chicken TBM.

Best
Turkey Light Sandwich
· 390 calories · 5 g fat · 827 mg sodium
· 62 g carbohydrates · 26 g protein

Worst
Meatball Pesto Flatbread Pizza · 992 calories · 57 g fat
· 1,766 mg sodium
· 102 g carbohydrates · 47 g protein

DAIRY QUEEN

D+ Dairy Queen has a taste for excess that rivals that of other fast-food failures such as Carl's Jr. and Hardee's. But unlike Carl's, DQ offers a whole slew of abominable ice cream creations to pair with its calorie-riddled savory bites. Here's a look at one hypothetical meal: a Mushroom Swiss Burger with Regular Onion Rings and a Small Snickers Blizzard—a staggering 1,650-calorie meal with 78 grams of fat.

SURVIVAL STRATEGY

Your best offense is a solid defense. Skip elaborate burgers, fried sides, and specialty ice cream concoctions. Order a Grilled Chicken Sandwich or an Original Burger, and if you must have a treat, stick to soft serve or a small sundae.

Best
Original Hamburger
· 350 calories · 14 g fat
  (7 g saturated, 0.5 g trans)
· 680 mg sodium

Worst
6-Piece Chicken Strip Basket with Country Gravy · 1,640 calories
· 74 g fat (12 g saturated, 1 g trans)
· 3,690 mg sodium

DENNY'S

D+ Too bad the adult menu at Denny's doesn't adhere to the same standard as the kids' menu. The famous Slam breakfasts all top 800 calories, and the burgers are even worse. The Double Cheeseburger is one of the worst in the country, with 116 grams of fat, 7 of which are trans fat.

SURVIVAL STRATEGY

The Fit Fare menu gathers together all the best options on the menu. Outside of that, stick to the sirloin, grilled chicken, or soups. For breakfast, order a Veggie Cheese Omelette or create your own meal from à la carte options such as fruit, oatmeal, toast, and eggs.

Best
Veggie Cheese Omelette with Egg Beaters · 410 calories · 22 g fat
  (7 g saturated) · 1,100 mg sodium
· 11 g carbohydrates · 39 g protein

Worst
Flat Jack Sizzlin Skillet
· 1,210 calories · 60 g fat
  (18 g saturated) · 2,590 mg sodium
· 126 g carbohydrates · 45 g protein

DOMINO'S

 The Bad News Pies on Domino's menu are the same as those at any other pizza purveyor: oversize crusts, fatty meats, and greasy shag carpets of cheese. But Domino's Crunchy Thin Crust cheese pizza is one of the lowest-calorie pies in America, which makes a sound foundation for a decent dinner. Just avoid the bread sticks and Domino's appalling line of pasta bread bowls and oven baked sandwiches.

SURVIVAL STATEGY

Domino's thin crust has fewer calories than any other pizza chain's. Show your appreciation by making it your go-to order. Want toppings? Stick to ham and pineapple or pure veggies.

Best

Thin Crust Pizza with Ham and Pineapple (2 slices, medium pizza)
· *310 calories · 14 g fat (5 g saturated)*
· *680 mg sodium · 32 g carbohydrates*

Worst

Chicken Bacon Ranch Oven Baked Sandwich · *890 calories*
· *45 g fat (16 g saturated, 1 g trans)*
· *2,210 mg sodium · 72 g carbohydrates*

DUNKIN' DONUTS

 The Dunkin' camp has made major improvements in recent years. The doughnut king cast out the trans fat in 2007, and they've been pushing the menu toward healthier options since—including the DDSmart Menu, which draws out the menu's nutritional champions and introduces the low-fat and protein-packed Flatbread sandwiches. Now there's no excuse to settle for bagels, muffins, or doughnuts, which are as nutritionally empty as ever.

SURVIVAL STRATEGY

Use the DDSmart Menu as a starting point, then stick to the sandwiches served on flatbread or English muffins. If you must order doughnuts, always opt for raised donuts over their cake counterparts.

Best

Egg White Turkey Sausage Flatbread Sandwich
· *280 calories · 6 g fat (2.5 g saturated)*
· *820 mg sodium · 37 g carbohydrates*

Worst

Sausage, Supreme Omelet & Cheese on Bagel · *690 calories*
· *31 g fat (13 g saturated)*
· *1,870 mg sodium · 78 g carbohydrates*

EINSTEIN BROS. BAGELS

This Einstein is no genius. Half of the items on this menu come served on or with a bagel—and each one comes loaded with twice as many carbs as a doughnut. And outside the bagel menu, not a wrap or specialty sandwich has fewer than 500 calories. An occasional bagel won't kill you, but a habit of these oversize sandwiches might be grounds for a new gym membership.

SURVIVAL STRATEGY

The best lunch option is the pairing of a half deli sandwich with a cup of soup. Add to that a side of fruit salad and a zero-calorie beverage and you'll have a well-rounded meal for around 400 calories.

Best

Half Deli Tuna Salad with cup of chicken noodle soup
· *340 calories · 11 g fat (2 g saturated)*
· *1,230 mg sodium*
· *39 g carbohydrates · 20 g protein*

Worst

Bros. Bistro Salad with Chicken
· *940 calories · 71 g fat (12 g saturated)*
· *810 mg sodium · 39 g carbohydrates*
· *30 g protein*

Marketing mischief
The food industry spends $30 billion a year on advertising—70 percent of it pitching convenience foods, candy, soda, and desserts.

FAZOLI'S

C When it comes to the kids' menu, you won't find a better Italian restaurant. Unfortunately, the grown-ups aren't treated with the same respect. An ill-formed pasta dish with a single bread stick might eat up 60 percent of your day's calories. What sets Fazoli's apart from the competition, however, is the option to order smaller portions and top your pasta with your choice of fresh vegetables and lean protein.

SURVIVAL STRATEGY

Among the small pasta bowls, there's not a single one with more than 520 calories. Give your noodles some extra protein and fiber by topping them off with peppery chicken and broccoli.

Best

Spaghetti Marinara with Grilled Chicken and Broccoli (small)
· 585 calories · 6 g fat (1 g saturated)
· 1,290 mg sodium · 95 g carbohydrates

Worst

Fettucine with Alfredo and Meatballs (regular) and a Garlic Bread Stick · 1,180 calories · 43 g fat (15.5 g saturated) · 2,590 mg sodium · 151 g carbohydrates

FIVE GUYS

C Without much more than burgers, hot dogs, and French fries on the menu, it's difficult to find anything nutritionally redeeming about Five Guys. The only option geared toward the health-conscious is the Veggie Sandwich, which also happens to be the only item on the menu to carry a load of trans fat. The burgers range from 480 to 920 calories, so how you order can make a big difference to your waistline.

SURVIVAL STRATEGY

The regular hamburger is actually a double, so order a Little Hamburger and load up on the vegetation. And if you must indulge somewhere, don't do it with the fries— the difference between a large and a small is 1,150 calories.

Best

Little Hamburger · 480 calories
· 26 g fat (11.5 g saturated)
· 380 mg sodium · 39 g carbohydrates

Worst

Bacon Cheeseburger
· 920 calories · 62 g fat (29.5 g saturated) · 1,310 mg sodium · 40 g carbohydrates

HÄAGEN-DAZS

D+ Häagen-Dazs doesn't provide nutritional information for the many in-house concoctions, but if its regular soft serve and packaged ice cream (the most caloric in the supermarket) are any indication, the numbers can't be good. And the many sundaes, shakes, and cakes on offer are surefire ways to double down on the danger. We do appreciate Häagen-Dazs' simplicity, but they'll need to adjust their sugar and cream ratios before we can proclaim this a safe place to eat.

SURVIVAL STRATEGY

The frozen yogurts all hover around the 200-calorie range, and the sorbets are closer to 120. Wander far from there and you'll be hovering in the 300-calorie range for a small scoop of ice cream.

Best

Mango Sorbet (1 scoop)
· 120 calories · 0 g fat · 36 g sugars

Worst

Belgian Chocolate Shake
· 1,260 calories · 79 g fat (47 g saturated) · 102 g sugars

HARDEE'S

C- A 1997 purchase by CKE Restaurants put Hardee's under the same parent company as Carl's Jr., and the adopted brothers are slowly coming to look like identical twins. Their penchant for oversize eats plays out most potently in the line of Monster Thickburgers. But while Hardee's elongated menu tips toward the heavy side, it also serves up more modest choices, which helps it earn a slightly less dismal grade than its big brother.

SURVIVAL STRATEGY

Choose a breakfast sandwich topped with ham or jelly and avoid anything served in a bowl or platter. Then for lunch, stick to single-patty burgers or ask for a Regular Roast Beef Sandwich.

Best

Small Cheeseburger
· 350 calories · 16 g fat (4 g saturated)
· 780 mg sodium · 36 g carbohydrates

Worst

⅔-Pound Monster Thickburger
· 1,420 calories · 108 g fat
  (43 g saturated) · 2,770 mg sodium
· 46 g carbohydrates

IHOP

 We knew IHOP was up to no good when it refused to reveal its nutritional information when we first asked in 2007. But not even our suspicions could prepare us for the numbers exposed when a New York City law forced them to post their calorie counts: 1,000-calorie crepes, 1,200-calorie breakfast combos, and 1,800-calorie Crispy Chicken Strips. The F is for its closed-door policy, but it might not score much better even if we crunched the numbers.

SURVIVAL STRATEGY

You'll have a hard time finding a regular breakfast with less than 700 calories and a lunch or dinner with less than 1,000 calories. Your only safe bet is to stick to the "IHOP for Me" menu, where you'll find the nutritional content for a small selection of healthier items.

Best

IHOP for Me Garden Scramble
· 440 calories

Worst

Big Steak Omelette
· 1,490 calories

IN-N-OUT BURGER

C+ In-N-Out's is the most pared down of all the burger-joint menus. Wander in and you'll find nothing more than burgers, fries, shakes, and sodas. While that's certainly nothing to build a diet on, In-N-Out earns major points for offering the Protein-Style burger, which replaces the carb-heavy bun with lettuce and saves you 150 calories.

SURVIVAL STRATEGY

A single cheeseburger and a glass of iced tea or H_2O make for a reasonable lunch, but if you want to opt for the formidable Double-Double, learn to say, "Protein Style, please." If not, you're looking at a nearly 700-calorie meal—and that's before you add fries and a drink.

Best

Protein-Style Hamburger
· 240 calories · 17 g fat (4 g saturated)
· 370 mg sodium · 11 g carbohydrates
· 13 g protein

Worst

Double-Double · 670 calories
· 41 g fat (18 g saturated, 1 g trans)
· 1,440 mg sodium · 39 g carbohydrates
· 37 g protein

JACK IN THE BOX

D+ This menu has plenty of suitable options, but where it fails, it fails in dangerous ways. At least half a dozen burgers surpass the detrimental 900-calorie mark, and everything that touches Jack's fryer emerges with a soggy load of trans fat. Order a side of Bacon Cheddar Potato Wedges, for instance, and you'll clog your arteries with 13 grams of trans fat, which is about 6 times the daily limit set by the American Heart Association.

SURVIVAL STRATEGY
Keep your burger small or order a Whole Grain Chicken Fajita Pita with a fruit cup on the side. For breakfast, order any Breakfast Jack without sausage. Whatever you do, don't touch the fried foods.

Best
Whole Grain Chicken Fajita Pita · *320 calories · 11 g fat (3.5 g saturated, 0.5 g trans) · 1,090 mg sodium · 33 g carbohydrates*

Worst
Double Bacon & Cheese Ciabatta Burger · *1,063 calories · 69 g fat (26 g saturated, 2 g trans) · 1,596 mg sodium · 64 g carbohydrates*

JAMBA JUICE

A− There's no doubt that smoothies can be part of a healthy diet, but there's an erroneous halo of health that seems to hang over all things smoothie-related. Make this your rule: If it includes syrup or added sugar, it ceases to be a smoothie. Jamba Juice makes more than a few faux-fruit blends, but their menu has plenty of real-deal smoothies. Just make sure you choose the right one.

SURVIVAL STRATEGY
For a perfectly guilt-free treat, opt for a Jamba Light or All Fruit Smoothie in a 16-ounce cup. And unless you're looking to put on weight for your new acting career, don't touch the Peanut Butter Moo'd or any of the other Creamy Treats.

Best
Berry Fulfilling Jamba Light (16 ounces) · *160 calories · 0.5 g fat · 26 g sugars*

Worst
Peanut Butter Moo'd (Power) · *1,170 calories · 30 g fat (7 g saturated) · 169 g sugars*

JIMMY JOHN'S

C Jimmy adheres to the bigger-is-better syndrome that pollutes countless sub shops the country over. Two slices of 7-Grain Wheat Bread run an unthinkable 390 calories, making healthy sandwich construction impossible. Good thing Jimmy John's preps the food in front of you; that way, you can play foreman while the sub crew constructs your perfect low-cal sandwich.

SURVIVAL STRATEGY
Start with the sub-size French bread, which has 140 fewer calories than its wheat cousin. Then build a sub from a single lean meat—ham, turkey, or roast beef—being sure to replace mayo with Dijon or avocado spread. And stay away from the Italian cold cuts!

Best
Totally Tuna Unwich (lettuce wrap) · *263 calories · 20 g fat (4 g saturated) · 603 mg sodium · 9 g carbohydrates*

Worst
The J.J. Gargantuan · *1,008 calories · 55 g fat (15 g saturated) · 3,783 mg sodium · 60 g carbohydrates*

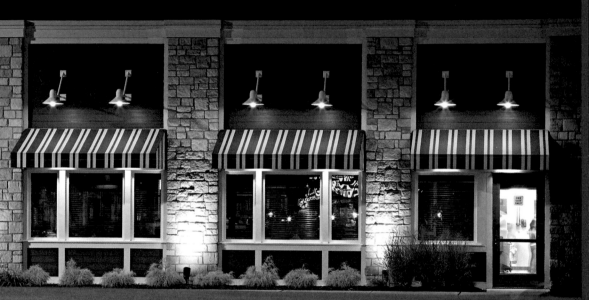

Calorie conundrums
We took to the streets with six of the worst
restaurant meals in America and asked
60 people to estimate the total calories in each.
Their average guess? Sixty-eight percent
fewer calories than what the dishes
actually contained.

KFC

 B+ Hold on a second! KFC gets a B+? KFC, the most vilified of the fried-chicken purveyors, has more than a few strong suits. The menu's crispy bird-bits are offset by skinless chicken pieces, low-calorie sandwich options, and a host of sides that go beyond the fryer. Plus, their recent introduction of grilled chicken to the menu shows they're determined to cast aside their Kentucky fried past.

SURVIVAL STRATEGY
Go the skinless route or pal up with a Chicken Stacker or a Toasted Sandwich. Then adorn your plate with one of the Colonel's healthy sides: Mashed Potatoes and Gravy, Corn on the Cob, Three-Bean Salad, or KFC Mean Greens.

Best
KFC Snacker with OR Strip and Buffalo Sauce · *240 calories · 7 g fat (2 g saturated) · 710 mg sodium · 29 g carbohydrates*

Worst
Chicken and Biscuit Bowl
· *780 calories · 37 g fat (14 g saturated, 1 g trans) · 2,440 mg sodium · 84 g carbohydrates*

KRISPY KREME

C− Unlike Dunkin' Donuts, which is expanding its menu to include more legitimate options, Krispy Kreme is stuck in the carb-heavy world of glazed, powdered, and jelly-filled dough rings. Their one dubious expansion move was to introduce Chillers, frozen beverages that can pack more than 1,000 calories into a 20-ounce cup. The good news is that Krispy Kreme has finally cut trans fat from its doughnuts. The bad news is a single doughnut can still carry more than half a day's saturated fat and more sugar than a Snickers bar.

SURVIVAL STRATEGY
Cap your sweet tooth at 1 filled or specialty doughnut or, worst case scenario, 2 glazed.

Best
Original Glazed Doughnut
· *200 calories · 12 g fat (6 g saturated) · 22 g carbohydrates · 10 g sugars*

Worst
Chocolate, Chocolate Chiller
(20 ounces) · *1,050 calories · 42 g fat (36 g saturated) · 170 g carbohydrates · 100 g sugars*

LITTLE CAESAR'S

C The quick-draw pizza maker has speed down to an art. Too bad efficiency has to come at the cost of options. Like Chuck E. Cheese's, Little Caesar's doesn't offer a thin-crust pie, which automatically puts them at a caloric disadvantage. And at least Chuck E. Cheese makes up for it with a salad bar. The Caesar might suffice in a pinch, but if you've got time, seek out a better option up the road.

SURVIVAL STRATEGY
Start with a few chicken wings to get some belly-filling protein into your system before moving on to pizza. Since Little Caesar's isn't selling thin crusts, you'll have to settle for a regular cheese pizza. Just be sure to close the box after 2 slices.

Best
Oven-Roasted Caesar Wings
(2 pieces) · *100 calories · 7 g fat (2 g saturated) · 300 mg sodium · 0 g carbohydrates*

Worst
Pepperoni Deep Dish Pizza
(2 slices) · *720 calories · 32 g fat (12 g saturated) · 1,220 mg sodium · 76 g carbohydrates*

LONG JOHN SILVER'S

C- Blame a stubborn reliance on partially hydrogenated oils for the sheen of trans fat that coats nearly everything to emerge from Long John's kitchen. The fish mogul has the healthy sides—Vegetable Medley, Corn Cobbettes—in place. But for now, it's not safe to eat fried food at a place where a snack-size box of Breaded Clam Strips means 7 grams of trans fat for your bloodstream.

SURVIVAL STRATEGY

The only fish to avoid the trans-fat oils are those that are grilled or baked. Pair one of those options with a healthy side. If you need some extra flavor, choose cocktail sauce or malt vinegar over tartar sauce.

Best
Baked Cod (1 piece) · *120 calories*
· *4.5 g fat (1 g saturated)*
· *240 mg sodium* · *1 g carbohydrates*
· *22 g protein*

Worst
Ultimate Fish Sandwich
· *530 calories* · *28 g fat*
  (8 g saturated, 5 g trans)
· *1,400 mg sodium*
· *49 g carbohydrates* · *21 g protein*

MANCHU WOK

C+ When analyzed individually, most of Manchu's entrée options hover in a respectable 200-calorie range. But factor in the inevitable side of empty, blood sugar—spiking carbs that comes with everything you order and it's hard to find a meal less than 500 calories. Lose the rice and noodles and win the battle of the bulge.

SURVIVAL STRATEGY

If you can't remember which chicken dishes are the best, just go with the red meat. Not a single beef dish has more than 180 calories per serving. More important, ask for vegetables instead of starch. This single move will save you 240 calories over white rice. If you must order a starch, choose the lo mein—easily the best carb on the menu.

Best
Pepper Steak · *170 calories*
· *12 g fat (2.5 g saturated)*
· *510 mg sodium* · *10 g carbohydrates*

Worst
Honey Garlic Chicken
· *430 calories* · *21 g fat (3.5 g saturated)*
· *940 mg sodium* · *50 g carbohydrates*

McDONALD'S

B+ The world-famous burger baron has come a long way since the days of *Fast Food Nation*—at least nutritionally speaking. The trans fat is mostly gone, the calorie bombs reduced, and there are more healthy options such as salads and yogurt parfaits. But don't cut loose just yet. Too many of the breakfast and lunch items still top the 500-calorie mark, and the dessert menu is a total mess.

SURVIVAL STRATEGY

The Egg McMuffin remains one of the best ways to start your day in the fast-food world. As for the later hours, you can splurge on a Big Mac or a Quarter Pounder, but only if you skip the fries and soda, which add an average of 590 calories onto any meal.

Best
Egg McMuffin · *300 calories*
· *12 g fat (5 g saturated)*
· *820 mg sodium* · *30 g carbohydrates*

Worst
Deluxe Breakfast with Large Biscuit, Syrup, and Margarine
· *1,370 calories* · *64.5 g fat*
  (21.5 g saturated) · *2,335 mg sodium*
· *161 g carbohydrates*

NOAH'S BAGELS

 Carb-loaded bagels are bad enough. But even outside the bagel menu, only one wrap or specialty sandwich has fewer than 450 calories. An occasional bagel won't hurt you, but a habit of these blood sugar—spiking breakfasts and oversize sandwich vehicles might earn you an oversize wardrobe. Throw in a disastrous dessert menu and a long list of heavily sweetened coffee drinks, and you've got way too many ways to fail.

SURVIVAL STRATEGY

The best lunch option is a half deli sandwich and a cup of soup. If you go with a full sandwich or wrap, be sure to pair it with a cup of fruit, not the potato salad or chips.

Best
Veggie Wrap · *460 calories*
· *17 g fat (6 g saturated)*
· *610 mg sodium*

Worst
City Salad with Chicken
· *950 calories · 66 g fat (12 g saturated)*
· *820 mg sodium*

OLIVE GARDEN

 We initially gave the Garden an F for failing to disclose their nutritional content. And we really appreciate the effort they've made to increase their transparency. But when a typical entrée packs an average of 905 calories (and that's before you factor in appetizers, sides, drinks, and desserts), it's not time to celebrate just yet.

SURVIVAL STRATEGY

While most pasta dishes are packed with at least a day's worth of sodium and more than 1,000 calories, the Linguine alla Marinara and Ravioli di Portobello are both reasonable options. As for chicken and seafood, stick with the Herb-Grilled Salmon, Parmesan Crusted Tilapia, or Shrimp and Asparagus Risotto.

Best
Herb-Grilled Salmon
· *510 calories · 26 g fat (6 g saturated)*
· *760 mg sodium · 5 g carbohydrates*

Worst
Chicken & Shrimp Carbonara
· *1,440 calories · 88 g fat*
  (38 g saturated) · 3,000 mg sodium
· *80 g carbohydrates*

ON THE BORDER

On the Border is a subsidiary of Brinker International, the same parent company that owns Chili's and Romano's Macaroni Grill. It should come as no surprise then that its food is just as detrimental to your health as its corporate brothers. The massive menu suffers from appetizers with 120 grams of fat, salads with a full day's worth of sodium, and taco entrées with no less than 1,100 calories. Hope you left your appetite at home.

SURVIVAL STRATEGY

The Border Smart Menu highlights 5 items with less than 600 calories and 25 grams of fat. Those aren't great numbers considering they average 1,600 milligrams of sodium apiece, but that's all you've got to work with.

Best
Pico Shrimp Tacos
· *490 calories · 5 g fat (1 g saturated)*
· *1,650 mg sodium*

Worst
Dos XX Fish Tacos with Creamy Red Chile Sauce
· *2,350 calories · 152 g fat*
  (31 g saturated) · 4,060 mg sodium

Risky investments

Americans spend half of their food dollars—about $500 billion a year—away from home.

OUTBACK STEAKHOUSE

You wouldn't order a meal if the restaurant refused to tell you the price, would you? Fat, calories, and sodium are all just as much a part of the overall cost of a meal as the dollar value. That's why we flunk Outback along with the rest of the nutritional holdouts. You don't show up for the test, you can't make the grade.

SURVIVAL STRATEGY

Curb your desire to order the 14-ounce rib eye (1,190 calories) by starting with the protein-rich Seared Ahi Tuna. Then move on to one of the leaner cuts of beef: the petite fillet or the prime rib. Assuming you skip the bread and house salad (590 calories) and choose steamed vegetables as your side, you might have a shot at escaping dinner for less than 1,000 calories.

Best

Prime Rib (8 ounces) with Seasonal Veggies and a Baked Potato
· *690 calories*

Worst
Bacon Cheese Burger
· *1,900 calories*

PANDA EXPRESS

 Oddly enough, it's not the wok-fried meat or the viscous sauces that cause this menu the most harm; it's the more than 400 calories of rice and noodles that form the foundation of each meal. Scrape these starches from the plate and Panda Express starts to look a lot healthier: Only one entrée item has more than 500 calories and hardly a trans fat on the menu. Gut-bloating problems arise when multiple entrées and sides start piling up on one plate, so bring your self-restraint.

SURVIVAL STRATEGY

Avoid these entrées: Orange Chicken, Sweet & Sour Chicken, Beijing Beef, and anything with pork. Then swap in Mixed Veggies for the ice cream scoop of rice.

Best
Mushroom Chicken with side of Mixed Veggies · *290 calories*
· *18 g fat (3.5 g saturated)*
· *765 mg sodium · 21 g carbohydrates*

Worst
Orange Chicken with Fried Rice
· *1,025 calories · 44 g fat (9 g saturated)*
· *1,640 mg sodium · 118 g carbohydrates*

PANERA BREAD

Artisan they may be, but some of the sandwiches push into quadruple digits, and a train-length list of brownies, pastries, and cookies almost qualifies Panera as a dessert shop. Pitfalls aside, the healthy selection of soups and salads offers a much-needed reprieve from the carb-heavy bagels and breads.

SURVIVAL STRATEGY

Breakfast options abound with refined carbohydrates, so cut your losses and order the Egg & Cheese breakfast sandwich. Skip the stand-alone sandwich lunch. Either pair together a soup and salad or take the soup and half-sandwich combo.

Best
Half Asian Sesame Chicken Salad with cup of Vegetarian Black Bean Soup · *405 calories*
· *15 g fat (2 g saturated)*
· *1,540 mg sodium · 48 g carbohydrates*

Worst
Chipotle Chicken Sandwich on Artisan French Bread
· *1,030 calories · 55 g fat
(13 g saturated, 1 g trans)*
· *2,540 mg sodium · 79 g carbohydrates*

PAPA JOHN'S

C Give Papa John's credit for being the only pizza franchise to offer a whole wheat crust, thus providing a viable, fiber-rich option to pizza lovers the country over. Combine that with an innovative list of healthy toppings—including the surprisingly lean Spinach Alfredo—and you start to see hope for Papa John's devotees. The chain loses big points for its line of treacherous dipping sauces, its belly-building bread sticks, and its 400-calorie-a-slice pan-crust pizza.

SURVIVAL STRATEGY
There are only two crust options to consider: thin and wheat. Ask for light cheese and cover it with anything besides sausage, pepperoni, or bacon.

Best
Garden Fresh Thin Crust Pizza (1 slice) · *210 calories*
· *11 g fat (2.5 g saturated)*
· *470 mg sodium · 23 g carbohydrates*

Worst
The Meats Pan Crust Pizza
(1 slice) · *440 calories · 26 g fat*
(8 g saturated) · 890 mg sodium
· *37 g carbohydrates*

P.F. CHANG'S

D+ A plague of quadruple-digit entrées turns Chang's menu into a nutritional minefield. Noodle dishes and foods from the grill all come with dangerously high fat and calorie counts, while traditional stir-fries aren't much better. Chang's does have a great variety of low-cal appetizers and an ordering flexibility that allows for easy substitutions and tweaks.

SURVIVAL STRATEGY
Order a lean appetizer like the Chicken Lettuce Wraps or the Seared Ahi Tuna for the table and resolve to split one of the more reasonable entrées between 2 people. Earn bonus points by tailoring your dish to be light on the oil and sauce.

Best
Wild Alaskan Salmon Steamed with Ginger (full serving)
· *250 calories · 28 g fat (4 g saturated)*
· *1,066 mg sodium · 18 g carbohydrates*

Worst
Combo Lo Mein (full serving)
· *1,968 calories · 96 g fat*
(12 g saturated) · 5,860 mg sodium
· *236 g carbohydrates*

PIZZA HUT

C In an attempt to push the menu beyond the ill-reputed pizza, Pizza Hut expanded into toasted sandwiches, pastas, and salads. Sound like an improvement? Think again. Every sandwich has at least 680 calories and 75 percent of your day's sodium. The salads aren't much better, and the pastas are actually worse. The thin crust pizzas and the Fit 'n Delicious offer redemption with sub-200-calorie slices. Eat a couple of those and you'll be doing just fine.

SURVIVAL STRATEGY
Start with a bowl of Tomato Basil Soup and then finish with a couple of slices. Turn to anything on the Fit 'n Delicious menu for slices as low as 150 calories.

Best
Ham, Red Onion & Mushroom Fit 'n Delicious Pizza (2 slices)
· *320 calories · 9 g fat (3 g saturated)*
· *1,100 mg sodium · 46 g carbohydrates*

Worst
Meat Lover's Personal Pan Pizza · *900 calories · 50 g fat*
(19 g saturated, 1 g trans)
· *2,250 mg sodium · 70 g carbohydrates*

POPEYE'S

 With the exception of the mayo-loaded Deluxe Sandwich, Popeye's menu isn't burdened by any items with more than 600 calories. Unless you go with all fried foods, the Louisiana kitchen makes it easy to get a nutritional bang for your caloric buck. The only dark spot on this chain's résumé is the trans fat lingering in its frying oil. The calories might be low, but everything with skin intact is carrying a load of the heart-clogging fats.

SURVIVAL STATEGY

The average piece of skinless chicken has 82 percent less fat than the regular crispy cuts. And when it comes to sides, mashed potatoes and the Cajun-specialty Crawfish Etouffee trounce plain ol' French fries. Stick with these and you'll be just fine.

Best

Po Boy Sandwich · *330 calories* · *17 g fat (3 g saturated)* · *560 mg sodium* · *36 g carbohydrates*

Worst

Deluxe Sandwich · *630 calories* · *31 g fat (8 g saturated, 1 g trans)* · *1,480 mg sodium* · *53 g carbohydrates*

QUIZNOS

Submarine sandwiches can only be so bad, right? We thought so, too, until we saw some of the bloated offerings on Quiznos' menu. The bigger subs can easily carry a full day's worth of saturated fat and close to 2 days of sodium, and the oversize salads aren't much better. Good thing Quiznos also provides an alternative. The sub shop's Sammies are served in flatbreads, and all fall between 200 and 300 calories apiece.

SURVIVAL STRATEGY

Avoid the salads, large subs, and soups that come in bread bowls. Stick with a small sub (at 310 calories, the Honey Bourbon Chicken is easily the best) or pair a Sammie with a cup of soup.

Best

Sonoma Turkey Flatbread Sammie

· *280 calories* · *14 g fat (4 g saturated)* · *740 mg sodium* · *26 g carbohydrates* · *12 g protein*

Worst

Roasted Chicken with Honey Mustard Flatbread Salad

· *1,070 calories* · *71 g fat (13.5 g saturated)* · *1,770 mg sodium* · *69 g carbohydrates* · *37 g protein*

RED LOBSTER

Like a lot of chain restaurants, Red Lobster has been slow in offering up its nutritional secrets—refusing to tell consumers what exactly they were eating. This past year, the chain relented—and they deserve credit for doing so. Turns out that with a strong roster of low-calorie, high-protein fish and seafood entrées, plus a number of healthy sides to boot, Red Lobster has earned the distinction of America's healthiest sit-down chain restaurant.

SURVIVAL STRATEGY

Avoid calorie-heavy Cajun sauces, combo dishes, and anything labeled "crispy." And tell the waiter to keep those biscuits for himself. You'll never go wrong with simple broiled or grilled fish and a vegetable side.

Best

Broiled Flounder · *280 calories* · *3 g fat (0.5 g saturated)* · *560 mg sodium* · *0 g carbohydrates*

Worst

Admiral's Feast · *1,506 calories* · *93 g fat (9 g saturated)* · *4,662 mg sodium* · *101 g carbohydrates*

Supersize you

For an average 17 percent more money, you get yourself 55 percent more calories when you supersize a fast-food meal. A bargain—if you consider flab a good investment.

ROMANO'S MACARONI GRILL

D- This fatty Italian spot serves some of the worst appetizers in the country, offers just 3 dinner entrées with less than 800 calories, and hosts no fewer than 40 menu items with more than a full day's recommended sodium intake. A select few menu items carry the restaurant's Sensible Fare logo, but unfortunately these can still carry up to 640 calories.

SURVIVAL STRATEGY
Take advantage of the build-your-own-pasta option. Ask for the marinara over a bed of the restaurant's whole wheat penne and then top it with grilled chicken and steamed vegetables. You can also order lunch-size entrées at both lunch and dinner.

Best
Pollo Magro "Skinny Chicken"
· *320 calories · 7 g fat (1.5 g saturated)*
· *1,950 mg sodium · 30 g carbohydrates*

Worst
Parmesan-Crusted Sole
· *2,190 calories · 141 g fat*
  (58 g saturated) · 2,980 mg sodium
· *145 g carbohydrates*

RUBY TUESDAY

D+ The chain earned its infamy off a hearty selection of hamburgers. The problem is that they average 76 grams of fat apiece—more than enough to exceed the USDA's recommended limit for the day. Even the veggie and turkey burgers have more than 900 calories! The chain rounds out its menu with a selection of appetizers that hover around 1,000 calories, a smattering of high-impact entrées like potpie and ribs, and an egregious selection of salads that are just as bad.

SURVIVAL STRATEGY
Solace lies in the three S's: steak, seafood, and sides. Sirloin, salmon, and shrimp all make for relatively innocuous eating, especially when paired with one of Ruby Tuesday's half-dozen healthy sides such as mashed cauliflower and baby green beans.

Best
Petite Sirloin · *285 calories*
· *15 g fat · 2 g carbohydrates*

Worst
Colossal Burger · *2,014 calories*
· *141 g fat · 95 g carbohydrates*

SBARRO

F Please welcome Sbarro to the list of restaurants that refuse to disclose their food facts. As of this writing, the nutritional information on Sbarro's Web site is frozen in a permanent state of "under construction." Sounds like a pizza pie to the face of anyone who cares about eating healthy. We'll be happy to revise the grade once Sbarro cleans up the scaffolding and jack hammers and reveals a site teeming with nutritional transparency. In the meantime, proceed with caution.

SURVIVAL STRATEGY
Sbarro serves up massive New York—style slices, so keep it to one and be sure to make it of the thin-crust variety. Round out the meal with a side of fruit or a tomato and cucumber salad.

Best
New York Style Thin Cheese Pizza (1 slice) · *460 calories*

Worst
Spaghetti with Chicken Parmigiana · *930 calories*

SCHLOTZSKY'S

C+ Although none of Schlotzsky's menu items cross the 1,000-calorie threshold, far too many of them come dangerously close. More than half of the small-size subs pack more than 500 calories, and there are small amounts of trans fat in everything from pizzas to paninis. The soups get it the worst—a bowl of Schlotzsky's Boston Clam Chowder has 5 grams of trans fat, not to mention 70 percent of your day's sodium.

SURVIVAL STRATEGY
Stay away from fancy, store-branded subs like the Original, Deluxe, and Albuquerque Turkey. Or, if you can't work it out, just order the Chipotle Chicken Sub or the Baby Spinach Salad Pizza.

Best
Small Chicken Breast Sandwich · *344 calories · 4 g fat*
(0 g saturated) · 1,343 mg sodium
· 52 g carbohydrates

Worst
Medium Albuquerque Turkey
· 972 calories · 51 g fat
(16 g saturated, 1 g trans)
· 2,432 mg sodium
· 80 g carbohydrates

SMOOTHIE KING

B- Smoothie King, the older and smaller of the two smoothie titans, suffers from portion problems. The smallest adult option is 20 ounces, which makes it that much harder to keep escalating sugar calories under the lid. Smoothie King does offer to cut out the turbinado sugar that sweetens most of its smoothies, which eliminates up to 100 empty calories. But why not remove the sugar entirely from the menu? Isn't fruit sweet enough?

SURVIVAL STRATEGY
Favor the Stay Healthy and Trim Down portions of the menu and be sure to stick to 20-ounce smoothies. No matter what you do, avoid anything listed under Indulge or anything with the word Hulk in the name.

Best
Youth Fountain (skinny, 20 ounces) · *153 calories · 0 g fat*
· 38 g carbohydrates · 31 g sugars

Worst
The Hulk Strawberry (40 ounces) · *2,088 calories · 70 g fat*
(32 g saturated)
· 314 g carbohydrates · 240 g sugars

SONIC

C For whatever it's worth, Sonic manages to keep all of its burgers under the 1,000-calorie threshold, but just barely. Its sides menu, with a fat-loaded lineup of fries, tots, and onion rings, will push you well beyond that. And if you settle on a shake or a sugar-spiked "fruit" drink to wash down your lunch, you may have just doubled your caloric intake. It's best to view Sonic as a quick-stop snack shop because full-on meals can be dangerous.

SURVIVAL STRATEGY
The Jr. Banana Split makes an awesome treat with only 180 calories. Besides that, there are a couple of staples that you should remember: the Jr. Burger, the Grilled Chicken Wrap, and the Grilled Chicken on Ciabatta.

Best
Grilled Chicken Wrap
· 380 calories · 11 g fat (3 g saturated)
· 1,440 mg sodium · 44 g carbohydrates

Worst
Super Sonic Cheeseburger with Mayo · *980 calories*
· 64 g fat (24 g saturated, 2.5 g trans)
· 1,430 mg sodium · 58 g carbohydrates

STARBUCKS

 Starbucks' signature line of drinks typically involves injecting espresso with massive loads of sugary syrup and milk, making 500 calories too common for comfort. Plus their selection of muffins and pastries leaves much to be desired. That said, Starbucks has recently begun offering more nutritious items such as oatmeal, specialty drinks made with skim milk, and in-store pamphlets instructing customers on how to cut calories from their favorite drinks.

SURVIVAL STRATEGY

There's no beating a regular cup of joe or unsweetened tea, but if you need a specialty fix, stick with skim milk, sugar-free syrup, and no whipped cream. As for food, go with Perfect Oatmeal or a Spinach, Roasted Tomato, Feta & Egg.

Best

Nonfat Cappuccino (Tall)

· 60 calories · 0 g fat · 8 g sugars

Worst

2% Peppermint White Chocolate Mocha (Venti) · 660 calories · 22 g fat (15 g saturated) · 95 g sugars

SUBWAY

 If Jared was able to shed 245 pounds on his own Subway diet, then surely you can find a decent meal to keep your gut in check. But beware of what researchers call the "health halo." Patrons who believe they're eating in a healthy place tend to reward themselves with extra cheese, mayonnaise, and soda, none of which would have helped Jared lose a single pound. Avoid the halo shine and you'll be fine at Subway.

SURVIVAL STRATEGY

Stick to 6-inch cold subs made with ham, turkey, roast beef, or chicken. Be sure to load up on veggies and skip the fattening sauces and dressings (calorie counts at Subway don't include cheese, mayo, or dressings).

Best

Ham Sandwich on 9-Grain with all the veggies you want

· 290 calories · 5 g fat (1.5 g saturated) · 1,260 mg sodium

Worst

Footlong Meatball with Cheese

· 1,260 calories · 54 g fat (22 g saturated) · 3,570 mg sodium

TACO BELL

 Here's the good news: The next time you run for the border, you don't have to run all the way home to burn off the calories. Taco Bell combines 2 things with bad nutritional reputations—Mexican food and fast food—but provides plenty of paths to keep your meal less than 500 calories. The best way to do it is to stick with the Fresco Menu, where no single item exceeds 350 calories.

SURVIVAL STRATEGY

Grilled Stuft Burritos, food served in a bowl, and anything prepared with multiple "layers" are trouble. Instead, order any combination of 2 of the following: crunchy tacos, bean burritos, or anything on the Fresco menu.

Best

Fresco Ranchero Chicken Soft Tacos (2)

· 340 calories · 8 g fat (3 g saturated) · 1,460 mg sodium

Worst

Fiesta Taco Salad · 840 calories · 45 g fat (11 g saturated, 1.5 g trans) · 1,780 mg sodium

T.G.I. FRIDAY'S

We salute Friday's for one thing and one thing only, and that's their smaller-portions menu. The option to order smaller plates ought be the new model to dethrone the dogmatic bigger-is-better principle that dominates chain restaurants. But no matter how small they shrink the entrées, we're still forced to fail this chain due to their strict policy of nutritional secrecy.

SURVIVAL STRATEGY

We realized just how dangerous Friday's menu was when a New York City ordinance forced them to cough up the numbers on their caloric bombs. Our advice: Stick to either their smaller-portions menu or check out the Lighter Side of Friday's menu, which promises to find you meals with around 500 calories apiece.

Best
Shrimp Key West · *370 calories*
Worst
Jack Daniel's Ribs and Shrimp
· *1,910 calories*

UNO CHICAGO GRILL

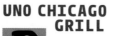

Uno has a number of serious strikes against it: They invented the deep-dish pizza, they encouraged gluttony with their one-time Bigger and Better menu, and in 1997, they faced false-advertising charges for erroneously claiming that some of their pizzas were low in fat. They've since increased nutritional transparency at all of their stores, but from appetizers to desserts, this menu is still riddled with belt-busting loads of calories.

SURVIVAL STRATEGY

Stick with flatbread over deep-dish pizzas—it could save you more than 1,000 calories in a sitting. Beyond that, turn to soups, grilled or baked fish dishes, and sirloin for nutritional salvation.

Best
Grilled Mahi-Mahi with Mango Salsa · *240 calories*
· *2 g fat (0 g saturated)*
· *980 mg sodium · 12 g carbohydrates*
Worst
Chicago Classic Deep Dish Pizza (individual pizza)
· *2,310 calories · 165 g fat*
  (54 g saturated) · 4,920 mg sodium

WENDY'S

Scoring a decent meal at Wendy's is just about as easy as scoring a bad one, and that's a big compliment for a burger joint. Options such as chili and mandarin oranges offer the side-order variety that's missing from less-evolved fast-food chains like Dairy Queen and Carl's Jr. Plus they offer a handful of Jr. Burgers that don't stray far over 300 calories. Where they err is in their expanded line of desserts and their roster of double- and triple-patty burgers, including the infamous Baconator.

SURVIVAL STRATEGY

The grilled chicken sandwiches and wraps don't exceed 320 calories. Or opt for a small burger and pair it with chili or a side salad.

Best
Single with Everything
· *430 calories · 20 g fat (7 g saturated)*
· *870 mg sodium*
Worst
Triple with Everything and Cheese · *960 calories · 60 g fat*
  (27 g saturated) · 2,010 mg sodium
· *39 g carbohydrates*

14 Restaurant
SURVIVAL STRATEGIES

Whether you find yourself in the drive-thru or the local sushi den, use these immutable rules to navigate the many nutritional land mines waiting for you in the restaurant world.

❶ Front-load with protein

So what's the best way to start the meal? Easy—you want something loaded with lean protein. A study published in *Physiology & Behavior* showed that people who ate a protein-heavy appetizer consumed an average of 16 percent fewer calories in their entrée than those who loaded up with carbohydrates. The effect is spoiled, though, if you wolf down a bunch of greasy chicken strips. Look for something like shrimp cocktail, which hasn't been deep-fried or slathered with cheese.

❷ Beware of the booze

We know life's rough, but here's the deal: The standard cocktail has anywhere from 200 to 500 calories, yet those who drink before a meal actually wind up eating more come chow time. Researchers in the Netherlands gave people a premeal treatment of booze, food, water, or nothing. Those who had the booze spent more time eating, began feeling full later in the meal, and consumed an average 192 extra calories.

❸ Beware of portion distortion

According to data collected by the Nationwide Food Consumption Survey, food portions are growing. Hamburgers, for instance, have grown by 97 calories since 1977. French fries have grown by 68 calories. The problem with this is, as the research points out, that people don't necessarily stop eating when they're full. Students at Cornell were given access to an all-you-can-eat buffet and told to go to town. Researchers took note of how much they ate; the following week, they served the same students portions of either equal size, 25 percent bigger, or 50 percent bigger. Those with 25 percent more food ate 164 more calories, and those with 50 percent more food ate 221 extra calories.

❹ Enjoy the conversation

It takes your stomach about 20 minutes to tell you that you're full. That means you need to eat slowly so you get the message before you've overeaten. That shouldn't be hard—just set your fork down every now and again and tell one of the many adventurous stories from your childhood. Told them already? Make up some new ones.

❺ Avoid handouts

Just because it doesn't cost money doesn't mean it doesn't have a price. Munch on a couple of Olive Garden's bread sticks or Red Lobster's Cheddar Bay Biscuits and you've just put down 300 calories before your meal arrives. A basket of chips at the Mexican joint? Expect a price tag around 500 calories, which can easily double the impact of an entrée. Not so free now, is it?

❻ Don't fall for combos

At every fast-food restaurant, as soon as you decide on an entrée, expect to face some variation of this question: "Would you like to make it a combo meal?" Of course, you're tempted. This is the modern-day equivalent of supersizing, wherein you get an average of 55 percent more calories for 17 percent more money. It's also the cheapest way to get fat in a hurry. Just say no.

❼ Drink responsibly

Sure, sure, you know all about the dangers of soda, but here's what you might not realize: A cup of sweet tea is only marginally better than Pepsi. Each glass you drink with dinner adds about 120 calories to your meal, and the same goes with juice. In fact, America's love affair with flavored drinks adds 450 calories to our daily diet, according to a study from the University of North Carolina. That's an extra 47 pounds of body mass to burn off (or not) each year. Switch to water, though, and it has the opposite effect: The more you drink, the more you shrink. Choose accordingly.

❽ Think big

Restaurants are not required to emblazon nutritional information on the side of their plates, which makes it nearly impossible to guess how many calories are in each meal. Care to venture a guess? Well, if you're like most people, you're not even in the ballpark. A 2006 study published in the *American Journal of Public Health* found that consumers given an obviously high-calorie restaurant meal still underestimated the caloric load by an average of 600 calories. Use that as the new barometer to gauge the heft of your dinner.

❾ Think thin

Want to know the easiest way to make a portly pizza? Here's a hint: It has nothing to do with toppings. Nope, the biggest problem facing your pie is the massive boat of oily crust hunkering along the bottom. Your best defense is to order it as thin as you can. Three deep-dish slices from a large Domino's pie, before toppings, will cost you 1,002 calories. Downsize that to a thin crust and you just burned off 420 calories without lifting a finger. Who knew losing weight was so easy?

❿ Invite the kids to the grown-up table

Speaking of pizza, how do you rein in the kids' growing affection for cheese and pepperoni? Not by ordering them a personal pan found on so many kids' menus across America. The mini pepperoni at Pizza Hut runs 660 calories, and even the kids' regular crust pizza at Uno Chicago Grill has 780. And it's not just pizza; from 873-calorie "mini" turkey burgers at Ruby Tuesday to 981-calorie nachos at On the Border, kids' menus are often cluttered with problematic foods. Massive portions like this help explain how today's little ones consume 180 more calories per day than their peers of 1989. That's a lot of girth over the course of childhood. Instead of ordering whole meals, combat the trend by feeding the small appetites with a little off your plate. A couple of slices of your thin pepperoni pizza, for instance, will cost only 400 calories. Half a cheeseburger? About 350 calories. Make this the norm and you'll save calories for them and yourself.

⓫ Side with sides

Some of the best of restaurant fare can be found in the side items section of the menu. Plates of black beans, roasted seasonal vegetables, and even skewers of "add-on" shrimp are prime fodder for a healthy meal. Stick to two and you can walk out feeling better for not having busted your calorie bank. (Oh, and you'll save cash, too—if you're into that kinda thing.)

⓬ Personalize your order

Think of the menu as a list of starting points. Any respectable joint in the country—even fast-food purveyors—will tailor to your wants, but only if you voice them. The caloric savings are as big as your imagination. Take a BLT—ask for mustard instead of mayo, then pick off a slice or two of bacon and you've just cut 250 to 400 calories from your sandwich. Use these to help you get the hang of it: Ask them to sub in whole-grain bread on your sandwich at Panera, to make your pasta with whole wheat noodles at Macaroni Grill, and to go light on the oil with your omelet at Denny's. There, wasn't that easy?

⓭ Order it to go

How many times have you finished your plate just because there wasn't enough to take home? Well, next time, make sure there's enough. Every time you order a full-size dinner entrée, ask the server to deliver a to-go box with your food. The food is easier to divide before you start eating, and you won't have to fight the temptation of a half-eaten manicotti sticking in your face.

⓮ Be a dessert dodger

When the food-industry research company Technomic surveyed 1,500 people on their dessert habits, not a single person reported that they never ate dessert. To contrast, 57 percent said they ate dessert frequently. Of course, there's no problem with an occasional treat, but there is a problem when it tacks on half a day's calories to the end of your meal. The average dessert at T.G.I. Friday's, for instance, packs 819 calories. So rather than order your own massive dessert, ask for an extra spoon and take a few bites from your tablemates' orders. You'll be doing everyone a favor.

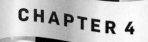

CHAPTER 4

The Best
(&Worst)
Breakfasts
in America

Eat This

McDonald's Egg McMuffin

300 calories
12 g fat
(5 g saturated)
820 mg sodium

Add a cup of joe, but pass on the hash browns. Those little potato pucks pack 150 empty carb calories.

Save 480 calories!
That means you could have 2 Egg McMuffins and still pocket an extra 180 calories to be used later in the day.

Save 39 g fat!
Plus you'll trim a heap of salt from the morning meal.

Not That!

Hardee's Loaded Breakfast Burrito

780 calories
51 g fat
(20 g saturated)
1,620 mg sodium

Hardee's breakfast menu reads like a blueprint of how not to start your day. Exhibit A: A massive tortilla swaddling a glut of ham, bacon, sausage, eggs, cheese, and hash browns. You might as well stay in bed.

Are you really ready to sacrifice an entire day's worth of saturated fat to a food made in the microwave?

"A hearty breakfast."

Perhaps no three more promising words have been as twisted and manipulated into meaninglessness (except perhaps, "If elected, I'll...").

A hearty breakfast ought to be, as the cliché goes, the most important meal of the day. Studies show that people who take time for a morning meal consume fewer calories over the course of the day, have stronger cognitive skills, and are 30 percent less likely to be overweight or obese. Beyond that, people who skip breakfast are more likely to drink alcohol and smoke, and they're less likely to exercise. Your morning meal, in other words, is like the foundation of your house—everything else rests on it. As long as you start your day with some fiber (from whole grains), lean protein (from eggs, low-fat dairy, or peanut butter), and some vitamins and minerals (from fruit), you're in great shape.

But when food marketers get their hands on it, "a hearty breakfast" turns into something more like "a heart-unhealthy breakfast." Because an unhealthy heart is exactly what many of the country's most popular breakfast joints are setting you up for, by peddling fatty scrambles, misguided muffin missiles, and pancakes that look like manhole covers. These foods are loaded with unhealthy fats, added sugars, and refined carbohydrates, which catapult your blood sugar, sap your energy levels, and tell your body to store fat. Start your day this way and you'll be ready for a second breakfast—and a nap—before 11 A.M.

To help you avoid the morning mishaps, we searched out the good, the bad, and the greasy and uncovered some of the best and worst breakfast foods in America. This one choice—what to start your day with—is both the easiest and the most important, as long as you know what to look for and what to avoid.

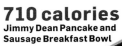

710 calories
Jimmy Dean Pancake and Sausage Breakfast Bowl

The emerging breakfast bowl trend is a troubling one for health-conscious eaters. It invariably involves a carb- and fat-riddled amalgamation of eggs, meat, pancakes, and potatoes—or some combination thereof.

The Worst Breakfasts in America

17 General Mills Reese's Puffs (1 cup)

- *150 calories*
- *4 g fat (1 g saturated)*
- *1.5 g fiber*
- *15 g sugars*

This cereal has more sugar than you'll find in a real Reese's Peanut Butter Cup and just a trace of fiber. Not all super-sweet cereals are terrible for you—consider General Mills Honey Nut Cheerios, which you can easily blend with regular Cheerios to lower the sugar content but hang on to the flavor.

Eat This Instead!
Honey Nut Cheerios (1 cup)
- *138 calories • 2 g fat (0 g saturated)*
- *2.5 g fiber • 11 g sugars*

WORST SUPERMARKET
BREAKFAST BAR

16 Kellogg's Special K Bliss Bar Raspberry (2 bars)

- *180 calories*
- *4 g fat (2 g saturated)*
- *< 1 g fiber*
- *18 g sugars*

Special K shrinks the bar down to half the normal size, but it's still nearly 40 percent sugar and doesn't even contain a whole gram of fiber. Choosing a cereal bar is just like choosing a cereal: Look for as much fiber and as little sugar as possible.

Eat This Instead!
Fiber One Oats & Chocolate (1 bar)
- *140 calories • 4 g fat (1.5 g saturated)*
- *9 g fiber • 10 g sugars*

WORST SUPERMARKET
"HEALTHY" CEREAL

15 Bear Naked All Natural Banana Nut Granola (½ cup)

- *280 calories*
- *14 g fat (4 g saturated)*
- *4 g fiber*
- *10 g sugars*

Granola may be the most overrated breakfast food of all time. What do you think is holding all those clumps together? Sugar and oil. And 4 grams of fiber just isn't enough to save this bowl. Studies have shown that if you eat more fiber at breakfast, you'll consume fewer calories throughout the day. Choose All-Bran, which is as fiber-rich as it gets.

Eat This Instead!
Kellogg's All-Bran Original (1 cup)
- *160 calories • 2 g fat (0 g saturated)*
- *20 g fiber • 12 g sugars*

WORST SUPERMARKET
BREAKFAST PASTRY

14 Otis Spunkmeyer Muffins Banana Nut (1 muffin)

- *460 calories*
- *22 g fat (3 g saturated)*
- *32 g sugars*
- *1 g fiber*

Otis Spunkmeyer is often the king of calorie- and sugar-packed breakfast pastries. Scarier still is the fact that this muffin sounds so harmless—bananas and nuts are usually considered health-food staples. But think of muffins as cupcakes without the icing and you'll understand why this particular breakfast bread contains as much sugar as you'll find in 14 Hershey's Kisses.

Eat This Instead!
Quaker Muffin Bars Banana & Oats (1 bar)
- *130 calories • 3.5 g fat (1 g saturated)*
- *11 g sugars • 4 g fiber*

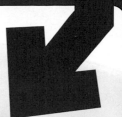

Anxious to know how much fat and sodium are packed into this beef and cheddar bomb? So are we, but unfortunately, IHOP is one of the few chain restaurants in the country that don't provide nutritional information for their menu items.

1,490 calories
IHOP The Big Steak Omelette

150 calories
General Mills Reese's Puffs

WORST DOUGHNUT

13 Dunkin' Donuts Blueberry Crumb Donut

- *470 calories*
- *14 g fat (8 g saturated)*
- *52 g sugars*

Most doughnuts hover in the 200- to 300-calorie range, but Dunkin' Donuts has broken new barriers with this doughy disaster. Ignore the blueberry bells and whistles: This one doughnut packs more calories than an Egg McMuffin and hash browns at McDonald's and nearly as much sugar as 5 bowls of Froot Loops. Always opt for raised doughnuts over cake doughnuts. The raised type pack plenty of yeast, which gives the doughnuts lift and reduces caloric density. Cake doughnuts, as the name suggests, are just dessert in the shape of a zero.

Eat This Instead!
Sugar Raised Donut
- *190 calories • 9 g fat (4 g saturated)*
- *4 g sugars*

WORST "HEALTHY" BREAFAST

`12` Dunkin' Donuts Multigrain Bagel with Reduced Fat Strawberry Cream Cheese

- 550 calories
- 19 g fat (7 g saturated)
- 800 mg sodium
- 80 g carbohydrates

The worst part about this breakfast is that scores of health-conscious eaters order this thinking they're making a smart choice. No matter how healthy the bagel or its toppings may appear, there is just no escaping the fact that bagels are bogus. You're unlikely to find any bagel combination that registers less than 400 calories, based almost entirely around refined carbs and low-grade fats.

Eat This Instead!
Egg and Cheese English Muffin Sandwich
- 320 calories • 13 g fat (5 g saturated)
- 730 mg sodium • 34 g carbohydrates

WORST FROZEN BREAFAST

`11` Jimmy Dean Pancake and Sausage Links Breakfast Bowl

- 710 calories
- 31 g fat (11 g saturated)
- 890 mg sodium
- 34 g sugars

A disastrous trifecta of refined carbs from the pancakes, saturated fat from the sausage, and added sugar from the syrup. Jimmy's got

The Great Cereal Spectrum

The average American consumes more than 160 bowls of cereal a year, so picking the right box could mean knocking 15 pounds off your waistline yearly and infusing your diet with massive doses of vital nutrients. Use our bowl-by-bowl breakdown to find the perfect cereal for you. Our criteria: the highest ratio of fiber to sugar, along with a respectable calorie count. Sidle up and grab a spoon!

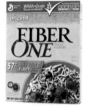

General Mills Fiber One Original
- 60 calories
- 1 g fat (0 g saturated)
- 14 g fiber
- 0 g sugars

The gold standard. Add sweetness with a bit of fresh fruit.

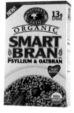

Nature's Path Organic Smart Bran
- 90 calories
- 1 g fat (0 g saturated)
- 13 g fiber
- 6 g sugars

You're getting 52 percent of your daily fiber in every bowl.

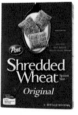

Post Shredded Wheat Original (spoon size)
- 170 calories
- <1 g fat (0 g saturated)
- 6 g fiber
- 0 g sugars

This one-ingredient cereal is the real breakfast of champions.

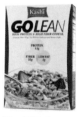

Kashi GoLean
- 80 calories
- 0.5 g fat (0 g saturated)
- 6 g fiber
- 3 g sugars

Low-cal, high-fiber, and a reasonable amount of sugar.

Figures are based on 30 grams of cereal.

The Worst Breakfasts in America

his name attached to more than a few solid breakfast choices, so find one less than 400 calories immediately and make the switch. Hint: Look to the breakfast sandwiches and the D-Lights line.

Eat This Instead!
Canadian Bacon, Egg White & Cheese Muffin Sandwich
· *230 calories · 6 g fat (3 g saturated)*
· *790 mg sodium*

WORST HANDHELD BREAKFAST

10 Hardee's Loaded Breakfast Burrito

· *780 calories*
· *51 g fat*
  (20 g saturated)
· *1,620 mg sodium*

Burritos are bad news in even the most capable hands, but give a giant tortilla to Hardee's and watch the mayhem ensue. Not surprisingly, they found a way to stuff ham, bacon, *and* sausage into the carb vessel, plus shredded cheddar and a pile of eggs. Your best strategy is to skip Hardee's lackluster breakfast fare altogether, but if you find yourself in a pinch, the Texas Toast sandwiches are your safest bet.

Eat This Instead!
Texas Toast Ham Breakfast Sandwich
· *390 calories · 18 g fat (6 g saturated)*
· *1,170 mg sodium*

The Great Cereal Spectrum—*Continued*

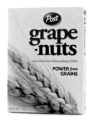

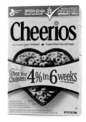

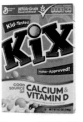

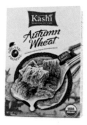

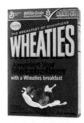

Post Grape-Nuts
· *103 calories*
· *0.5 g fat (0 g saturated)*
· *4 g fiber*
· *2 g sugars*

A small serving of these breakfast pellets should carry you until lunch.

General Mills Cheerios
· *107 calories*
· *2 g fat (0 g saturated)*
· *3 g fiber*
· *1 g sugars*

It's hard to beat the ubiquitous yellow box and its admirable balance of fiber and sugar.

General Mills Kix
· *110 calories*
· *1 g fat (0 g saturated)*
· *3 g fiber*
· *3 g sugars*

As far as the sweet cereals go, this is about as good as it gets.

Kashi Autumn Wheat
· *105 calories*
· *0.5 g fat (0 g saturated)*
· *3 g fiber*
· *4 g sugars*

A semisweet bowl without the risk of a sugar spike.

General Mills Wheaties
· *111 calories*
· *0.5 g fat (0 g saturated)*
· *3 g fiber*
· *4 g sugars*

Sure, they get athletic sponsors, but still lose out to a lot more nutritionally stacked cereals.

Figures are based on 30 grams of cereal.

9 Jack in the Box Hearty Breakfast Bowl

- *780 calories*
- *60 g fat*
  (20 g saturated, 6 g trans)
- *1,346 mg sodium*

The American Heart Association recommends that people not eat more than 2 grams of cholesterol-raising trans fat a day. This bowl alone contains nearly 3 times that limit. When in doubt, opt for the breakfast sandwich with ham; it's a strategy that works nearly everywhere—especially Jack's. And since it's available all day, consider it a smart way to avoid the dreary lunch and dinner options on the menu.

Eat This Instead!

Breakfast Jack

- *287 calories • 12 g fat*
  (4 g saturated, 0 g trans)
- *742 mg sodium*

8 Au Bon Pain Sausage, Egg, and Cheddar on Asiago Bagel

- *810 calories*
- *47 g fat*
  (23 g saturated, 0.5 g trans)
- *1,540 mg sodium*

A healthy breakfast sandwich has a low carbohydrate-to-protein ratio. That means the bread or bun holding the meat and eggs together should be

---

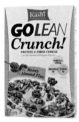

Kashi Go Lean Crunch! Honey Almond Flax

- *113 calories*
- *3 g fat (0 g saturated)*
- *5 g fiber*
- *7 g sugars*

Lose half the sugar and this would be a superlative cereal.

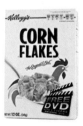

Kellogg's Corn Flakes

- *107 calories*
- *0 g fat*
- *1 g fiber*
- *2 g sugars*

The calorie count is okay, but the second ingredient is sugar. And where's the fiber?

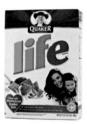

Quaker Life Cereal Original

- *112.5 calories*
- *1 g fat (0 g saturated)*
- *2 g fiber*
- *6 g sugars*

Seemingly harmless, but Life could do without the Yellow #5.

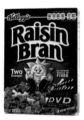

Kellogg's Raisin Bran

- *96 calories*
- *0.7 g fat (0 g saturated)*
- *3.5 g fiber*
- *10 g sugars*

Raisins are sweet enough naturally, so why coat them in sugar?

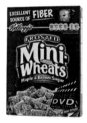

Kellogg's Frosted Mini-Wheats Maple & Brown Sugar

- *109 calories*
- *0.5 g fat (0 g saturated)*
- *3 g fiber*
- *7.5 g sugars*

For a sweetened cereal, Mini-Wheats at least deliver some fiber.

The Worst Breakfasts in America

minimized. A bagel, as one of the most carbohydrate-packed breads in the food chain, makes the worst vessel for any sandwich. Opt for English muffins as often as possible—they have less than half the calories and carbs of an average bagel.

Eat This Instead!

Egg and Cheddar Salsa Verde Sandwich

- *450 calories* • *22 g fat*
  (12 g saturated)
- *1,080 mg sodium*

WORST BREAKFAST PASTRY

7 Atlanta Bread Company Pecan Roll

- *860 calories*
- *59 g fat*
  (10 g saturated, 7 g trans)
- *34 g sugars*
- *72 g carbohydrates*

This pecan roll suffers from the sugar equivalent of 3 scoops of Bob Evans vanilla ice cream and the caloric equivalent of 3 Snickers bars. Overloading on carbohydrates

and sugar first thing in the morning will make you hungry again well before lunchtime. But if you're really in the mood for carbs, choose one of their muffin tops—about half the calories and sugar of a whole muffin but just as delicious.

Eat This Instead!

Blueberry Muffin Top

- *250 calories* • *12 g fat*
  (2 g saturated, 0 g trans)
- *20 g sugars* • *31 g carbohydrates*

The Great Cereal Spectrum—*Continued*

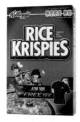

Kellogg's Rice Krispies
- *118 calories*
- *0 g fat*
- *0 g fiber*
- *4 g sugars*

Fiber is cereal's one true virtue, so why start your day with a bowl utterly devoid of it?

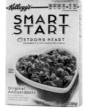

Kellogg's Smart Start
- *114 calories*
- *0 g fat (0 g saturated)*
- *2 g fiber*
- *8 g sugars*

Don't be lured in by the buzzwords. This is anything but an intelligent start to your day.

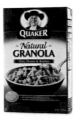

Quaker Natural Granola Oats, Honey & Raisins
- *123.5 calories*
- *3.5 g fat (2 g saturated)*
- *2 g fiber*
- *9 g sugars*

Most granolas are only a small step above sugary kids' cereals.

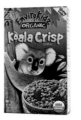

Nature's Path EnviroKidz Organic Koala Crisp
- *110 calories*
- *1 g fat (0 g saturated)*
- *2 g fiber*
- *11 g sugars*

Don't let the flowery label lead you astray—this cereal is no good.

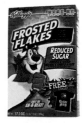

Kellogg's Reduced Sugar Frosted Flakes
- *116 calories*
- *0 g fat*
- *<1 g fiber*
- *8 g sugars*

The sugar decrease is minimal and the fiber offering is abysmal.

Figures are based on 30 grams of cereal.

WORST BREAKFAST BISCUIT

6 Arby's Sausage Gravy Biscuit

- *1,040 calories*
- *60 g fat*
  (22 g saturated, 2 g trans)
- *4,700 mg sodium*
- *107 g carbohydrates*

This one bloated biscuit has the caloric equivalent of 7 Hostess Twinkies and the sodium equivalent of 13 large orders of McDonald's French fries. Surprisingly enough,

Arby's is one of the few chains that have figured out how to bake some of their biscuits without the use of trans fat. This may be one of the first times we've ever recommended eating any biscuit, but the bacon option will save you 700 calories and 39 grams of fat.

Eat This Instead!

Bacon Biscuit

- *340 calories · 21 g fat*
  (6 g saturated, 0 g trans)
- *1,028 mg sodium · 29 g carbohydrates*

WORST BREAKFAST SMOOTHIE

5 Smoothie King Grape Expectations II (large)

- *1,096 calories*
- *0 g fat*
- *250 g sugars*

This 40-ounce industrial-strength sugar explosion easily makes it onto our list of the most sugar-packed foods in America. It's got the same amount of sweet stuff as you'd find in 10

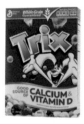

General Mills Trix

- *112 calories*
- *1 g fat (0 g saturated)*
- *<1 g fiber*
- *11 g sugars*

Let the rabbit have them for you; they're no good.

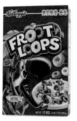

Kellogg's Froot Loops

- *113 calories*
- *1 g fat (0.5 g saturated)*
- *<1 g fiber*
- *12 g sugars*

The sugar rush will throw you for a loop.

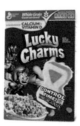

General Mills Lucky Charms

- *122 calories*
- *1 g fat (0 g saturated)*
- *1 g fiber*
- *12 g sugars*

A rainbow of artificial colors with a pot of sugar at the end.

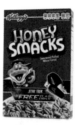

Kellogg's Honey Smacks

- *111 calories*
- *0.5 g fat (0 g saturated)*
- *1 g fiber*
- *17 g sugars*

The fiber-to-sugar ratio is alarming—this is essentially a bowlful of pure sucrose.

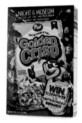

Post Golden Crisp

- *122 calories*
- *0 g fat*
- *<1 g fiber*
- *15.5 g sugars*

Sugar is the first ingredient.

The Worst Breakfasts in America

packs of Peanut M&Ms or 54 Oreo cookies! Add to that the fact that you'll slurp up half a day's calories through a little straw in a matter of minutes. Thankfully, Smoothie King offers plenty of legitimately healthy smoothies for any time of day, including anything in their low-carb line. Just keep it to a small, okay?

Drink This Instead!
Low-Carb Strawberry Smoothie (small)
· *268 calories* · *9 g fat (4 g saturated)*
· *3 g sugars*

WORST BREAKFAST BURRITO
4 Bob Evans Border Scramble Burrito

· *1,101 calories*
· *64 g fat*
  (24 g saturated, 1 g trans)
· *2,298 mg sodium*
· *81 g carbohydrates*

The problem here starts and stops with the massive tortilla conveyance, which not only packs on the calories but also provides a spacious home for excessive amounts of eggs, cheese, and salty breakfast meat. Whether they're called wraps or burritos, foods that rely on a giant vessel of refined carbohydrates to ensure their structural integrity should be cut out of your diet entirely. The menu at Bob Evans is overflowing with atrocious breakfast foods, and unfortunately this isn't even the worst offender.

Eat This Instead!
Border Scramble Omelet with Bob Evans Egg Lites
· *493 calories* · *31 g fat*
  (13 g saturated, 0 g trans)
· *1,187 mg sodium* · *14 g carbohydrates*

WORST ALL-INCLUSIVE BREAKFAST
3 McDonald's Deluxe Breakfast (large biscuit) with Syrup and Margarine

· *1,370 calories*
· *64.5 g fat (21.5 g saturated)*
· *2,340 mg sodium*
· *161 g carbohydrates*

This deluxe platter comes with nearly three-quarters of your day's allotment of calories and an entire day's worth of sodium. What's even scarier is that it's one of McDonald's most popular items. Make sure you get this most important meal of the day right—an Egg McMuffin and a cup of coffee definitely qualifies.

Eat This Instead!
Egg McMuffin
· *300 calories* · *12 g fat (5 g saturated)*
· *820 mg sodium* · *30 g carbohydrates*

WORST BREAKFAST OMELET
2 IHOP The Big Steak Omelette

· *1,490 calories*

We're not sure what's more concerning: IHOP's never-ending stacks of margarine-slathered sweets or their reckless attempts at covering the savory side of breakfast with entrées like this one. With close to three-quarters of a day's worth of calories folded into its eggy shell (thanks to a heaping portion of fatty beef), you're committing to eating rice cakes for your next 2 meals when you start your morning off with this bomblette. Why not enjoy the substantial Garden Scramble and 2 more real meals instead?

Eat This Instead!
IHOP for Me Garden Scramble
· *440 calories*

1 Bob Evans Stacked and Stuffed Caramel Banana Pecan Hotcakes

- *1,543 calories*
- *77 g fat*
  (26 g saturated, 9 g trans)
- *2,259 mg sodium*
- *198 g carbohydrates*
- *109 g sugars*

This appalling platter is stacked and stuffed with the sugar equivalent of 7 Twinkies, the caloric equivalent of 8 Dunkin' Donuts glazed doughnuts, the sodium equivalent of 6½ large orders of McDonald's French fries, and 4½ times your daily limit of trans fat. It's made numerous lists in this book, including Worst Foods, Most Sugar-Packed Foods, and Trans-Fattiest Foods. Above all of these dubious distinctions, it's the undisputed Worst Breakfast in America.

Eat This Instead!

3 Scrambled Egg Lites with 2 slices of bacon and fresh fruit

- *502 calories* · *19 g fat (7 g saturated)*
- *832 mg sodium* · *21 g carbohydrates*
- *19 g sugars*

1,543 calories
Bob Evans Stacked and Stuffed Caramel Banana Pecan Hotcakes

We took this train wreck to the street and asked people how many calories they thought it contains. The average estimate came in at 470 calories below the staggering reality.

The Best Breakfasts

START YOUR DAY WITH ONE OF THESE EARLY-MORNING ALL-STARS

BEST DOUGHNUT
Dunkin' Donuts Sugar Raised Donut

- 190 calories
- 9 g fat (4 g saturated)
- 4 g sugars

As vessels for refined carbohydrates and fat and little else, doughnuts probably should be denied induction into any hall of fame. But there comes a time when everyone craves a sweet start to the day. When such a mood strikes you and a doughnut is the only answer, you will find no "better" O-shaped breakfast pastry in America. Enjoy.

BEST BALANCED BREAKFAST
Bob Evans 3 Scrambled Egg Lites with 2 slices of bacon and fresh fruit

- 502 calories
- 19 g fat
  (7 g saturated)
- 832 mg sodium
- 21 g carbohydrates

Bob Evans is responsible for some of the worst nutrition crimes ever perpetrated during the morning hours, but we have to give credit where credit is due. The eggs and the bacon provide a solid shot of metabolism-spiking protein, while the fruit pitches in with belly-filling fiber and a host of antioxidants. So go to Bob Evans for breakfast if you must, but don't stray far from this dish.

BEST YOGURT
Fage Total 2%

- 150 calories
- 4.5 g fat
  (3 g saturated)
- 19 g protein
- 9 g sugars

We love Greek-style yogurt. Manufacturers like Fage and Stony-field's Oikos (another of our favorites) skim off the watery whey from their yogurts, yielding a thicker, richer product with more than twice the amount of protein you'll find in other popular brands. And why 2 percent and not fat free? Because research shows that a little bit of fat can have a strong effect on satiety.

BEST OMELET
Atlanta Bread Company Tomato Bacon Omelette

- 360 calories
- 27 g fat
  (12 g saturated)
- 1,000 mg sodium

Research published in the *International Journal of Obesity* found that people who start their day with eggs lose weight up to 65 percent faster than those who favor refined carbohydrates (like bagels). You'll be hard-pressed to find an omelet anywhere less than 400 calories, including at Atlanta Bread, where the Three Cheese Omelette weighs in at a staggering 1,100 calories. Consider this a diamond in the rough.

in America

BEST PACKAGED BREAKFAST

Jimmy Dean D-Lights Canadian Bacon, Egg White & Cheese Muffin Sandwich

- *230 calories*
- *6 g fat*
  (3 g saturated)
- *790 mg sodium*

It's an Egg McMuffin in a box instead of a to-go bag. Nearly 40 percent of the calories come from protein, which is exactly the type of percentage you need first thing in the morning. Just add a piece of fruit and a cup of hot coffee and you have everything you need to fire up your metabolism and begin to conquer the day.

BEST DRIVE-THRU BREAKFAST

McDonald's Egg McMuffin

- *300 calories*
- *12 g fat (5 g saturated)*
- *820 mg sodium*

With 18 grams of protein in a portable, handheld package, it's hard to beat McDonald's ubiquitous breakfast offering. Just don't veer away from the classic version with Canadian bacon; switching to sausage will tack on a useless 150 calories and 15 grams of fat.

Protein is never more important than in the morning hours, when your metabolism needs a jump start. Here are two great options rich in the macronutrient, one for home and one for when you're out and about.

230 calories
Jimmy Dean D-Lights
Canadian Bacon,
Egg White & Cheese
Muffin Sandwich

502 calories
Bob Evans 3 Scrambled Egg Lites with
2 slices of bacon and fresh fruit

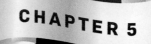

CHAPTER 5

The Best
(& Worst)
Salads
in America

Eat This

Panera Bread Asian Sesame Chicken Salad

(half portion) with Reduced-Sugar Asian Sesame Vinaigrette

255 calories
14 g fat (2 g saturated)
640 mg sodium

Save 1,105 calories!
Or go for the full-size salad and still cut 850 calories out of your lunch routine.

Make this one simple swap just once a week and you'll save more than 16 pounds in a year!

Not That!

T.G.I. Friday's Pecan Crusted Chicken Salad

1,360 calories*

*Friday's refuses to reveal the full nutritional data on their menu. We can only imagine why.

Health-imposter salads like this one are part of a nutritional scourge on the loose in this country's chain restaurants. Turn the page for another 10 frightening examples you must avoid.

Medical professionals

have a code they have been living by since the fourth century B.C. It's the motto of Hippocrates: First, do no harm. Never do something to a healthy patient that can make the person unhealthy.

Sadly, the Hippocratic oath does not apply to America's food marketers. No meal on the planet starts out healthier than salad. And when a salad is done right—when it is loaded with vitamins and minerals and fiber, is low in fat and sodium, and offers a wide array of tastes and textures—nothing can beat it as a weight-loss tool.

But today's "food doctors" get in there and, like Joan Rivers's plastic surgeons, keep tinkering until what comes out is nearly unrecognizable. Most of today's salad entrées aren't healthy at all, and your local salad bar is more like a jungle, where those once-tender leaves are drenched in a toxic rain of fat and sodium.

The most troubling thing about today's salad entrées is that those of us who really care about eating healthy are being lulled into the trap over and over again. Reports from the National Restaurant Association and the USDA show salad sales up by as much as 50 percent over the past decade, as more and more of us become health conscious in our food choices. But often, that dinner salad is as bad as—or worse than—anything else on a restaurant's menu. Today's fresh produce increasingly is freighted with more crumbled cheese, greasy bacon, and oily dressing. And often, what should be a cornucopia of crisp produce is reduced to wilted iceberg and some semifrozen peas.

With that in mind, we've developed a lineup of the most egregious veggie offenders, along with a few great salads that can guide your own green revolution.

910 calories
Quiznos Classic Cobb Flatbread Salad

The harmless-looking flatbread that comes with every salad actually packs 310 calories and 590 milligrams of sodium. Ditch it and go extra light on the dressing and this salad has a shot at being healthy.

The Worst Salads in America

WORST FAST FOOD SALAD
11 Wendy's Chicken BLT Salad with Honey Dijon Dressing and Croutons

- *790 calories*
- *53.5 g fat (14 g saturated)*
- *1,735 mg sodium*

A little bacon on your salad is one thing, but this bowl of lettuce packs the saturated equivalent of 14 crispy strips of swine. Not the model of health most people bargain for when they opt for a pile of greens. You can improve matters significantly (to the tune of 160 calories and 18 grams of fat) by swapping the recommended Honey Dijon for Balsamic Vinaigrette. Better yet, opt out of this salad entirely and grab the more reasonable Mandarin Chicken Salad. Or a burger; believe it or not, most burgers on Wendy's menu are considerably better for you than this bowl.

Eat This Instead!
Mandarin Chicken Salad with Balsamic Vinaigrette
- *470 calories • 22 g fat (2.5 g saturated)*
- *1,270 mg sodium*

WORST COBB SALAD
10 Quiznos Classic Cobb Flatbread Salad

- *910 calories*
- *58 g fat (12.5 g saturated, 0.5 g trans)*
- *1,890 mg sodium*
- *61 g carbohydrates*

Cobb salads are popular because they're so tasty. And it's no wonder—they're packed with bacon, egg, and tomatoes. Together they bring protein and other important nutrients to the table, but in the case of Quiznos' Cobb, they team up with the pile of flatbread to bring a reckless flood of calories. When 4 Krispy Kreme original glazed doughnuts have fewer calories than a pile of greens, you know something is wrong. All entrée-size salads from Quiznos are problematic, so stick with the smaller serving or pick up a few Sammies instead.

Eat This Instead!
Side Salad with Raspberry Chipotle Dressing
- *225 calories • 6 g fat (1 g saturated)*
- *515 mg sodium • 43 g carbohydrates*

WORST BISTRO SALAD
9 Einstein Bros. Bistro Salad with Chicken

- *940 calories*
- *71 g fat (12 g saturated)*
- *810 mg sodium*

Chicken, mixed greens, walnuts, raspberry vinaigrette: Sounds like good eating, right? Too bad the walnuts are candied, the leaves are strewn with salty hunks of Gorgonzola cheese, and the dressing alone has 14 grams of fat. All told, this salad packs the caloric equivalent of 6 Twinkies and gobbles up half of your day's recommended intake of saturated fat. As is too often the case with chain restaurants, you'll need to order a half salad just to ensure you don't blow half a day's worth of calories on what should be a stellar lunch option.

Eat This Instead!
Half Chicken Chipotle Salad
- *360 calories • 21 g fat (4.5 g saturated)*
- *970 mg sodium*

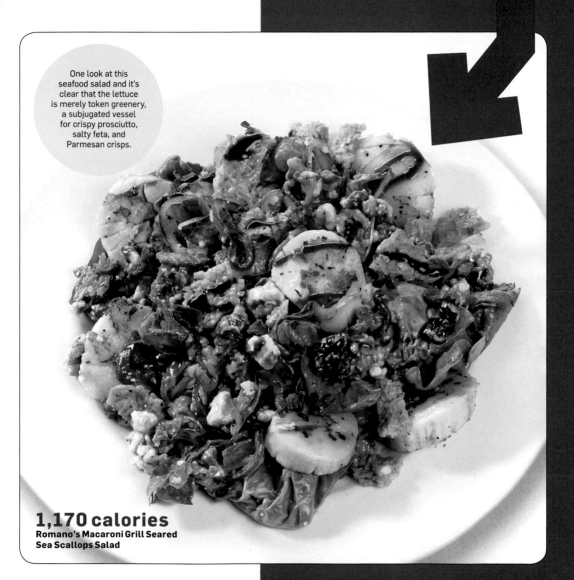

One look at this seafood salad and it's clear that the lettuce is merely token greenery, a subjugated vessel for crispy prosciutto, salty feta, and Parmesan crisps.

1,170 calories
Romano's Macaroni Grill Seared Sea Scallops Salad

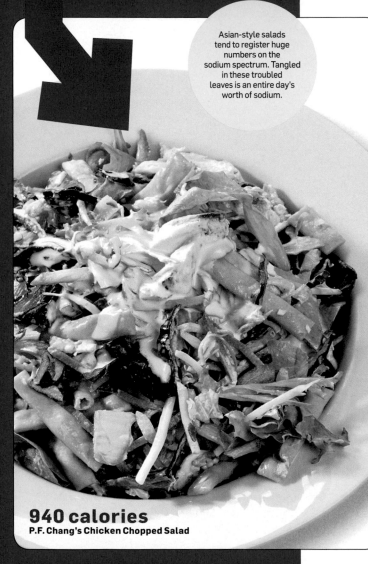

Asian-style salads tend to register huge numbers on the sodium spectrum. Tangled in these troubled leaves is an entire day's worth of sodium.

940 calories
P.F. Chang's Chicken Chopped Salad

8 P.F. Chang's Chicken Chopped Salad
with Ginger Dressing

- *940 calories*
- *68 g fat (10 g saturated)*
- *2,225 mg sodium*

The ginger dressing gives this salad a tangy Asian-style kick; it also packs in a whole day's worth of sodium. Order this salad as a starter and you'll be consuming the caloric equivalent of 3½ Snickers bars before your main meal even hits the table.

Eat This Instead!
Spinach Stir-Fried with Garlic (large)
- *136 calories • 6 g fat (1 g saturated)*
- *895 mg sodium*

7 Chili's Boneless Buffalo Chicken Salad

- *1,070 calories*
- *77 g fat (15 g saturated)*
- *4,380 mg sodium*

This twisted concoction earns the dubious distinction of being America's Saltiest Salad, packing more sodium in a single bowl than you'll find in 58 cups of Pop-Secret

Movie Theater buttered popcorn. It's a feat accomplished by mixing fried chicken with some of the food world's most sodium-riddled conspirators: wing sauce, crumbled bacon, blue cheese, and fried tortilla strips.

Eat This Instead!
Side Salad Caesar
· 350 calories · 31 g fat (6 g saturated)
· 550 mg sodium

WORST SEAFOOD SALAD

6 Romano's Macaroni Grill Seared Sea Scallops Salad

· 1,170 calories
· 94 g fat (27 g saturated)
· 2,680 mg sodium

Macaroni Grill manages to take two normally healthy foods—salad and seafood—and turn them into the caloric equivalent of 26 Chicken McNuggets. Not to mention more than 1 day's worth of sodium, fat, and saturated fat. The Caprese offers a delicious reprieve from the Mac Grill mayhem.

Eat This Instead!
Mozzarella Alla Caprese (3)
· 250 calories · 21 g fat (7 g saturated)
· 410 mg sodium

Buy This, Not That!
THE BEST AND WORST BOTTLED DRESSINGS

The Best
Annie's Naturals Organic Buttermilk (2 Tbsp)
· 70 calories
· 7 g fat
  (1 g saturated)
· 210 mg sodium

Ranch's rich flavor and creamy texture, but with fewer than half the calories.

Maple Grove Farms of Vermont Fat Free Honey Dijon (2 Tbsp)
· 40 calories
· 0 g fat
· 200 mg sodium

Not one in this great line of fat-free dressings has more than 40 calories per serving.

Kraft Roasted Red Pepper Italian with Parmesan (2 Tbsp)
· 40 calories
· 2 g fat
  (0 g saturated)
· 440 mg sodium

This is about as low-cal as Italian gets.

Newman's Own Natural Salad Mist Tuscan Italian (10 sprays)
· 10 calories
· 1 g fat
  (0 g saturated)
· 100 mg sodium

Spraying ensures minimum calories and maximum distribution.

The Worst
Hidden Valley The Original Ranch (2 Tbsp)
· 140 calories
· 14 g fat
  (2.5 g saturated)
· 260 mg sodium

Ranch is one of the most dangerous things you can keep in your kitchen.

Ken's Steak House Thousand Island (2 Tbsp)
· 140 calories
· 13 g fat
  (2 g saturated)
· 300 mg sodium

This dubious dressing cancels out a salad's benefits.

Kraft Golden Italian (2 Tbsp)
· 150 calories
· 14 g fat
  (2 g saturated)
· 630 mg sodium

This is as salt-soaked as dressing gets: 2 tablespoons pack 25 percent of your sodium quota.

Newman's Own Creamy Caesar Dressing (2 Tbsp)
· 150 calories
· 16 g fat
  (1.5 g saturated)
· 450 mg sodium

As much as we like many of Newman's products, this isn't one of them. In fact, we never met a Caesar dressing we did like.

The Worst Salads in America

WORST CAESAR SALAD
5 IHOP's Grilled Chicken Caesar Salad

• *1,210 calories**

IHOP serves up plenty of savory bites beyond the breakfast hour, and unfortunately, most of them hover in the same stratospheric calorie range. (How does an 1,850-calorie plate of chicken strips sound for a nice evening out with the family?) The salad section may be the worst section of the entire menu (noticing a trend here?). Caesars, with their fatty dressing deluges and Parmesan flurries, are never a good idea, but this particular heap of greens is as bad as we've seen (blame it on the elephantine portion). In fact, hailing Caesar or any other salad at IHOP will get you into trouble; opt for a chicken sandwich instead.

Eat This Instead!
Simple Chicken Sandwich
• *460 calories**

*IHOP refuses to disclose the full nutritional content of the food they're serving you.

WORST STEAK SALAD
4 Baja Fresh Charbroiled Steak Tostada Salad

• *1,230 calories*
• *63 g fat*
  (17 g saturated, 2 g trans)
• *2,380 mg sodium*

While the charbroiled steak doesn't do this salad any favors, it's the calorie-heavy Mexican-theme add-ins that really sink it into a nutritional void. The 2 grams of trans-fatty acids meet your daily limit of the heart-harming junk, and there's as much salt as you'll find in 9 orders of McDonald's French Fries tangled up in this leafy loser. Choose a Baja Ensalada over a Tostada Salad and opt for the salsa verde as a dressing, instead of the fat-spiked ranch or vinaigrette.

Eat This Instead!
Baja Ensalada Charbroiled Shrimp Salad with Fat-Free Salsa Verde
• *245 calories • 6 g fat (2 g saturated)*
• *1,480 mg sodium*

WORST CHICKEN SALAD
3 T.G.I. Friday's Pecan Crusted Chicken Salad

• *1,360 calories**

Turns out Friday's monster salads aren't much better than their burgers. Six out of the 7 we analyzed topped out with more than 900 calories, which means that lunchtime can be the start of something big—namely, your belly.

Eat This Instead!
Cobb Salad
• *590 calories**

*Friday's refuses to disclose the full nutritional content of the food they're serving you.

WORST MEXICAN SALAD
2 Chevy's Fresh Mex Tostada Grande Salad with Chicken

• *1,551 calories*
• *94 g fat (37 g saturated)*
• *2,840 mg sodium*

Steer clear of Mexican-theme salads; they invariably suffer from the caloric impact of fried tortillas, shredded cheese, and ice-cream-size scoops of sour cream. This particular mess has nearly 2 days' worth of saturated fat and more than an entire day's sodium, putting it on par with the brackish bites that round out our list of the 20 Saltiest Foods in America.

Eat This Instead!

Santa Fe Chopped Salad (no cheese or bacon)

• *318 calories* • *11 g fat (2 g saturated)*
• *412 mg sodium*

WORST SALAD IN AMERICA

1 On the Border Grande Taco Salad with Taco Beef and Chipotle Honey Mustard Dressing

• *1,700 calories*
• *124 g fat (37.5 g saturated)*
• *2,620 mg sodium*

The dismal dawn of the 1,700-calorie salad is upon us. With as much saturated fat as 37 strips of bacon and more calories than 11 Taco Bell Fresco Beef Tacos, this abdomen expander earns a well-deserved spot on our list of the Worst Foods in America (page 10).

Eat This Instead!

House Salad with Fat-Free Mango Citrus Vinaigrette

• *255 calories*
• *12 g fat (3.5 g saturated)*
• *280 mg sodium*

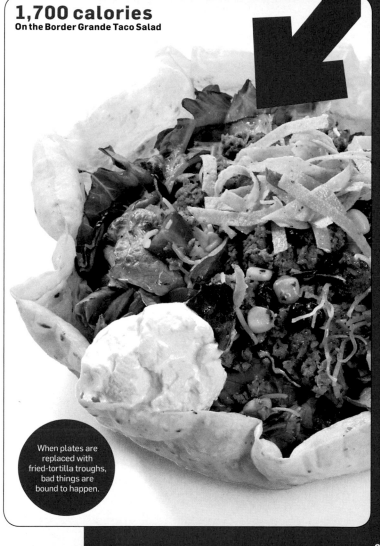

1,700 calories
On the Border Grande Taco Salad

When plates are replaced with fried-tortilla troughs, bad things are bound to happen.

The Best Salads in A

MAKE FRIENDS WITH THIS IMPRESSIVE LINEUP OF LEAFY GREENS

BEST CLASSIC SALAD

T.G.I. Friday's Cobb Salad

- *590 calories*

Compared with the rest of Friday's salads, this take on the American standby is a nutritional dream come true. Loaded with chopped egg, tomato, avocado, and lean grilled chicken, it's one of the few entrée-size salads in America substantial enough to make a meal and low-cal enough to consume in good conscience. Still, go light on the dressing. We recommend the old fork trick: Ask for dressing on the side, then dip your tines in before each bite.

BEST SUBSTANTIAL SALAD

Chipotle Steak Salad with Black Beans and Tomato Salsa

- *340 calories*
- *8 g fat (2 g saturated)*
- *1,045 mg sodium*

Chipotle's salad option is one of its few virtues, as long as you forgo the dressing, which adds 260 calories, 25 grams of fat, and 700 milligrams of sodium to your creation. Instead, top the leaves with a chunky tomato salsa and a hefty scoop of steak and black beans and end up with 39 grams of protein and 13 grams of fiber. If you need more lubrication than that, grab a side of the 15-calorie green tomatillo salsa.

BEST VEGETARIAN SALAD

Così Lighten Up! Signature Salad Light

- *371 calories*
- *19 g fat*
- *485 mg sodium*

Packed with pistachios, Gorgonzola, and a battery of fruit (pears, grapes, and cranberries), this salad makes for a perfect meatless lunch. Take advantage of Così's new Lighten Up! option, which translates into a restrained application of the high-impact ingredients (here, the Gorgonzola) and a lower-calorie option for the dressing.

BEST LIGHT LUNCH

Panera Bread Asian Sesame Chicken Salad (half portion) with Reduced-Sugar Asian Sesame Vinaigrette

- *255 calories*
- *14 g fat (2 g saturated)*
- *640 mg sodium*

Panera entrée-size salads are hulking, so even a half portion could stand in as a meal for most hungry eaters. This one comes laced with chunks of citrus-herb chicken, mandarin oranges, heart-healthy almonds, and a light, low-sugar, low-sodium vinaigrette. Even if you go with the full-size order, you'll be lapping nearly every other misinformed salad eater in America.

590 calories
T.G.I. Friday's Cobb Salad

Finally a salad to celebrate. Friday's, home to a host of atrocious attempts at healthy bowls of greens, finally gets one right with this classic mix of vegetables and lean protein.

Salad Bar Survival Gu

OIL AND VINEGAR
Your best bet, since you control the ratio. Slick your salad with equal parts oil and vinegar, but be sure to add only enough to lightly coat the greens.

VINAIGRETTES
Now you're getting warmer. Assuming the vinaigrette is based on olive oil, you'll be getting a big dose of mono-unsaturated fats. Even so, since most vinaigrettes abide by the three parts oil to one part vinegar ratio, you're still looking at 100 calories per serving.

CHICKPEAS
Like all legumes, chickpeas bring to the table both protein and fiber, the sultans of satiety. Add to that a healthy dose of antioxidants and you have the makings of a salad-topping superstar.

TUNA
Tuna fish on a salad, as opposed to tuna salad swimming in mayonnaise, will provide protein and heart-helping omega-3 fats without the heavy caloric price.

BLUE CHEESE
Delicious blue cheese comes at a caloric price. If you absolutely must have it, limit yourself to just one meat or other protein and load up on the low-cal veggies we've mentioned.

RANCH/ BLUE CHEESE/ CAESAR
The type of dressing you use is the single most important decision you make at the salad bar. These three represent the most destructive dressings, clocking in around 150 calories and 15 grams of fat per serving.

FRENCH/ CATALINA/ THOUSAND ISLAND
The trio of orange dressings are only marginally less problematic than their white counterparts. That's because they're based on low-grade oils and excess sugar. Expect at least 150 calories for 2 tablespoons of one of these.

SHREDDED CHEDDAR
The worst cheese at the salad bar. Not only is it high in calories and sodium, but the minuscule shreds tend to bury themselves in the bowl, making portion control a challenge.

CHICKEN
Lean protein is the key to making filling salads, and none come much leaner than chicken. If you're banking on the bird, though, remember that a healthy portion is the size of a deck of cards.

BACON
Bacon's gotten some bad press over the years, but one strip has only 40 calories and less than 200 milligrams of sodium. So a pinch of bacon bits is permissible; a handful, however, is not.

RAISINS OR CRAISINS
They're fruit, yes, but they're likely to be coated in sugar. Opt for fresh fruit whenever possible.

CORN
There are too many nutritionally superior vegetables at the salad bar to invest the calories on corn.

FETA CHEESE
A smarter pick than blue, being that feta provides that same crumbly bite for fewer calories and less sodium. Still, only in moderation and only with a colorful crew of vegetables to back it up.

HARD-BOILED EGG
Sick of chicken? Turn to the egg for another great source of protein. Mix with chickpeas, avocado, and red peppers for the closest thing to salad perfection.

ide

CARROTS
You'll love them for their sweet crunch and their vision-boosting beta-carotene.

MIXED GREENS
The diversity of leaves assures you a bowl filled with a wide variety of nutrients and active compounds. The delicate nature of these little lettuces, though, means they don't hold up as well to heavy ingredients and dressings.

SPINACH
Pick darker greens for the base. Spinach, on the greenest side of the spectrum, has more vitamins and nutrients than can fit on this page, including folate, which helps ward off mental decline, and beta-carotene, which helps protect your eyes and skin.

ICEBERG
The least healthy of common salad bar lettuces. Its high water content makes for a low nutrient density. If you can't skip it, mix it in with darker, healthier greens.

TOMATOES
Throw some on for lycopene, which has been linked to reduced risk of cancer and heart disease. Tomatoes also provide vitamins A, C, and K.

ROMAINE
Compared with iceberg, romaine contains 3 times more folate, 6 times more vitamin C, and 8 times the beta-carotene. Makes a good, sturdy bed for more substantial salads.

ALFALFA SPROUTS
These feathery salad additions have a cache of vitamins unrivaled by nearly anything else you can put in your body. Get in the habit of topping off your salad with these.

AVOCADO
Avocados provide a ton of heart-healthy fats and a rich, creamy bite to any salad. But just because monounsaturated fats are good for your heart doesn't mean they won't still make you fat. Try to choose between avocados and nuts.

CROUTONS
Think of these oil-soaked, enriched flour cubes as salad bar grenades— they'll blow your healthy salad away.

SUNFLOWER SEEDS
One of nature's finest sources of vitamin E, a fat-soluble antioxidant that helps fight inflammation and lower cholesterol.

BEETS
The scarlet crusaders help to lower blood pressure, maintain your memory, and fight cancer.

RED OR YELLOW PEPPERS
Pick red and yellow over green peppers, which contain half the amount of vitamin C. The more colorful your salad, the greater variety of nutrients you'll take in.

BROCCOLI
Vitamin C, fiber, calcium, and few calories. Need we say more?

WALNUTS
Yes, they are absolutely jacked with omega-3s and antioxidants, but they're incredibly dense with calories. Keep it down to a tablespoon or two.

CONSUMPTION KEY
● Feel free to scarf
○ Show some restraint
● Avoid at all costs

101

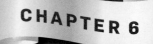

CHAPTER 6

The Best
(&Worst)
Burgers
in America

Eat This

McDonald's Big N' Tasty

460 calories
24 g fat
(8 g saturated)
720 mg sodium

Trim 60 g fat!
Plus cut out over a day's worth of saturated fat.

HAVE IT... It gets the first part of its name from a patty of sizzling 100% beef and a second from fresh onions and a firm, plump tomato. And you, lucky diner, get it all.

i'm lovin' it®

Save 790 calories!
Make this swap once a week and you'll shed nearly 12 pounds this year without changing anything else about the way you eat.

Not That!

Burger King Triple Whopper

with Cheese and Mayo

1,250 calories
84 g fat
(32 g saturated, 3.5 g trans)
1,600 mg sodium

Burger King reps claim the fast-food chain went trans fat free in November 2008, but their burgers are still riddled with the cholesterol-spiking junk. Until they replace their patties with more honest beef, proceed with caution.

In the battle of the burger bigs, the King gets trounced on account of its triplex of trans fat and genre-bending calorie counts.

Burgers are an American birthright.

Think of Wimpy, gladly paying Popeye Tuesday for a hamburger today. Or Jughead, ignoring the allures of Betty and Veronica for the more compelling siren call of a cheeseburger. Or Richie, Potsie, and Ralph, bonding over girls and burgers and rock 'n' roll at Arnold's Drive-in. Or your own family backyard BBQ, where fishing out burnt chunks of ground meat that have fallen through the rack is as much a part of the Fourth of July as fireworks and sparklers and Uncle Chuckie having one too many beers and falling into the pool.

But like a lot of other things that are all-American—like blue jeans, country music, and baseball stadiums—hamburgers have been seized by megacorporations who have tweaked and manipulated and supersized them until they've lost much of what made them quaint and cool—and relatively healthy—to begin with. Indeed, the average hamburger now packs nearly 100 more calories than the burgers that Wimpy, Jughead, and the *Happy Days* boys enjoyed—and some are 1,500 calories more! Like designer jeans, they're all tricked out, and they're costing us a whole lot more.

The funny thing is, a hamburger isn't, by itself, a terrible nutritional choice. Topped with some lettuce and tomato, ketchup and mustard, and a relatively small bun, a burger is a high-protein treat that shouldn't pack too much fat or calories. But just as country music went from skinny little Hank Williams playing honkytonks to Garth Brooks touring stadiums—and just as baseball went from wiry Jackie Robinson stealing home to muscle-bound Barry Bonds stealing homers—so have our burgers evolved from lean and simple to very fat and very complicated. How hard has it become to decode the once-simple hamburger? Get a load—literally—of these.

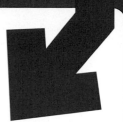

1,358 calories
Ruby Tuesday Bacon Cheddar Minis

Unless you can limit yourself to one or two, sliders make for a consistently calamitous menu choice. That's because the burger to bun ratio is low and the novelty factor is high, both of which have been shown to encourage excess eating.

The Worst Burgers in America

WORST "HEALTHY" BURGER
10 Ruby Tuesday Veggie Burger

- *1,007 calories*
- *53 g fat*
- *73 g carbohydrates*

If anyone is capable of turning a veggie burger into an assault on your waistline and overall well-being, it's Ruby Tuesday. After all, these are the burger barons who brought you the 1,088-calorie turkey burger, the 1,358-calorie Bacon Cheddar "mini" burgers, and, of course, the 2,014-calorie catastrophe they call the Colossal Burger. But this is the most shocking of them all: a meatless burger with the same number of calories you'd find in 3 Ruby Tuesday sirloin steaks. Like most restaurants, Ruby Tuesday has an anemic roster of vegetarian options, so if you're looking for a meatless meal, you'll have to piece together a few side dishes.

Eat This Instead!
Creamy Mashed Cauliflower with Premium Baby Green Beans and Sautéed Baby Mushrooms
- *395 calories • 27 g fat*
- *41 g carbohydrates*

WORST FUSION BURGER
9 Carl's Jr. Guacamole Bacon Six Dollar Burger

- *1,040 calories*
- *70 g fat*
  (25 g saturated)
- *2,240 mg sodium*
- *53 g carbohydrates*

Carl's Jr. bills this burger as a great deal—what's better than gourmet eats for a fast-food price? Not so fast. That chump change is also buying you half of your day's worth of calories and an entire day's worth of sodium. Guacamole may have healthy fat, giving it an edge over the empty calories in mayo, but it still packs a major caloric punch. The Big Hamburger and Jalapeno Burger have the least, but if you want to skip the junk entirely (and you should), try the 550-calorie Charbroiled Chicken Club sandwich.

Eat This Instead!
Big Hamburger
- *460 calories • 17 g fat (8 g saturated)*
- *1,090 mg sodium • 54 g carbohydrates*

WORST TRIPLE BURGER
8 Burger King Triple Whopper Sandwich
with Cheese and Mayo

- *1,250 calories*
- *84 g fat*
  (32 g saturated, 3.5 g trans)
- *1,600 mg sodium*

This Triple Whopper is triple trouble. You could remove 2 patties and still be looking at more calories than you should tussle with in one sitting. And the fact that it's got more trans fat than you should eat in a day only adds insult to injury. The problem with BK burgers is that not a single one comes without the heart-harming trans-fatty acids, despite their long-standing promise to (someday) make their menu trans fat free. Your best bet when dealing with the King is to choose a chicken sandwich, instead.

Eat This Instead!
Tendergrill Chicken Sandwich with mayo
- *490 calories • 21 g fat*
  (4 g saturated, 0 g trans)
- *1,220 mg sodium*

Big Mouth? More like retractable jaw. If you can actually manage to get your gullet around this burger, you'll be "rewarded" with nearly 2,000 calories—not to mention roughly 25 percent of your daily sodium in every bite.

1,901 calories
Chili's Smokehouse Bacon
Triple Cheese Big Mouth Burger

The Worst Burgers in America

7 Ruby Tuesday Bacon Cheddar Minis (4 burgers)

- *1,358 calories*
- *86 g fat*
- *75 g carbohydrates*

Diminutive dishes are one of the hottest trends in the restaurant world right now (probably since most are looking for ways to stretch a buck), and you'd think that would serve health-conscious eaters well. But not under the reckless watch of the burger barons at Ruby Tuesday, who manage to turn 4 "mini" burgers into the caloric equivalent of 7 Dunkin' Donuts Sugar Donuts. We're really not trying to pick on Ruby Tuesday, but with a burger menu cluttered with so many nutritional losers, they're lucky to only make 3 appearances on this list.

Eat This Instead!
Turkey Minis (2)
- *529 calories • 29 g fat*
- *40 g carbohydrates*

6 Hardee's ⅔-Pound Monster Thickburger

- *1,420 calories*
- *108 g fat (43 g saturated)*
- *2,770 mg sodium*
- *46 g carbohydrates*

Hardee's and Carl's Jr. take misplaced pride in their shamelessly caloric approach to everything they put under a heat lamp, which is probably reason enough for some to find another place to eat. Need more motivation? Many of their burgers break the perilous 1,000-calorie barrier; their worst bun-buster has nearly 75 percent of your entire day's calories and as much fat as a dozen Taco Bell soft beef tacos. If you're on the West Coast, the Carl's Jr. Double Six Dollar Burger is the Thickburger's evil twin, so beware.

Eat This Instead!
⅓-Pound Low Carb Thickburger
- *420 calories • 32 g fat (12 g saturated)*
- *1,010 mg sodium*

5 Red Robin A.1. Peppercorn Burger

- *1,440 calories*
- *97 g fat (unknown grams saturated)*
- *5,784 mg sodium*
- *93 g carbohydrates*

As their motto (almost) goes: uniquely created to be insanely caloric. There's hardly a burger on Red Robin's menu that slips under the 1,000-calorie threshold. More troubling than the caloric impact with the A.1. burger, though, is the 2½ days' worth of sodium slammed between its buns. There are myriad factors to blame for the sodium deluge, including cheese, bacon, the bed of fried onion straws, and the namesake spread, which contains a staggering 507 calories and 3,894 milligrams of sodium. It took Red Robin years to give up the nutritional goods on their "gourmet burgers"; now we know why.

Eat This Instead!
Lettuce-Wrap Cheeseburger
- *422 calories • 27 g fat*
- *562 mg sodium • 8 g carbohydrates*

The Burger Topping Selector

Whether you're grabbing a burger at the local diner or crafting your own masterpiece at home, it's always a good idea to know what type of caloric investment you're really making. Learn to approximate the calorie, fat, and sodium counts for any burger that crosses your path with this comprehensive list of burger components.

	CALORIES	FAT	SODIUM	PROTEIN	CARBS	SUGARS	FIBER
MEAT							
Ground chuck, 80% lean (4 oz)	278	18g (7g saturated)	94mg	27g			
Ground sirloin, 90% lean (4 oz)	231	12g (5g saturated)	85mg	29g			
Ground bison (4 oz)	202	10g (4g saturated)	86mg	28g			
Ground turkey (4 oz)	193	11g (3g saturated)	88mg	22g			
Bacon (2 slices)	84	6g (2g saturated)	384mg	6g			
Ground lamb (4 oz)	32	22g (9g saturated)	92mg	28g			
BUNS							
Ciabatta roll	230	3g (2g saturated)	620mg		43g		2g
Kaiser roll	167	2.5g (0.5g saturated)	310mg		30g		1.5g
Plain white bun	120	2g (0g saturated)	206mg		21g		1g
Whole wheat bun	113	3g (0.5g saturated)	197mg		19g		2g
PRODUCE							
Onions (1 thick slice)	15	0g fat	1mg		4g		1g
Tomatoes (2 thick slices)	10	0g fat	3mg		2g		
Sautéed mushrooms (25 g serving, about ¼ c)	6	0g fat	100mg		1g		1g
Iceberg lettuce (½ c shredded)	5	0g fat	4mg		1g		0.5g
Dill pickles (4 slices)	3	0g fat	245mg		0.5g		0g
SAUCES							
Mayonnaise (1 Tbsp)	103	12g (2g saturated)	73mg			0g	
Pesto (1 Tbsp)	63	6g (1g saturated)	110mg			1g	
Special sauce (Thousand Island, 1 Tbsp)	59	6g (1g saturated)	138mg			2g	
Guacamole (1 oz)	37	3g (0.5g saturated)	48mg			0.5g	1.5g
Barbecue sauce (1 Tbsp)	26	0g fat	196mg			4g	
Ketchup (1 Tbsp)	15	0g fat	167mg			3g	
Yellow mustard (1 Tbsp)	10	0g fat	179mg			0g	
CHEESE (1 slice, about 1 oz)							
Blue cheese	85	7g (4.5g saturated)	335mg	5g			
Cheddar	70	6g (4g saturated)	108mg	4.5g			
Pepper jack	69	6g (4g saturated)	106mg	4g			
Swiss	66	5g (3g saturated)	47mg	5g			
Mozzarella	61	4g (2.5g saturated)	149mg	6g			
American	58	4.5g (3g saturated)	325mg	3.5g			

The Worst Burgers in America

TRANS-FATTIEST BURGER
4 Denny's Double Cheeseburger

- *1,540 calories*
- *116 g fat*
  (52 g saturated, 7 g trans)
- *3,880 mg sodium*

Add this to our ever-expanding list of the Trans-Fattiest Foods in America—this burger has more than 3 days' worth of the stuff. In fact, with as much saturated fat as 52 strips of bacon and more sodium than 21 small bags of Lay's potato chips, this burger also belongs on the salt-packed list of 14 Foods Your Cardiologist Won't Eat.

Eat This Instead!
BLT
- *570 calories* • *37 g fat (9 g saturated)*
- *850 mg sodium*

WORST SPECIALTY BURGER
3 Outback Steakhouse Blooming Burger

- *1,880 calories*

By fusing one of the worst appetizers in America with an already-bruising line of burgers, the corporate cooks behind this faux-Aussie establishment have birthed a monster of a burger with more calories than 9 Krispy Kreme original glazed doughnuts. With no burger less than 1,530 calories, you'll have to turn to chicken if you want to eat at Outback and not spend the next day on the treadmill.

Eat This Instead!
Grilled Chicken and Swiss Sandwich
- *760 calories*

WORST BACON BURGER
2 Chili's Smokehouse Bacon Triple Cheese Big Mouth Burger with Jalapeño Ranch Dressing

- *1,901 calories*
- *138 g fat (47 g saturated)*
- *4,201 mg sodium*

Any burger whose name is 21 syllables long is bound to spell trouble for your waistline. This burger packs almost an entire day's worth of calories and 2$^1/_2$ days' worth of fat. Chili's burger menu rivals Ruby Tuesday's for the worst in America, so you're better off with one of their reasonable Fajita Pitas to silence your hunger.

Eat This Instead!
Fajita Pita Beef
- *489 calories* • *21 g fat (4 g saturated)*
- *1,543 mg sodium*

WORST BURGER IN AMERICA
1 Ruby Tuesday Colossal Burger

- *2,014 calories*
- *141 g fat*
- *95 g carbohydrates*

They've truly outdone themselves with this new offering, a massive double burger that defies all nutritional (and architectural) odds. This terror of beef comes with its own steak knife. "To divide and conquer" brags the menu. You could conquer 6 hamburgers at Dairy Queen and get the same number of calories. We'd love to give you a better burger alternative, but not one (!) burger here—whether crafted from beef, buffalo, chicken, fish, or even vegetables—contains less than 800 calories. The blackened fish burger is the lesser of all evils. Otherwise, seek solace in sirloin.

Eat This Instead!
Blackened Fish Burger
- *861 calories* • *53 g fat*
- *44 g carbohydrates*

2,014 calories
Ruby Tuesday Colossal Burger

Ruby Tuesday is home to a long line of jaw-droppingly bad burgers, but this sordid specimen stands alone in the annals of atrociousness. You'd be better off eating 3 pounds of Ruby Tuesday sirloin steaks.

The Best Burgers in

CUT CALORIES AND BOOST NUTRITION BY MAKING PALS WITH THESE

DQ Original Hamburger

- *350 calories*
- *14 g fat*
  (7 g saturated)
- *680 mg sodium*

Just a simple, straightforward classic from Dairy Queen, a chain known more for sweets than meat. Don't wander far from here when seeking out savory sustenance, though, since nearly every other burger, fried chicken strip, and chili fry creation will get you into trouble, fast.

In-N-Out Burger Protein-Style Cheeseburger

- *330 calories*
- *25 g fat (9 g saturated)*
- *720 mg sodium*

In-N-Out may have only a handful of items on their menu—hamburger, Double-Double, French fries—but their secret menu allows hungry eaters to custom fit their burger to their appetite and nutritional needs. Long before the Atkins craze spread across America, these guys were wrapping burgers in big, crispy leaves of iceberg lettuce, and it's still the healthiest way to enjoy their justly famous eats today.

Wendy's ¼-Pound Single

- *430 calories*
- *20 g fat*
  (7 g saturated)
- *870 mg sodium*

When we want a burger, we want a *burger*, and this substantial creation from Wendy's most definitely qualifies. Four ounces of fresh ground beef and a heaping pile of produce for minimal caloric investment make this one of our favorite burgers in America.

McDonald's Big N' Tasty

- *460 calories*
- *24 g fat*
  (8 g saturated)
- *720 mg sodium*

Created to compete with the Whopper, this generous patty edges out the iconic BK burger by a full 210 calories and brings a nice balance of protein, fat, and carbs to the table. Mickey D's has never been a big fan of loading their burgers with vegetation, but the Big N' Tasty breaks with tradition, donning a sprightly wardrobe of lettuce, onions, tomatoes, and pickles.

America

SUPERLATIVE PATTIES

Burger King
Whopper Jr.
without mayo

- *290 calories*
- *12 g fat
  (4.5 g saturated)*
- *500 mg sodium*

BK burgers leave plenty to be desired, but the Whopper Jr. is the one ray of hope in an otherwise murky menu. Consider this for a hearty midday snack in a pinch or add a side salad and call it lunch.

430 calories
Wendy's ¼-Pound Single

Take advantage of Wendy's extensive list of sides and skip the ubiquitous order of fries. A mandarin orange cup, a side salad, even a bowl of chili make for a considerably healthier way to round out your next meal.

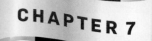

CHAPTER 7

The Best
(&Worst)
Pizzas
in America

Eat This

Pizza Hut 12" Fit and Delicious

Diced Red Tomato, Mushrooms, and Jalapeño (2 slices)

300 calories
8 g fat
(3 g saturated)
1,220 mg sodium
46 g carbohydrates

Save 30g fat!
Plus eliminate half a day's worth of saturated fat.

Save 340 calories!
Eat pizza twice a week and these savings translate into 10 fewer pounds you'll have to worry about a year from now.

It might not taste like a slice of Naples, but *this*— thin crust, light cheese, balanced topping distribution—is closer to the Italian ideal than *that*.

Not That!

740 calories
38 g fat
(12g saturated)
1,320 mg sodium
78 g carbohydrates

Papa John's Pan Crust Garden Fresh Pizza

(2 slices)

Gardens aren't always what they're cracked up to be. (Just ask Adam.)

When it comes to having your pizza and eating it too, the first and most important consideration is crust. Thick, deep dish, or pan crust slices will generally pack 40% more calories than regular slices, thin crust 40% less.

Garlic

119

We all love the image of a hard-working Italian chef/athlete/juggler in the back kitchen of the local pizzeria,

twirling a delicious disk of dough over his head like some kind of culinary Harlem Globetrotter, sprinkling it with fresh cheese and just the right amount of red sauce and then whisking the flat little wheel of wonderment into the oven, where it bakes to perfection—and arrives at your doorstep with a chilled six-pack, just in time for kickoff.

In reality, pizza isn't always quite so magical—and not just because the delivery guy came late and the game was a blowout. A lot of pies aren't at all what the Italian chefs first imagined as a low-calorie appetizer. As for sit-down restaurants, many offer pizzas that are closer to leaden manhole covers than the original subdued Neapolitan delicacy. And what's in your freezer section is usually better for Ultimate Frisbee than for dinner.

What's the problem? Thin, healthy crusts have gotten thicker, more bloated with cheap carb calories. Toppings have gotten gimmicky, so healthy mozzarella and tomato sauces are sometimes replaced with things like burger meat, ziti, and other insults to Italians everywhere. And serving sizes—especially for "individual" pizzas—have taken these pies to a new level of caloric callousness.

But, that said, there really is nothing like a pizza, a cold beer, and a great group of friends. So let's indulge—but let's be smart about it!

350 calories
Mama Celeste Original Cheese Pizza

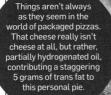

Things aren't always as they seem in the world of packaged pizzas. That cheese really isn't cheese at all, but rather, partially hydrogenated oil, contributing a staggering 5 grams of trans fat to this personal pie.

The Worst Pizzas in America

9 Mama Celeste Original Cheese Pizza

- *350 calories*
- *17 g fat*
  (4 g saturated, 5 g trans)
- *1,090 mg sodium*
- *39 g carbohydrates*

This pizza didn't make our list because of a glut of calories or sodium; it made our list because the second ingredient on the label is imitation mozzarella. The first ingredient in imitation mozzarella? Partially hydrogenated soybean oil—hence the 2½ days of trans fat. Blech! When buying pizzas from the freezer aisle, always check the ingredients lists. You're better off sacrificing a few calories than sacrificing the strength of your ticker.

Eat This Instead!

Palermo's Primo Thin Margherita (⅓ pizza)

- *260 calories • 12 g fat (5 g saturated)*
- *520 mg sodium • 26 g carbohydrates*

8 CiCi's Pizza Buffet Macaroni and Cheese 15" Pizza (2 slices)

- *460 calories*
- *8 g fat (3 g saturated)*
- *660 mg sodium*
- *78 g carbohydrates*

Macaroni and cheese pizza? While it might seem like the best idea ever to kids the world over, this cute concept is potentially disastrous for your health—and your children's. Why top an already carbohydrate-heavy dish with more carbs, not to mention fat? While the calorie count doesn't register as high as most problematic pies on this list, that's only because the slices are tiny; believe us, in CiCi's all-you-can-eat environment, the damage can add up quickly. But if you bring one of their pizzas home, celebrate their smaller slices as built-in portion control.

Eat This Instead!

CiCi's Olé 12" (2 slices)

- *220 calories*
- *6 g fat (2 g saturated)*
- *580 mg sodium • 40 g carbohydrates*

7 Red Lobster Lobster Pizza

- *720 calories*
- *30 g fat (13 g saturated)*
- *1,390 mg sodium*
- *69 g carbohydrates*

It's a cool concept (certainly more appetizing than your grandfather's old anchovies habit), but it makes for a heavy meal that's stuffed with more sodium than you should eat in one sitting. Fare from the sea is typically a healthy way to go, but sprinkle it over a bed of starchy dough and fatty cheese and you have a different story altogether. Billed as a starter, this Lobster Pizza is the only pizza on Red Lobster's menu—luckily it shares space with one of the world's greatest appetizers: shrimp cocktail.

Eat This Instead!

Chilled Jumbo Shrimp Cocktail

- *120 calories • 1 g fat • 590 mg sodium*
- *9 g carbohydrates*

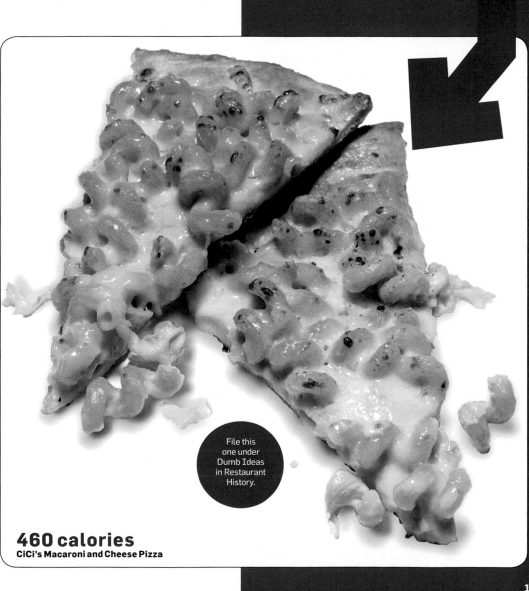

File this one under Dumb Ideas in Restaurant History.

460 calories
CiCi's Macaroni and Cheese Pizza

The Worst Pizzas in America

6 Papa John's Pan Crust Garden Fresh Pizza (2 slices)

- *740 calories*
- *38 g fat (12 g saturated)*
- *1,320 mg sodium*
- *78 g carbohydrates*

You'll read this statement over and over again in this book because it bears repeating: Just because it's topped with veggies doesn't make it healthy. The real problem here isn't the toppings, though; it's the excessively thick, greasy pan crust that sinks this veggie-strewn ship. Two slices of this garden-fresh pie will set you back the caloric equivalent of more than 8 Rice Krispies Treats. Save more than 300 calories by switching from the 12" pan slice to a larger pie (14") with a thinner crust. Just another example of why crust is king when trying to find a healthy pie.

Eat This Instead!
Thin Crust Garden Fresh Pizza (2 slices)
- *420 calories • 22 g fat (5 g saturated)*
- *940 mg sodium • 46 g carbohydrates*

5 Sbarro Stuffed Pepperoni Pizza

- *960 calories**

Sbarro's individual pizza slices are oversized to begin with, but throw in an entire extra layer of cheese, sauce, and toppings and you're looking at this single worst slice of pizza in America—the equivalent of almost 4 pepperoni slices from Pizza Hut. It should go without saying that the word "stuffed," in whatever culinary context, is a clear indicator of excess calories. Downsize this massive wedge for Fresh Tomato Pizza (which is plenty large in its own right) and be sure to limit yourself to just one.

Eat This Instead!
Sbarro Fresh Tomato Pizza (1 large slice)
- *450 calories**

*Sbarro doesn't offer other nutritional information.

4 Romano's Macaroni Grill Sicilian Mio Pizza and Insalata Blu

- *1,080 calories*
- *88 g fat (25 g saturated)*
- *2,660 mg sodium*
- *72 g carbohydrates*

Consuming more than half of your daily calories at lunch is just asking for a 3 P.M. desktop snooze (not to mention belt buckle difficulties). Macaroni Grill boasts about their lunch combos as if supersized individual pizzas and high-calorie "side" salads are a good thing. Plus, recent research found people underestimate portion sizes when their meals have more variety in them—so you're likely to eat more when you have more pieces on your plate. So skip the Mac Grill combo meals and choose a simpler lunch instead. (But beware: Chicken Cannelloni and Pasta Pomodoro are 2 of only 4 pastas with fewer than 1,000 calories.)

Eat This Instead!
Chicken Cannelloni Lunch
- *590 calories • 29 g fat (17 g saturated)*
- *1,710 mg sodium • 41 g carbohydrates*

The Ultimate Pizza Topping Decoder

If your favorite pizza joint or delivery service isn't one of the three or four national titans, then you probably don't have access to reliable nutritional information for the pies you love most. Fear not; this comprehensive topping breakdown will allow you to calculate the caloric heft of your next slice in a matter of seconds. Just choose a crust, sauce, type of cheese, and a range of toppings and the next time you order up a pizza, you'll know exactly what you're biting into.

	CALORIES	FAT	FIBER	PROTEIN	SODIUM	CARBS	SUGARS
Crusts (¼ of 12" pizza)							
Hand-tossed	120	1g	2g		240 mg	24g	
Pan/deep-dish	160	7.5g (1g saturated)	3g		260 mg	30g	
Thin	80	0.5g	0.5g		27 mg	15g	
Whole wheat	130	1.5g	4g		240 mg	24g	
Sauces							
Marinara (2 Tbsp)	20		0.5g		170 mg		3g
Alfredo (2 Tbsp)	55	5g (2g saturated)	0g		200 mg		1g
Cheeses (About ½ ounce per 12" slice)							
Mozzarella	35	2g (1.5g saturated)		3.5g	87 mg		
Cheddar	56	4.5g (3g saturated)		3.5g	87 mg		
Provolone	46	3.5g (2.5g saturated)		3.5g	123 mg		
Parmesan	66	3g (3g saturated)		6g	228 mg		
Meats							
Pepperoni (10g/6 slices)	50	4g (1g saturated)		3g	170 mg		
Sausage (10g)	40	3g (1g saturated)		2g	110 mg		
Ham (12g)	10	0.5g		2g	120 mg		
Ground beef (10g)	30	3g (1g saturated)		2g	60 mg		
Chicken (10g)	17	0.5g		2g	90 mg		
Bacon (10g)	40	3g (1g saturated)		3g	100 mg		
Anchovies (7g)	5	0g		1g	150 mg		
Veggies and Fruit							
Green peppers (9g)	1	0g	0.5g		0mg	0g	
Onions (10g)	3	0g	0g		0mg	1g	
Mushrooms (10g)	2	0g	0g		0mg	0g	
Olives (7g)	10	1g	0g		60mg	1g	
Tomatoes (9g)	2.5	0g	0g		0mg	0.5g	
Pineapple (12g)	5	0g	0.5g		0mg	2g	

The Worst Pizzas in America

3 Pizza Hut Meaty P'Zone Pizza

- 1,480 calories
- 66 g fat
  (30 g saturated, 2 g trans)
- 3,680 mg sodium
- 152 g carbohydrates

The word *calzone* is, in fact, an ancient Roman term meaning "Help, I can't see my feet." Okay, no it's not. But it is a word that should sound alarm bells for anyone interested in watching his or her weight. The worst part is that Pizza Hut brags about their massive P'Zone like it's something to be proud of: The Web site reads "Over 1 pound of pizza goodness." Why is it over a pound? Because it's a regular-sized 12" pizza folded over onto itself and stuffed with meat and cheese. Unless you are pledging a fraternity, there's nothing impressive about eating an entire pizza by yourself.

Eat This Instead!

Meat Lover's 12" Pan Pizza (1 slice)

- 330 calories • 18 g fat (7 g saturated)
- 820 mg sodium • 27 g carbohydrates

2 Uno Chicago Grill Pizza Skins

- 2,400 calories
- 155 g fat (45 g saturated)
- 3,600 mg sodium
- 195 g carbohydrates

How are pizza skins different from an actual pizza? Well, they're not—they just come topped with crumbly processed bacon bits and a big fat dollop of sour cream. The only reason this didn't make it to our number one worst pizza spot is because it's supposed to be an appetizer, to be split (in theory) among a crew of hungry cohorts. But even if you're traveling with a party of 5, it makes no sense to order what's essentially a family-sized pizza before your meal. To put it in perspective, a medium 12" pepperoni pizza from Pizza Hut only racks up 1,840 calories. That's nearly 600 fewer calories than you'll find in this one appetizer! Disgusting.

Eat This Instead!

Crispy Cheese Dippers

- 840 calories • 48 g fat (18 g saturated)
- 2,490 mg sodium

1 Uno Chicago Grill Chicago Classic Deep Dish Individual Pizza

- 2,310 calories
- 165 g fat (54 g saturated)
- 4,920 mg sodium
- 120 g carbohydrates

The problem with deep dish pizza (which Uno's knows a thing or two about since they invented it back in 1943) is not just the extra empty calories and carbs from the crust, it's that the thick doughy base provides the structural integrity to house extra heaps of cheese, sauce, and greasy toppings. The result is an individual pizza with more calories than you should eat in a day and more sodium than you would find in 27 small bags of Lays Potato Chips. Oh, did we mention it has nearly 3 days' worth of saturated fat, too? The key to success at Uno's lies in their flatbread pies.

Eat This Instead!

Cheese and Tomato Flatbread Pizza (1/2 pizza)

- 405 calories
- 16.5 g fat (7.5 g saturated)
- 1,065 mg sodium • 46 g carbohydrates

2,310 calories
Uno Chicago Grill Classic Deep Dish Pizza

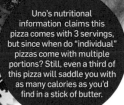

Uno's nutritional information claims this pizza comes with 3 servings, but since when do "individual" pizzas come with multiple portions? Still, even a third of this pizza will saddle you with as many calories as you'd find in a stick of butter.

The Best Pizzas in Am

SATISFY YOUR PIZZA CRAVING WITH THESE SUPER SLICES

BEST VEGGIE PIZZA
Pizza Hut 12" Fit and Delicious Diced Red Tomato, Mushroom, and Jalapeño (2 slices)

· 300 calories
· 8 g fat (3 g saturated)
· 1,220 mg sodium
· 46 g carbohydrates

Vegetable pizza is too often an excuse for pizza makers to pile on extra cheese and sauce. But Pizza Hut takes a truly purist approach to this veggie iteration, leaving you with a 2-slice combo that boasts the antioxidant benefits of tomato and mushroom, plus the metabolism-charging upside of the capsaicin found in jalapeños.

BEST HAWAIIAN PIZZA
Domino's Thin Crust Ham and Pineapple Pizza (2 slices)

· 310 calories
· 14 g fat (5 g saturated)
· 680 mg sodium
· 32 g carbohydrates

Pepperoni may be the country's most popular topping, but it's also one of the absolute worst. That's why we love the Hawaiian pie so much: It adds substance to your slice without dramatically affecting the calorie count (in the case of Domino's, ham and pineapple add just 15 calories to a slice, versus 40 for a few disks of oily pepperoni).

BEST INDIVIDUAL PIZZA
Chuck E. Cheese Individual Cheese

· 540 calories
· 19 g fat (8 g saturated)
· 1,255 mg sodium
· 69 g carbohydrates

Chuck's may be better known for the quality of their video games than the quality of their pizzas, but they do happen to offer one of the only individual pizzas worth ordering in this country. Normally, personal pies mean more calories and fat than you bargained for, but in this case, opting for your own pizza might just save you the heartache of having to fight for a slice with a dozen rambunctious kids at your son's next birthday party.

BEST MEAT-LOVER'S PIZZA
Pizza Hut Meat Lover's 12" Pan Pizza (1 slice)

· 330 calories
· 18 g fat (7 g saturated)
· 820 mg sodium
· 27 g carbohydrates

Meat-muddled pizzas are generally best to skip entirely—the shower of sausage, pepperoni, bacon, and ground beef can double up the calories on a single slice in a flash. But if you can't imagine a slice without at least 3 different sources of protein, then Pizza Hut's sparing hand with toppings will keep the increased caloric cost to a minimum.

erica

BEST FROZEN PIZZA
Palermo's Primo Thin Margherita
(⅓ pizza)

- 260 calories
- 12 g fat (5 g saturated)
- 520 mg sodium
- 26 g carbohydrates

Frozen pizza normally packs a wallop. Most modest pies—ones that a hungry eater could eat alone—easily top the 1,000-calorie threshold, once you add up the 3 or 4 servings on the nutritional label. Palermo's is our favorite line because their cracker-thin crust keeps the calorie count low and the taste true to the authentic pies of Naples.

BEST FUSION PIZZA
CiCi's Pizza Buffet Olé 12" (2 slices)

- 220 calories
- 6 g fat (2 g saturated)
- 580 mg sodium
- 40 g carbohydrates

CiCi's flattened the taco into a pizza slice, with surprisingly good results. Who would have thought ground beef, cheddar, lettuce, and beans could come so low in calories?

BEST PIZZA INNOVATION
Papa John's Whole Wheat Crust

In 2008, Papa John's became the first major pizza purveyor to offer up a whole-grain crust option for all of their pies, bringing to each slice more than twice the fiber of a regular pizza.

310 calories
Domino's Thin Crust Ham and Pineapple Pizza

Considering your town's average delivery joint is pushing pies with about 300 calories a slice, consider this a tasty three-for-one. Nobody makes a lower calorie thin crust slice than the boys in blue.

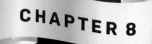

CHAPTER 8

The Best (&Worst) Sandwiches in America

Eat This

Chili's Fajita Pita Chicken

455 calories
13 g fat (2 g saturated)
1,401 mg sodium
52 g carbohydrates

Unlike wraps, pitas are usually a good sign of a healthy menu item. At Chili's, the Fajita Pitas reign supreme.

Save 66g fat!
Cut the fat equivalent of 6 scoops of ice cream before you even make it to dessert.

Save over 900 calories!
And you don't even need to leave the restaurant to do it. Just choose the right chicken and cash in on the huge savings.

Hot or cold, crusty or chewy, a sandwich is nothing more than

some meat and vegetables getting a big soft hug from something that is, or looks like, bread. And so it's no wonder sandwiches are among our favorite go-to comfort foods: Mom's grilled cheese or PB&J or Dad's burgers and dogs hot off the grill are hallmarks of our early days, when our nutritional needs were met by the people who love us.

Now, here's the bad news: If you're ordering a sandwich from a chain restaurant or picking one up from your grocery store, your nutritional needs are being met by people who not only don't love you but don't know you from Adam. Or, more clearly, they only know you from George, as in Washington, as in the guy who's tucked away in your wallet.

And that's what makes the worst sandwiches in this book such terrible weapons of nutritional sabotage. The sandwich is the go-to for lunch and, as our lives become increasingly fast paced and furious, the go-to for breakfast and sometimes dinner as well. (When you don't have time for napkins and utensils, you're saddled with a sandwich, right?)

And these once-simple meals are getting more complicated: Now we have not just sandwiches but something called "wraps" and yet another entry into the sweepstakes called a "panini." What's up with these? And whereas once we had three choices— white, wheat, or rye— now we have a whole armada of doughy choices, from ciabatta to semolina to sourdough. Which are good for you? Which will deliver protein and other nutrients and help you stay in fighting trim? And which ones will break apart your diet the way Jack Nicholson broke down that bathroom door in *The Shining*? Here's a hint: Some of the worst offenders carry innocent-sounding words like "chicken" or "salad" or even "vegetarian" in their names. Before you pick up a sandwich, make sure you know just what's lurking below those innocent-looking loaves.

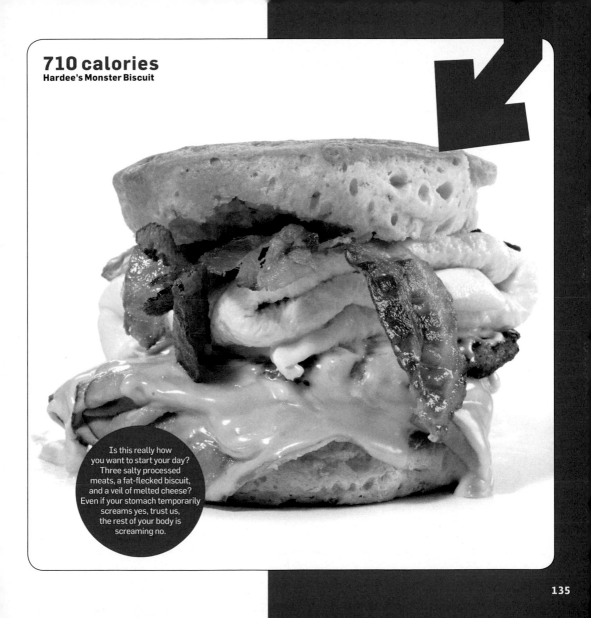

710 calories
Hardee's Monster Biscuit

Is this really how you want to start your day? Three salty processed meats, a fat-flecked biscuit, and a veil of melted cheese? Even if your stomach temporarily screams yes, trust us, the rest of your body is screaming no.

The Worst Sandwiches in America

12 Hardee's Monster Biscuit

- *710 calories*
- *51 g fat (17 g saturated)*
- *2,250 mg sodium*

The only thing worse than Hardee's abysmal lineup of burgers and afternoon atrocities is their breakfast menu. More than 60 percent of the entrées contain at least half a day's worth of saturated fat and only 3 items have less than 1,000 milligrams of sodium. Blame two constants: the Southern loyalty to the biscuit, and the penchant for piling multiple breakfast meats into a single dish. Here, that means ham, sausage, and bacon, plus a melted cheddar blanket. While Hardee's doesn't offer up trans fat counts, we suspect there are some of those nasty hydrogenated lipids lurking in this biscuit. You deserve a better start to your day.

Eat This Instead!

Texas Toast Breakfast Ham Sandwich

- *390 calories · 18 g fat (6 g saturated)*
- *1,170 mg sodium*

WORST TURKEY SANDWICH

11 Atlanta Bread Company Turkey Bacon Rustica

- *960 calories*
- *56 g fat (19 g saturated)*
- *2,480 mg sodium*
- *62 g carbohydrates*

Even turkey can be tainted when placed in the wrong hands. That's because the meat in your sandwich is never as important as the condiments. Here, the triple threat of mayo, pesto, and bacon takes a perfectly lean meat and turns it into the headliner for one of America's most underachieving sandwiches.

Eat This Instead!

Turkey on 9 Grain

- *370 calories · 6 g fat (2 g saturated)*
- *1,240 mg sodium · 50 g carbohydrates*

WORST BBQ SANDWICH

10 Bob Evans Knife and Fork Pulled Pork BBQ Sandwich

- *1,004 calories*
- *36 g fat (10 g saturated)*
- *1,377 mg sodium*
- *112 g carbohydrates*

Any sandwich that requires a knife and fork to eat it is bound to threaten your waistline. Bob Evans offers 2 barbecue sandwiches, and not surprisingly, the one that comes without silverware has 350 fewer calories and nearly half the sodium and carbs. Our recommendation: Pick up the knife and fork and wave them at the waitress when she tries to bring this sandwich to your table.

Eat This Instead!

Bob-B-Q Pulled Pork Sandwich

- *655 calories · 30 g fat (5 g saturated)*
- *788 mg sodium · 68 g carbohydrates*

WORST ITALIAN SANDWICH

9 Panera Full Italian Combo on Ciabatta Bread

- *1,050 calories*
- *47 g fat (18 g saturated, 1 g trans)*
- *3,050 mg sodium*
- *94 g carbohydrates*

Beware the dreaded Italian sub—its combination of fatty meats and salty cheeses makes it the ticking time bomb of the deli counter. Panera's odious ode to Italy packs as much salt as 4 medium orders of Burger King Onion Rings and as

1,186 calories
Blimpie Special Vegetarian sub

A certified catastrophe for those who enjoy their meals meat-free. Blame the calories on a cheese overload, plus an unhealthy dose of oil. Blimpie even offers an "off menu" addition of crushed Doritos to this already-sullied sandwich.

many calories as 2 Big Macs. No matter how bad some of Panera's full-size sandwiches may be, all of them come in half portions and can be paired up with soup or salad for a decent lunch. Take advantage.

Eat This Instead!
Smoked Turkey Breast on Sourdough

• *470 calories*
• *17 g fat (2.5 g saturated, 0 g trans)*
• *1,680 mg sodium • 49 g carbohydrates*

WORST SALAD SANDWICH

8 Noah's Deli Chicken Salad Sandwich

• *1,150 calories*
• *95 g fat*
  (14 g saturated, 1.5 g trans)
• *1,190 mg sodium*

If anything, the word "salad" should raise your nutritional guard, not slacken it. Here, salad translates into a heaping scoop of mayonnaise, polluting an otherwise lean serving of chicken with empty calories. (Warning: Noah's cousin Einstein Bros.' chicken salad sandwich is nearly as bad.) If you want a truly healthy sandwich, stick with the chicken, just ditch the "salad."

Eat This Instead!
California Chicken Sandwich

• *360 calories • 7 g fat (2 g saturated)*
• *840 mg sodium*

WORST VEGGIE SANDWICH

7 Blimpie Special Vegetarian (12")

• *1,186 calories*
• *60 g fat (19 g saturated)*
• *3,532 mg sodium*
• *131 g carbohydrates*

"Vegetarian" doesn't automatically translate to "healthy." Sure, this sandwich has vegetables, but it also has 3 different kinds of cheese and a deluge of oil tucked into a hulking 12" roll. No wonder it contains more than half a day's worth of calories and a cascade of carbs. For a truly healthy pile of vegetables, try the garden salad. If a sandwich is the only thing that will do, you'll have to settle for the small VeggieMax, still far from a model of meatless eating.

Eat This Instead!
VeggieMax on Wheat (6")

• *499 calories • 21 g fat (6 g saturated)*
• *1,212 mg sodium*
• *50 g carbohydrates*

The Ultimate Sandwich Selector

Hoagies, heroes, grinders, subs, po'boys, zeppelins: Whatever you call them in your town, sandwiches are undeniably an American food. We may not lay claim to their invention (that vaunted distinction may belong to England's Earl of Sandwich), but we've done plenty to advance them over the years. Problem is, we've done plenty to distort them, too, turning humble creations into caloric catastrophes (see Quiznos' 1,760-calorie Tuna Melt for reference) weighted down by reckless condiments, bloated breads, and an excess of ill-chosen toppings. As our contribution to America's long-standing love affair with the sandwich, we've broken the sub down into its many components, laying out the nutritional goods on the meat, produce, cheese, and condiments you're most likely to squeeze between 2 slices of bread. We've even thrown in a few surprises. Consider this a blueprint for a tastier, more nutritious future.

	CALORIES	FAT	PROTEIN	FIBER	SODIUM	CARBS	SUGARS
THE FOUNDATION (Two 35-g slices, unless otherwise noted)							
Whole grain pita (small, 28 g)	74	1g (0g saturated)	3g	2g	149mg	15.5g	
Whole wheat	182	2.5g (0.5g saturated)	7.5g	5g	264mg	8g	
Sprouted wheat	160	2g (0g saturated)	10g	6g	330mg	34.5g	
French roll (75 g)	207	3g (1g saturated)	7g	2.5g	445mg	37.5g	
Ciabatta roll (69 g)	153	2g (0g saturated)	5.5g	1.5g	453mg	29g	
Rye	180	2.5g (0.5g saturated)	6g	3g	462mg	34g	
Sourdough (73 g)	202	1.5g (0.5g saturated)	8g	1.5g	454mg	39.5g	
100% whole wheat English muffin (57 g)	127	1g (0g saturated)	5g	2.5g	315mg	5.5g	
THE FILLING (48 g, unless otherwise noted)							
Turkey breast	54	1.5g (0g saturated)	6.5g		576mg		
Roast beef (¾ cup)	60	2g (0.5g saturated)	10g		450mg		
Tuna salad (¾ cup)	360	32g (4.5g saturated)	18g		460mg		
Smoked salmon	99	3.5g (1g saturated)	17g		288mg		
Grilled chicken breast	55	1.5g (0.5g saturated)	10.5g		285mg		
Pastrami	70	3g (1.5g saturated)	10.5g		25mg		
Ham	63	2g (1g saturated)	8g		626mg		
Bacon (4 slices)	168	13g (4g saturated)	12g		767mg		
THE VEGETATION (⅓ cup)							
Tomatoes	16			1g		1g	
Romaine	4			0.5g		0.5g	
Sliced avocado	117	11g (1.5g saturated)		1.5g		5g	
Red onions	9					0.5g	
Arugula	2			0.5g			
Pickles	9			1g	872mg		0.5g
Roasted red peppers	19			0.5g		1g	
Peperoncini	18			1g		0.5g	
THE DAIRY (48 g, unless otherwise noted)							
American cheese	116	8.5g (5.5g saturated)	7g		650mg		
Brie	117	10g (6g saturated)	7.5g		220mg		
Fresh mozzarella	105	8g (4.5g saturated)	7.5g		147mg		
Pepper jack	138	11g (6.5g saturated)	7.5g		212mg		
Fresh goat cheese	128	10.5g (7g saturated)	7.5g		180mg		
Cheddar	141	11.5g (7.5g saturated)	9g		217mg		
Swiss	133	9.5g (6g saturated)	9.5g		95mg		
Egg (medium)	63	4.5g (1.5g saturated)	5.5g		62mg		
THE ACCENTS (1 tablespoon)							
Salsa	5			1g	60mg		2g
Tapenade	40	4g (0.5g saturated)			290mg		
Oil and vinegar	72	8g (1.5g saturated					
Mayonnaise	103	11.5g (1.5g saturated)			73mg		
Grainy mustard	16	1g (0g saturated)			68mg		
Pesto	45	3.5g (1g saturated)			95mg		
Cranberry sauce	26				5mg		6.5g
Hummus	25	1.5g (0g saturated)	1g	1g	57mg		

The Worst Sandwiches in America

6 Subway Footlong Meatball with Cheese

- *1,260 calories*
- *54 g fat (22 g saturated)*
- *3,570 mg sodium*
- *142 g carbohydrates*

Okay, really—you couldn't see this coming? Subway's shining health halo blinds most people from the fact that their menu is still riddled with belt-breaking options. And none breaks more belts than this 12" marinara-slathered behemoth. There are only 2 things that will get you into trouble at Subway: footlongs and hot sandwiches. Solve both problems by sticking to a 6" ham, turkey, or roast beef. Really hungry? Then double up on the protein for a mere 50 to 80 calories more.

Eat This Instead!
Subway 6" Double Roast Beef
- *400 calories · 7 g fat (2.5 g saturated)*
- *1,410 mg sodium · 47 g carbohydates*

5 Chili's Cajun Crisper Bites Sandwiches

- *1,412 calories*
- *79 g fat (18 g saturated)*
- *3,986 mg sodium*
- *126 g carbohydrates*

Think these cute little miniature sandwiches are harmless? Think again. At Chili's, the words "bites" and "crisper" translate into calorie-packed sauces and a bucket of frying oil, respectively. Put them between 2 slices of bread and you've got one of the worst sandwiches—4 of them, to be exact—we've found on all counts, with the equivalent of 120 saltine crackers and the same number of calories as you'll find in 28 Krispy Kreme original glazed doughnut holes. Taste the same bold flavors and save nearly 1,000 calories and more than 2,500 milligrams of sodium by opting for the Fajita Pita instead.

Eat This Instead!
Fajita Pita Chicken
- *455 calories · 13 g fat (2 g saturated)*
- *1,401 mg sodium*

4 Quiznos Prime Rib Cheesesteak Sub (large)

- *1,490 calories*
- *92 g fat*
  (22.5 g saturated, 2 g trans)
- *2,620 mg sodium*
- *102 g carbohydrates*

At 670 calories, even the small version of this sub is pushing the bounds of reasonable consumption. Tussle with the big guy, though, and you're taking in a day's worth of saturated fat, plus as many calories as you'd find in 2 whole sticks of butter. A survival strategy for eating at Quiznos: If you're going to order a sub, order it small, skip the dressing, and load up on the vegetables. Better yet, skip the subs altogether in favor of the more restrained Sammies. You'd be better off with 2 of them than with most regular-size sandwiches at Quiznos.

Eat This Instead!
Bistro Steak Melt Flatbread Sammie
- *280 calories · 13 g fat (4 g saturated)*
- *645 mg sodium · 26 g carbohydrates*

Looks kinda healthy from here, no? But judging by the calorie count, not to mention the 133 grams of fat, this sub is more mayo than tuna. If you want to keep it around 500 calories at Quiznos, keep it to a small, or 2 Sammies.

1,760 calories
Quiznos Large Tuna Melt

The Worst Sandwiches in America

3 Applebee's Oriental Chicken Rollup

• *1,550 calories**

Applebee's should call this handheld disaster what it is: an oversized burrito with the caloric heft of 10 Taco Bell Fresco Beef Tacos. Add the fries that comes with it and you're sacrificing your entire day's caloric allowance. Yikes. The Chicken and Portobello, one of Applebee's best options, will save you more than 1,000 calories in one sitting.

Eat This Instead!

Italian Chicken Portobello Sandwich

• *360 calories**

**Applebee's refuses to release full nutritional data on the foods they serve.*

WORST GRILLED CHEESE

2 Romano's Macaroni Grill Formaggio Melts

• *1,590 calories*
• *125 g fat (49 g saturated)*
• *2,370 mg sodium*
• *68 g carbohydrates*

We thought the 1,090-calorie Grilled Chicken and Arti-choke was bad, but then Macaroni Grille dropped these ticking time bombs. The menu description boils it down to toasted cheese, tomatoes, and basil, but the end result—part of a wave of mini-food disasters spreading across the country—packs more saturated fat than you'll find in a dozen Dunkin' Donuts Chocolate Frosted doughnuts. If it's cheese, tomatoes, and basil you seek, switch over to the Moz-zarella Alla Caprese. It might

---

Super Sandwiches AT-HOME RECIPES THAT WILL POWER UP YOUR DIET—AND YOUR DAY

The Sunrise Sammie
for energy and weight loss

Whole wheat English muffin, ham, romaine, tomato, Cheddar, egg

Studies show that people who choose quality protein over refined carbs for breakfast are able to burn 65 percent more calories and maintain higher levels of energy throughout the day.

The Gladiator
for muscle power

Whole grain pita, roast beef, romaine, tomato, fresh mozzarella, hummus

This baby is bursting at the seams with lean protein, with chicken, chickpeas, and mozza-rella completing the trifecta. Not only is this a good postworkout option, it's great at any time of day for firing up your metabolism.

The Gobbler
for cancer-fighting

Rye, avocado, turkey, Brie, arugula, cranberry sauce

Can sandwiches cure cancer? Of course not, but few fruits pack more antioxidants than cranberries, and with a dose of cell-protecting flavonols from the pile of arugula, this nutrient-dense creation certainly can't hurt the cause.

The Einstein
for brain power

Sprouted wheat, smoked salmon, red onion, avocado, goat cheese, pesto

Omega-3 fatty acids (from the salmon) and anthocyanidins (from the red onion) are pivotal in both building and preserving our frazzled minds.

The Sure Shot
for nerves

Rye, turkey, egg, arugula, red onion, grainy mustard

Big doses of magne-sium from the rye and mustard, along with the calming powers of tryptophan from the turkey and egg, make for a seriously sooth-ing sandwich.

not be melted, but it will save you more than 1,000 calories and 88 grams of fat.

Eat This Instead!
Mozzarella Alla Caprese
• *440 calories* • *37 g fat (12 g saturated)*
• *770 mg sodium* • *9 g carbohydrates*

WORST SANDWICH IN AMERICA

1 Quiznos Tuna Melt (large)

• *1,760 calories*
• *133 g fat*
  (25 g saturated, 1.5 g trans)
• *2,120 mg sodium*

In almost all other forms, tuna is a nutritional superstar, so how did it end up as the headliner for America's Worst Sandwich? Blame an absurdly heavy hand with the mayo the tuna is mixed with, along with Quiznos' larger-than-life portion sizes. Even though they've managed to trim this melt down from the original 2,000-plus calorie mark when we first tested it, it still sits squarely at the bottom of the sandwich ladder.

Eat This Instead!
Sonoma Turkey Flatbread Sammie
• *280 calories* • *14 g fat (4 g saturated)*
• *760 mg sodium*

1,590 calories
**Romano's Macaroni Grill
Formaggio Melts**

The average homemade grilled cheese contains about 400 calories. The average deli grilled cheese ups the ante to 600 calories. This cheesy calamity blows past all of those, sandwiching more than 2 days' worth of fat between the bread.

The Best Sandwiches

MAKE THESE HANDHELD HEROES PART OF YOUR EAT-OUT ROSTER

BEST RESTAURANT SANDWICH

Applebee's Italian Chicken Portobello Sandwich

- *360 calories*

Applebee's may have the most polarized menu in America, filled with nutritional black holes but punctuated by some surprisingly good fare—none better than this sandwich. The lean chicken breast is grilled, the portobello adds a layer of meaty intensity, and the traditional high-calorie spreads are replaced with a chunky marinara sauce. Oh, and it comes with a side of fresh fruit, making for a well-rounded meal with 1,380 fewer calories than a basket of Riblets.

BEST SUB

Subway 6" Double Roast Beef

- *400 calories*
- *7 g fat (2.5 g saturated)*
- *1,410 mg sodium*

Subway's double protein option is a tremendous way to add substance to a smaller sandwich without significantly upping the calorie commitment. Ultimately, 80 calories is a pretty small price to pay for an extra shot of lean protein—especially if those 80 calories will help fend off the urge to order the full footlong. As for the meat, turkey, ham, and roast beef—at least in the deli space—have nearly identical nutritional profiles, so order the one you enjoy most.

BEST SANDWICH ALTERNATIVE

Chili's Fajita Pita Chicken

- *455 calories*
- *13 g fat (2 g saturated)*
- *1,401 mg sodium*

We love this sandwich as much for what it is as for what it is not: It's not another 1,800-calorie Chili's entrée, and it's not just another member in the massive group of sit-down sandwiches that double as nutritional nightmares. Seriously, it's a challenge to find a chain sandwich with fewer than 800 calories, which makes this offering—with its 31 grams of protein and heap of fresh produce—all the more impressive (even if it is high in the sodium department).

BEST SANDWICH TO WAKE UP TO

Dunkin' Donuts Egg White Turkey Sausage Flatbread

- *280 calories*
- *6 g fat (2.5 g saturated)*
- *820 mg sodium*

In an effort to bring a tinge of health to a brand tainted by breakfast pastries, Dunkin' fired up their line of flatbread sandwiches in 2008. Not a moment too soon, either, since most of the breakfast options there are dubious at best. But this modest sandwich brings 19 grams of protein to the start of your day, for fewer calories, carbs, and sodium than you'll find in any other breakfast sandwich in the country.

in America

400 calories
Subway 6" Double Roast Beef

Subway's real strength doesn't lie in the much-publicized list of sandwiches with "under 6 grams of fat"; it's in their vast supply of fresh produce and the ability to double up on lean protein for an extra 40 to 80 calories. This sandwich takes advantage of both.

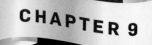
The Best (& Worst) Sushi in America

Imagine it's 1959.

You and your hepcat friends and your swingin' dolls hop into the T-Bird, crank up the AM to catch Wolfman Jack spinning some Little Richard, and split Dullsville to chase a little excitement downtown. And the first place you come to on the corner of Main Street and Daddy-O Boulevard is...

A sushi restaurant? Wait . . . *who* won WWII?

Fifty years ago, finding sushi for sale in most areas of the US of A was about as likely as finding an alien spaceship on the mall in front of the high school. In fact, up until the 1980s, this Japanese import was incredibly exotic—the kind of food only daring cosmopolitan types and your older sister's "interesting" friends from college would even think of eating. But today you can find it on offer in just about any strip mall within a day or two's drive of the coasts, and even many supermarkets now have part-time sushi chefs whacking raw fish

and prepping it for the hungry masses. In fact, sushi consumption in the United States has increased by 70 percent in the last 20 years, and even folks who can't fathom eating raw fish have discovered the allure of tempura, vegetable rolls, and skewers of chicken and beef teriyaki.

But while reams of scientific studies continue to show that fish—especially when it's unadorned by glazes, sauces, or breading—is an incredible source of heart-strengthening, inflammation-reducing, brain-boosting, life-lengthening nutrients,

just walking into a sushi restaurant and properly pronouncing the word "uni" doesn't guarantee you're eating well. Yes, you're in great shape when you order most

The Raw Fish Rundown

Ever wonder what all those mysterious pieces of colorful flesh behind the sushimaster's glass case really are? Well, we'll tell you exactly that, plus all of the nutritional information you need to make informed decisions next time you belly up to the bar.

Few foods pack more flavor and vital nutrition for fewer calories than sushi. Ladies and gents, grab your chopsticks.

Forget about sitting at a table—the sushi bar is the place to be. Get to know the knife-wielding wonder preparing your sushi and he'll clue you in on the day's freshest catch, plus he just might pass along a few of those rare bites he's been saving for special customers.

Salmon (wild, 1 ounce)
Japanese name: sake

- 40 calories (fish only)
- 2 g fat
- 6 g protein
- 565 mg omega-3 fatty acids

sushi or sashimi (sushi means a piece of fish sitting on a rice pillow; sashimi is just the fish, totally naked) or even a sushi roll. As a general rule, the combination of rice, seaweed, seafood, and vegetables (often avocado or cucumber) makes for a low-calorie, high-protein meal that will fill you up and, depending on the type of seafood you choose, provide a healthy dose of heart-helpful omega-3 fatty acids.

That said, not all of these fish dishes will be kind to your waistline. Some sushi rolls come laced with mayo and cream cheese, and not all the meat is actually "real"—imitation crab comes with only 40 percent of the protein of the real deal and offers almost no omega-3s. Check out the following sashimi and sushi roll nutrition breakdowns—whether constructing your own Japanese masterpiece or ordering a popular roll, you'll know which ones are worth choosing and which are secret diet destroyers.

The Four Forms of Sushi

Nigiri: Fish or roe draped over balls of rice

Maki: Ubiquitous sushi roll cut into 6 to 8 bite-size pieces

Temaki: Cone-shaped handheld sushi roll

Sashimi: Raw fish served without rice

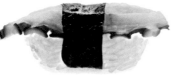 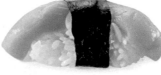

Octopus (1 ounce)
Japanese name: tako

- 23 calories
- 0 g fat
- 4 g protein
- 45.5 mg omega-3 fatty acids

Giant Scallop (1 ounce)
Japanese name: hotategai

- 25 calories
- 0 g fat
- 5 g protein
- 60 mg omega-3 fatty acids

Squid (1 ounce)
Japanese name: ika

- 26 calories
- 0 g fat
- 4 g protein
- 140 mg omega-3 fatty acids

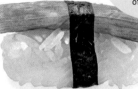

Each little tuft of rice used in nigiri sushi contains approximately 24 calories and 5.5 grams of carbs.

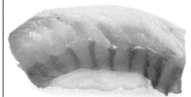

Flounder (1 ounce)
Japanese name: hirame

- *26 calories*
- *0 g fat*
- *5 g protein*
- *71.5 mg omega-3 fatty acids*

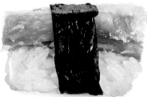

King Crab (real, 1 ounce)
Japanese name: kani

- *27 calories*
- *0 g fat*
- *5 g protein*
- *128 mg omega-3 fatty acids*

Krab/Crab Stick
(fake, 1 ounce)
Japanese name: kani (surimi)

- *27 calories*
- *0 g fat*
- *2 g protein*
- *236 mg sodium*
- *8 mg omega-3 fatty acids*

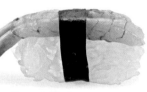

Sweet Shrimp (1 ounce)
Japanese name: ama-ebi

- *30 calories*
- *0 g fat*
- *6 g protein*
- *151 mg omega-3 fatty acids*

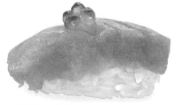

Yellowtail (1 ounce)
Japanese name: hamachi

- *31 calories*
- *0 g fat*
- *7 g protein*
- *69 mg omega-3 fatty acids*

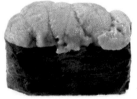

Sea Urchin (1 ounce)
Japanese name: uni

- *34 calories*
- *1 g fat*
- *3 g protein*
- *96 mg omega-3 fatty acids*

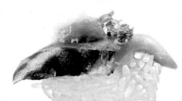

Mackerel (1 ounce)
Japanese name: saba

- *39 calories*
- *2 g fat (1 g saturated)*
- *5 g protein*
- *413 mg omega-3 fatty acids*

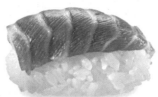

Salmon (wild, 1 ounce)
Japanese name: sake

- *40 calories*
- *2 g fat*
- *6 g protein*
- *565 mg omega-3 fatty acids*

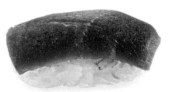

Bluefin Tuna (1 ounce)
Japanese name: maguro

- *40 calories*
- *1 g fat*
- *7 g protein*
- *363 mg omega-3 fatty acids*

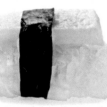

Japanese Omelet
(1 piece)
Japanese name: tamago

- *45 calories*
- *2 g fat*
- *2 g protein*

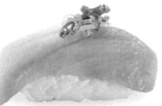

Albacore
(White tuna, 1 ounce)
Japanese name: shiro maguro

- *49 calories*
- *2 g fat*
- *7 g protein*
- *72 mg omega-3 fatty acids*

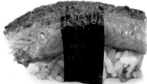

Eel (1 ounce)
Japanese names: anago, unagi

- *52 calories*
- *3 g fat (1 g saturated)*
- *5 g protein*
- *183 mg omega-3 fatty acids*

The Ultimate Sushi Roll Selector

Unlike the Japanese, who favor sashimi and nigiri-style sushi, the vast majority of sushi consumed in this country comes in roll form. And nowhere does the potential for seriously healthy eats or nutritional negligence oscillate so wildly than in these rice-stuffed seaweed bites. Better take a second to digest our version of a roll call, listed from best to worst. (Nutrition stats are for an entire 6 to 8 piece roll.)

Rainbow Rolls are essentially California Rolls topped with the chef's choice of sashimi.

For a superior Rainbow Roll, ask the sushi chef to make it with real crab. They may charge a bit more, but the extra flavor and nutrition make it a worthy upgrade.

Rainbow Roll

Nori, rice, avocado, surimi, plus a variety of raw fish arranged on top

- *476 calories*
- *16 g fat*
- *33 g protein*
- *6 g fiber*
- *50 g carbohydrates*

Higher in calories than most rolls you'll find, but loaded as this is with substantial portions of myriad raw fish, most of those calories are the good kind. Rainbow rolls are typically large, so a single order and a bowl of miso soup make a filling dinner.

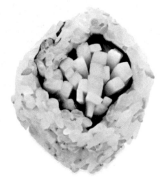

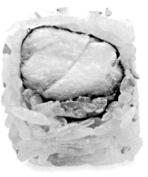

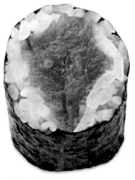

Cucumber Roll
Nori, rice, cucumber

- *136 calories*
- *0 g fat*
- *6 g protein*
- *3.5 g fiber*
- *30 g carbohydrates*

It's hard to go wrong with cucumbers and seaweed. Though not a nutritional powerhouse, cucumbers are a low-calorie delivery system for vitamins A and C, fiber, and silica, a compound that has been shown to foster healthy skin.

Avocado Roll
Nori, rice, avocado

- *140 calories*
- *5.5 g fat*
- *2 g protein*
- *6 g fiber*
- *28 g carbohydrates*

Most of the calories in this vegetarian roll come from healthy monounsaturated fats. Avocado makes a great addition to any roll, since a sushi-size portion also contains about 3 grams of fiber.

Tuna Roll
Nori, rice, tuna

- *184 calories*
- *2 g fat*
- *24 g protein*
- *3.5 g fiber*
- *27 g carbohydrates*

More than half of the calories in this simple, classic roll come from protein, making it a great light meal or a snack with substance.

As a general sushi strategy, less is more. Menu words like "spicy" and "crunch" usually denote untraditional add-ons like mayo, cream cheese, and tempura batter that can boost calories by 50 percent.

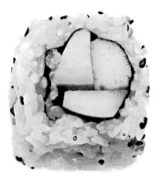

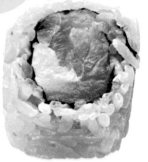

California Roll
Nori, rice, avocado, surimi

- *255 calories*
- *7 g fat*
- *9 g protein*
- *6 g fiber*
- *38 g carbohydrates*

The ubiquitous fusion roll is a great beginner's foray into the potential of sushi, since there's no raw fish involved. There are also no real healthy fats either (aside from the avocado, of course), since the fake crab (made from a variety of processed and compressed fish) has $^1/_{15}$ the amount of omega-3s as the real stuff.

Spicy Tuna Roll
Nori, rice, tuna, mayo, chili sauce

- *290 calories*
- *11 g fat*
- *24 g protein*
- *3.5 g fiber*
- *26 g carbohydrates*

In the world of sushi, "spicy" means a spoonful of mayo spiked with an Asian chili sauce. The calorie counts can climb higher than this, depending on how heavy a hand the sushi chef has with the spicy stuff. Either way, you're better off satisfying your need for heat with a touch of wasabi.

Philadelphia Roll
Nori, rice, salmon, cream cheese, cucumber

- *290 calories*
- *12 g fat (5 g saturated)*
- *14 g protein*
- *2 g fiber*
- *28 g carbohydrates*

Just like the mayo adds empty calories to an otherwise reliable spicy tuna roll, cream cheese blankets perfectly fine salmon and cucumber with an unnecessary measure of fat.

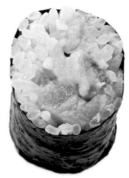

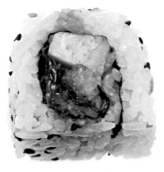

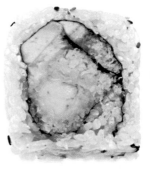

Salmon and Avocado Roll
Nori, rice, salmon, avocado

- *304 calories*
- *8.5 g fat*
- *13 g protein*
- *6 g fiber*
- *42 g carbohydrates*

High in calories, but nearly all of those calories come from the one-two punch of healthy fats found in the salmon and the avocado.

Eel and Avocado Roll
Nori, rice, avocado, eel

- *372 calories*
- *17 g fat*
- *20 g protein*
- *6 g fiber*
- *31 g carbohydrates*

Eel brings a solid helping of omega-3s to the sushi bar, but unfortunately, it's almost always covered in a gloppy, sugary brown sauce that masks both the nutrition and the delicate natural flavor of this wily sea creature. If you opt for this roll, make it your only one of the night.

Shrimp Tempura Roll
Nori, rice, shrimp, tempura batter, oil for frying

- *508 calories*
- *21 g fat*
- *20 g protein*
- *4.5 g fiber*
- *64 g carbohydrates*

Why take a perfectly good piece of lean shrimp and ruin it with thick batter and a hot oil bath? The joy of fried food—the crunch—is snuffed out by the moist rice, so this one doesn't make sense from either a flavor or a nutritional perspective.

To find out more about the most contaminant-free, environmentally friendly fish in the ocean, log on to montereybayaquarium.org.

The *Eat This, Not That!* Fish Finder

You know you should be eating more fish, but do you know which kind is healthiest? Fresh or frozen, wild or farmed, local or imported: The challenges and nuances of the industrial food complex have made choosing the right fish more complicated than string theory. To simplify matters, we've analyzed a dozen of the most popular fish choices and ranked them from best to worst. Our favorite sea creatures are rich in omega-3s; relatively low in mercury, PCBs, and dioxins; and ecologically sustainable.

Here's the catch: A high level of mercury in your fish will undo any heart-health benefit the fish might provide, according to Finnish scientists. That's because mercury impairs arterial flexibility.

FISH	OMEGA-3S (mg per 3 oz serving)	PROTEIN (g per 3 oz serving)	CONTAMINANTS *	ENVIRONMENTAL FRIENDLINESS **
Wild Alaskan Salmon	1,253	18	low	✔✔
Farmed Rainbow Trout	838	18	low	✔✔
Pacific Halibut	444	18	low	✔✔
Farmed Catfish	391	13	medium	✔✔
Farmed Tilapia	185	17	low	✔✔
Yellowfin Tuna	207	20	medium	✔
Farmed Salmon	1,705	17	high	—
Mahimahi	104	16	low	✔
Swordfish	701	17	high	✔
Grouper	227	16	medium	—
Atlantic Cod	166	15	medium	—
Chilean Sea Bass	570	16	medium	—

*Based on Environmental Defense's analysis of mercury and PCB data.
**Based on each fish's sustainability, as monitored by Monterey Bay Aquarium's Seafood Watch

Ingredients Selector

SUSHI ISN'T JUST LOW CALORIE—ITS INGREDIENTS CAN ACTUALLY HELP YOUR HEALTH

Key

California roll ●
Veggie roll ●
Alaskan roll ●
Spicy yellowtail roll ●
Rainbow roll ●
Boston roll ●

* Krab is used in California rolls but you can substitute real crab for a healthy alternative.

Avocado
Nutrient: Lutein
Benefit: Eye health and cancer protection
● ● ● ● ●

Carrots
Nutrient: Vitamin K
Benefit: Promotes healthy blood clotting
●

Cucumber
Nutrient: Vitamin C
Benefit: Strengthens bones
● ● ● ● ●

Crab* **(not krab)**
Nutrient: Zinc
Benefit: Fights infections
●

Romaine lettuce
Nutrient: Folic acid
Benefit: Prevents clogged arteries
●

Salmon
Nutrient: Vitamin B_{12}
Benefit: Maintains healthy nerve and red blood cells
● ●

Shrimp
Nutrient: Selenium
Benefit: Lowers risk of prostate cancer
●

Tuna
Nutrient: Vitamin B_6
Benefit: Helps reduce risk of colon cancer
●

Yellowtail
Nutrient: Niacin
Benefit: Improves good cholesterol levels
● ●

Sushi 101

There are dozens of different ways to enjoy sushi, but if you want to be a true zen master of raw fish consumption, there are rules that are worth knowing and following. Avoid another sashimi-gobbling faux pas by brushing up on some basic sushi etiquette.

● When you're not using your chopsticks, place them parallel to each other in the holder or on the dish. Never stick your chopsticks into your rice and leave them sticking up.

● When passing food from one plate to another, use the opposite end of your chopsticks to make the delivery, not the part you eat with.

● You can eat sushi rolls and nigiri with your hands, but you should eat sashimi with chopsticks. And forks should never enter the picture; sushi chefs don't want their creations tainted with the metallic tang of silverware.

● Eat sushi in one bite, especially sashimi and nigiri. The flavors and textures come in small packages for a reason—so that you can experience them all at once. There are a few exceptions, especially in the United States, where specialty rolls can be as big as cannons; you'll know an exception when you see it.

● The sliced ginger is for cleaning your palate in between different tastes, not for draping all over the delicate fish before you.

● As fun as it might be to evoke the nasal-clearing effects of wasabi overdose, that pile of concentrated Japanese horseradish is supposed to be used sparingly—if at all. A good sushi chef applies the correct amount of wasabi to his creations, meaning all you need to do is be ready to deliver them from plate to mouth.

● Rice-making is a craft that takes sushi chefs years to master, so don't go mucking up their perfect grains by drowning them in soy. If you want to dip, dip the fish side of the sushi into the sauce, not the rice side. The rice will soak up the soy like a sponge, compromising flavor and texture and leaving you with a surplus of sodium in your belly.

Anatomy of a Sushi Roll

Whereas sashimi and nigiri are about the simple elegance of the fish, rolls in America tend to favor bolder flavor combinations and, at times, unconventional ingredients. Mango-macadamian fried calamari roll, anyone? But there are a few constants in all maki rolls. Use this piece-by-piece blueprint to break down the nutritional value of nearly any roll you encounter.

TOBIKO
These tiny fish eggs contain about 50 calories per tablespoon, mostly from healthy fat.

RAW FISH
Good sushi spots will source their fish fresh daily. Ask the manager how often they get their fish deliveries.

SESAME SEEDS
Request them on any roll for a punch of brain-boosting magnesium.

KRAB
Not good. Krab sticks, also called surimi, are made from processed and compressed hake and pollock.

RICE
Rice in the average piece contributes approximately 15 calories and 3 grams of carbohydrates.

The best strategy when eating sushi is to maximize the quantity of raw fish and fresh vegetables and minimize the amount of empty carbs (i.e., rice) and unnecessary embellishments. The best way to do that? Favor nigiri and sashimi over rolls.

NORI
These dried seaweed sheets used to wrap sushi are high in protein and packed full of vitamins.

159

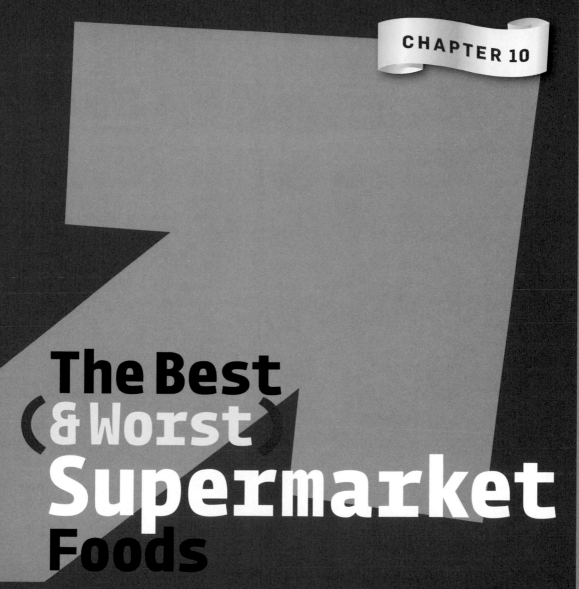

CHAPTER 10

The Best
(&Worst)
Supermarket
Foods

Eat This

Marie Callender's Oven Baked Chicken

320 calories
12 g fat (3 g saturated)
990 mg sodium

Save 840 calories!
Make this swap just once a week and save more than 12 pounds in a year.

Save 54 g fat!
Plus you'll knock off an entire day's worth of saturated fat.

Not That!

Stouffer's White Meat Chicken Pot Pie

Large Size

1,160 calories
66 g fat (26 g saturated)
1,780 mg sodium

Avoid the freezer burn: It's best to keep this potpie from ever defrosting.

The components of these two dishes are nearly identical—lean chicken, vegetables, creamy carbs—but the potpie loses in dramatic fashion as a result of its oil-soaked crust and the viscous tide of buttery sauce found within.

They say that the squeaky wheel gets the grease, and nowhere is that more true than in today's supermarkets.

As you push your little metal cart through the endless aisles of foodstuffs, you're taking a tour of an obscene amount of grease (and sugar and salt and unnecessary calories), all brought to you courtesy of today's food manufacturers.

It doesn't have to be this way. In the battle to stay lean and healthy, the supermarket should be your lair—your Bat Cave, your Situation Room, your personal nutritional workshop. And supermarkets really do carry everything you need to feed yourself and your family perfectly, while still saving yourself a ton of money. But this nutritional workshop is also filled with rusty nails and sharp edges, and you need to navigate your way through it with caution.

Many of the worst offenders are obvious— if it says "double chocolate" anywhere on the label, you don't get to claim nutritional ignorance. But a lot of the greasiest, saltiest, most sugary products on the shelves come with deceptive labels, touting keywords that seem to signal healthy choices: words like "all-natural" or "multigrain" or "lite."

Indeed, food packaging can be so deceptive that you often have no way of knowing which foods will lead you to a lifetime of leanness and which will undermine every effort you make to control your body—and your life.

But that's about to change. Because we've decoded the worst offenders in the super-market and given you the perfect swaps to start dropping pounds fast.

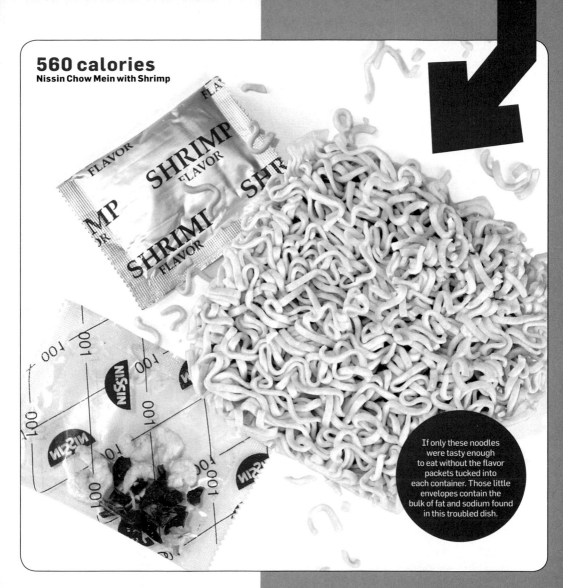

560 calories
Nissin Chow Mein with Shrimp

If only these noodles were tasty enough to eat without the flavor packets tucked into each container. Those little envelopes contain the bulk of fat and sodium found in this troubled dish.

The Worst Supermarket Foods

20 Quaker Quakes Ranch Rice Snacks
(20 cakes)

- 140 calories
- 5 g fat (0 g saturated)
- 0 g fiber
- 400 mg sodium

In general, rice snacks offer little besides empty calories; they contain no fiber and scarcely a shred of protein. And to make a bad product worse, Quaker bakes in some decidedly deleterious ingredients such as partially hydrogenated oil and monosodium glutamate (MSG), a food additive that has been linked to nerve cell damage and the worsening of asthma symptoms. You're better off with potato chips.

Eat This Instead!
GeniSoy Garlic & Onion Soy Crisps (17 crisps)
- 100 calories • 2 g fat (0 g saturated)
- 2 g fiber • 280 mg sodium

WORST DRESSING

19 Marie's Creamy Italian Garlic **(2 Tbsp)**

- 180 calories
- 19 g fat (3 g saturated)
- 135 mg sodium

Two tablespoons of soybean oil, the fat that goes into this dressing, contain about 240 calories. Yet somehow, even after Marie blends in the nonfat buttermilk, garlic, and vinegar, this dressing is still about 75 percent pure fat. That's a perilous waistline hazard unmatched by either ranch or blue cheese dressing. Try Bolthouse dressings instead; they're made with yogurt instead of pure oil.

Eat This Instead!
Bolthouse Farms Creamy Italian Yogurt Dressing (2 Tbsp)
- 70 calories • 7 g fat (1.5 g saturated)
- 105 mg sodium

WORST NUTRITION BAR

18 Powerbar Performance Chocolate Peanut Butter **(1 bar)**

- 240 calories
- 3.5 g fat (1 g saturated)
- 9 g protein
- 1 g fiber
- 26 g sugars

Powerbar's Performance line isn't the most caloric on the shelf, but it posts the most dismal numbers by far. The protein is too low, the fiber is virtually nonexistent, and there's as much added sugar as 2 chocolate pastries from Panera Bread. Think this is going to help with your "performance"? Only if you're entered in a get-fat-quick competition.

Eat This Instead!
Kashi GoLean Roll Protein & Fiber Chocolate Peanut (1 bar)
- 190 calories • 5 g fat (1.5 g saturated)
- 12 g protein • 6 g fiber • 14 g sugars

WORST PACKAGED COOKIE

17 Oreo Cakesters **(2 cookies)**

- 250 calories
- 12 g fat (2.5 g saturated)
- 24 g sugars

The only thing Oreo got right with their Cakesters is the name; each one's basically 2 small slices of birthday cake fused together with a sticky layer of sugar and fat. That's how they manage to pack 125 calories into each individual "cookie." Unless it's your birthday, stick to normal-size treats.

Eat This Instead!
Late July Organic Dark Chocolate (3 cookies)
- 150 calories • 6 g fat (3 g saturated)
- 9 g sugars

It's hard to believe that a grilled chicken pasta could contain the saturated fat equivalent of 22 strips of bacon, but if there's one thing the packaged food industry has taught us, it's that anything is possible.

710 calories
Bertolli Grilled Chicken Alfredo & Fettuccine Skillet Meal

520 calories
Toll House Ice Cream Chocolate Chip Cookie Sandwich

WORST ICE CREAM

16 Häagen-Dazs Chocolate Peanut Butter (1/2 cup)

- *360 calories*
- *24 g fat (11 g saturated)*
- *24 g sugars*

We've scoured the freezers of America in search of fattier ice cream, and we can safely say there's none to be found. Although we applaud Häagen-Dazs for keeping the number of ingredients to a minimum, it wouldn't hurt them to cut back on the cream and sugar just a bit. Maybe then this tiny carton wouldn't pack in more calories than 4 of Wendy's Jr. Bacon Cheeseburgers.

Eat This Instead!

Edy's Slow Churned Peanut Butter Cup (1/2 cup)

- *130 calories • 6 g fat (3 g saturated)*
- *13 g sugars*

WORST "HEALTHY" PANTRY ITEM

15 Pop-Tarts Whole Grain Brown Sugar Cinnamon (2 pastries)

- *400 calories*
- *12 g fat (4 g saturated)*
- *24 g sugars*

We've said over and over again that the words "whole grain" are important to look for. But it takes a lot more than whole wheat to cover up the damage done by the glut of vegetable oil and 7 different sugars that are buried inside each Pop-Tart. Switch to whole-grain mini bagels and sprinkle on a little cinnamon and brown sugar yourself.

Eat This Instead!

Pepperidge Farm 100% Whole Wheat Mini Bagels (1 bagel)

- *100 calories • 0.5 g fat (0 g saturated)*
- *3 g sugars*

WORST MACARONI & CHEESE

14 Kraft The Cheesiest Macaroni & Cheese (about 1 cup prepared with margarine and 2% milk)

- *410 calories*
- *19 g fat (5 g saturated, 4 g trans)*
- *710 mg sodium*

Somehow Kraft has determined that it takes a half stick of margarine to get these noodles sufficiently "cheesy." When you follow that advice, the outcome is a pot of noodles *with more*

trans fat than an entire family of 4 should eat in a day. If you must succumb to the blue-box allure, please do so responsibly. Replace the margarine with real butter.

Eat This Instead!

Pasta Roni Cheddar Macaroni (1 cup prepared)

- *210 calories • 3 g fat (1.5 g saturated)*
- *560 mg sodium*

WORST BAKED GOOD

13 Otis Spunkmeyer Banana Nut Muffins (1 muffin)

- *460 calories*
- *22 g fat (3 g saturated)*
- *2 g fiber*
- *32 g sugars*

Despite popular belief, muffins are very rarely healthy. Case in point: The first ingredient in this muffin is sugar. The result is metabolic mayhem: Blood sugar climbs, the pancreas goes into overdrive, and the body begins storing sugar as fat. Shortly after, you'll feel sluggish and crave more sugar. Instead, find a fibrous baked good that doesn't have more sugar than 3 Krispy Kreme original glazed doughnuts.

Eat This Instead!

Quaker Banana & Oats Muffin Bar (1 bar)
• 130 calories • 3.5 g fat (1 g saturated)
• 4 g fiber • 11 g sugars

WORST PACKAGED SIDE

12 Kraft Caesar Pasta Salad

• 493 calories
• 29 g fat
  (5 g saturated, 0.5 g trans)
• 867 mg sodium

Here's a good lesson in how to cram a quarter of a day's calories into one side dish. First you need a box of refined carbohydrates that have been pumped full of various fats and sugars, and then you must smother them in a bucket full of mayonnaise. Then feed it to your enemies to derail their plans of ever being thin.

Eat This Instead!

Kraft Pasta Salad Vinaigrette with Basil
• 293 calories • 11 g fat (1.5 g saturated)
• 787 mg sodium

WORST FROZEN TREAT

11 Toll House Ice Cream Chocolate Chip Cookie Sandwich

• 520 calories
• 23 g fat (9 g saturated)
• 44 g sugars

Considering so few frozen ice cream treats creep above the 300-calorie threshold, we're astounded that Nestlé stuffs this sandwich with nearly as many calories as a Big Mac. You can have 2 Toll House Chocolate Chunk cookies and a scoop of Breyers All Natural Vanilla ice cream and still save 110 calories. Or you could just switch to the Oreo option and use the 340 calories you save on something better.

Eat This Instead!

Breyers Oreo Ice Cream Sandwich
• 160 calories • 6 g fat (2 g saturated)
• 13 g sugars

The Ultimate Supermarket Label Decoder

Confused by all that bold chatter on your box of cereal? Stumped by the claims crying out from your carton of eggs? You're not the only one. Processed food manufacturers love to confuse and distract shoppers with label claims that are as bold as they are ambiguous and misleading. Some of these terms are regulated by the USDA; others are not. Use our encyclopedia of packaged proclamations to discover the truth behind all your favorite pantry staples.

Antibiotic free

Often livestock are given routine doses of antibiotics so that they can retain a semblance of health while living in polluted environments. This is especially worrisome with beef. Commercial cattle are generally fed a diet consisting of mostly corn, but because their stomachs are designed to digest grass, they need a treatment of antibiotics to fight off ulcers and potentially fatal liver abscesses. The problem for you is that corn-fed beef has nearly twice as much fat as grass-fed cows and lower concentrations of omega-3 fats. Look to the "antibiotic free" claim for meats that are healthier and more humane.

10 Hostess Chocolate Pudding Pie

- *520 calories*
- *24 g fat (12 g saturated)*
- *40 g sugars*

Pudding and pie, as 2 separate entities, are nowhere near as dangerous as Hostess's attempt to combine the 2 using a viscous dovetail of hydrogenated oil. This cold pocket o' pudding has as much sugar and more fat than 3 Little Debbie Marshmallow Pies, which makes it an unacceptable treat even by the most decadent of standards. Look for treats that satisfy your sweet tooth without bombing your blood sugar.

Eat This Instead!

Pepperidge Farm Dark Chocolate Almond Crunchy Granola Cookie

- *130 calories • 7 g fat (2.5 g saturated)*
- *8 g sugars*

---

9 Nissin Chow Mein with Shrimp (1 container)

- *560 calories*
- *28 g fat (10 g saturated)*
- *1,440 mg sodium*

Nissin lists the serving size as half of this bowl. What do they think, that you're going to eat half and put the rest in the fridge for later? While certainly a solid strategy with any problematic packaged food, it's not realistic. Sticking this bowl in the microwave is a commitment to sucking down 60 percent of your day's sodium and half of your day's saturated fat in the form of murky fried noodles and the scary foil spice packet that accompanies them.

Eat This Instead!

Thai Kitchen Garlic & Vegetable Instant Rice Noodles

- *190 calories • 3 g fat (0.5 g saturated)*
- *740 mg sodium*

Hormone free

A worthwhile claim when it appears on beef; about two-thirds of US cows are treated with growth hormones, and it's a contentious debate as to how these hormones affect humans. Fears of premature development in girls, breast cancer, and lower sperm count in men prompted the European Union in 1988 to ban the import of hormone-treated beef. When this claim appears on nonbovine meats, however, it's usually bunk. The USDA strictly prohibits the use of hormones for pigs and chickens. That means this claim could legally adorn every poultry and bacon package in the country and it wouldn't mean a thing.

Free range

Not as idyllic as it sounds. The USDA requires free-range birds to have access to the outdoors for only 51 percent of their lives, and "access" might be no more than a small parcel of dirt. Furthermore, many chickens are too nervous to leave their cages after having spent the better part of their lives in total captivity.

Excellent source of...

Packaging claim used to highlight a specific nutrient, such as in "excellent source of vitamin C." This might also be expressed as "high in vitamin C" or "rich in vitamin C." What it means is that the product contains 20 percent or more of your daily requirement for the mentioned nutrient.

The Worst Supermarket Foods

WORST BREAKFAST SANDWICH

8 Jimmy Dean Sausage and Cheese on a Croissant with Diced Apples & Hash Browns Breakfast Entrée

- *560 calories*
- *30 g fat*
  (10 g saturated, 3 g trans)
- *1,050 mg sodium*

Jimmy's croissant sandwiches are bad enough on their own—they don't need lousy sides weighing them down. The hash browns have been fried in partially hydrogenated oil (hence the trans fat), and the apples are buried under a Twinkie's worth of sugar. There are too many great ways to get a quick breakfast to rely on this thing for A.M. sustenance.

Eat This Instead!
Jimmy Dean D-Lights Turkey Sausage, Egg White & Cheese Sandwich

- *260 calories • 7 g fat (3.5 g saturated)*
- *790 mg sodium*

WORST HANDHELD MEAL

7 Hot Pockets Four Meat & Cheese Calzone

- *580 calories*
- *24 g fat (10 g saturated)*
- *1,660 mg sodium*

Think an Italian chef would approve of this thing? Only if he'd had a few too many grappas. If it's a grab-and-go meal you're looking for, you're better off with a McDonald's Quarter Pounder. That will save you 170 calories and cut your sodium by more than half. Go ahead and get a Fruit 'n Yogurt Parfait while you're at it; you'll still be saving calories. Better yet, have a Kashi Pocket and pocket the 310 calories you save for a better use later.

Eat This Instead!
Kashi Turkey Fiesta Pocket Bread

- *270 calories • 6 g fat (1 g saturated)*
- *660 mg sodium*

The Ultimate Supermarket Label Decoder—*Continued*

Good source of...
This packaging claim is of slightly less importance than "excellent source of." It means that the product contains between 10 and 19 percent of your daily requirement for the mentioned nutrient. In other words, you would have to eat between 5 and 10 servings to get your full day's value.

Light
This means either the number of calories has been reduced by one-third or the total fat has been reduced by half. The exception is with high-fat foods, which can only use this claim if they reduce fat by half.

Lightly sweetened
A frequently abused claim with no formal definition, this appears most often in the cereal aisle, and many of the boxes it adorns are actually loaded with various sweeteners. Need proof? Look at Kellogg's Smart Start. It claims to be "lightly sweetened," yet it has more sugar per cup than a full serving of Oreo cookies!

Multigrain
This simply means that more than one type of grain was used in processing (e.g., wheat, rye, barley, and rice). It doesn't, however, make any claim about the degree of processing used on those grains. The only trustworthy claim for whole grains is "100 percent whole grain."

6 Celentano Eggplant Parmigiana

- *660 calories*
- *44 g fat (10 g saturated)*
- *960 mg sodium*

The only way this meal is acceptable is if you split it into the 2 tiny servings the package suggests. Unfortunately, frozen dinners don't lend themselves very well to splitting, which means that this represents another resounding reason "vegetarian" doesn't automatically mean "nutritious."

Eat This Instead!
Cedarlane Eggplant Parmesan

- *320 calories*
- *16 g fat (6 g saturated)*
- *780 mg sodium*

---

5 Jimmy Dean Pancake and Sausage Links Breakfast Bowl

- *710 calories*
- *31 g fat (11 g saturated)*
- *890 mg sodium*

There's a reason that this meal has been a standby on our various Worst Lists, and it's because the supermarket provides no worse option for starting the day on the wrong foot. Eat this thing in the morning and you will have managed to wolf down more than half of your day's saturated fat limit before stepping foot out the door— not to mention a glut of refined carbohydrates.

Eat This Instead!
Jimmy Dean Sausage and Cheese Omelet

- *270 calories • 22 g fat (8 g saturated)*
- *570 mg sodium*

---

4 Bertolli Grilled Chicken Alfredo & Fettuccine Skillet Meal for Two (½ package)

- *710 calories*
- *42 g fat (22 g saturated)*
- *1,370 mg sodium*

Bertolli makes some of the

Wheat bread
Unless it's "whole wheat bread," this is an empty term. In order to be called wheat bread, a loaf must simply be made from wheat flour, which might very well be refined and colored with molasses to appear darker. Look at the ingredient list; if the first ingredient isn't "whole-grain wheat," then it isn't what you want.

Natural
This term is used almost entirely at the discretion of food processors. With the exception of meat and poultry products, the USDA has set no definition and imposes no regulations on the use of this term, making it essentially meaningless.

Reduced sodium
This packaging claim can be used when the sodium level is reduced by 25 percent or more. This claim is less meaningful than "low sodium," which can be used only when the product contains no more than 140 milligrams per serving.

Trans-fat free
Food processors can make this claim so long as their product contains less than 0.49 gram of trans fat per serving. Considering the American Heart Association recommends capping daily intake at 2 grams, this is no small amount. It's not "free" if shortening or partially hydrogenated oil is on the back label.

The Worst Supermarket Foods

worst (and a few of the best) meals in the freezer case. This one, which gets 28 percent of its calories from saturated fat, falls decidedly into the worst category. There are plenty of healthy stir-fry options in the freezer. Grab just about anything but this.

Eat This Instead!
Birds Eye Steamfresh Meals for Two Grilled Chicken in Roasted Garlic Sauce ($^1/_2$ package)
• *340 calories* • *13 g fat (5 g saturated)*
• *880 mg sodium*

WORST FROZEN PIZZA

3 DiGiorno For One Supreme Pizza (1 pizza)

• *790 calories*
• *36 g fat*
  (14 g saturated, 3.5 g trans)
• *1,460 mg sodium*

Pizza for one? The amount of fat—in all of its nebulous forms—in this pie makes it barely acceptable as a pizza for 2. (And if you happen to find the rare For One pizza made on a garlic bread crust, just know that it's even worse.) Personal pizzas usually mean trouble, but

for those who feel strongly about brand allegiance, DiGiorno's new line of Thin Crust single-serving pizzas makes for a solid alternative to its regular grease trap.

Eat This Instead!
DiGiorno For One Thin Crust Grilled Chicken and Vegetable Pizza (1 pizza)
• *520 calories* • *17 g fat (8 g saturated)*
• *850 mg sodium*

WORST FROZEN ENTRÉE

2 Hungry-Man Classic Fried Chicken

• *1,040 calories*
• *59 g fat (13 g saturated)*
• *1,610 mg sodium*

Hungry-Man? More like Lonely-Man, if you bulk up on enough of these calorie-fests. There's no way a single man needs a pound of fatty fried chicken, oily potatoes, and a brownie in one sitting. But if that one man were to eat this meal, he'd be wolfing down a foodlike substance that consists of more than 50 percent pure fat. Stouffer's offers a near-identical meal for a fraction of the calories.

Eat This Instead!
Stouffer's Fried Chicken Breast
• *360 calories* • *18 g fat (4.5 g saturated)*
• *880 mg sodium*

WORST PACKAGED FOOD IN AMERICA

1 Stouffer's White Meat Chicken Pot Pie (large size)

• *1,160 calories*
• *66 g fat (26 g saturated)*
• *1,780 mg sodium*

Within the walls of this pie's oily, white-flour crust, there's enough cream and margarine to contribute a full day's worth of fat for an adult. There's nearly enough saturated fat to get a person through a day and a half. Yet, remarkably, there's not a ton of protein. And fiber? Less than a single gram. It's this abundance of bad nutrients and curious lack of decent nutrients—combined with a staggering number of calories—that earns this pie the distinction of Worst Packaged Food in America.

Eat This Instead!
Amy's Shepherd's Pie
• *160 calories* • *4 g fat (0 g saturated)*
• *590 mg sodium*

"Hungry-Man is the name you can trust" goes the tagline. But we're not sure what makes them so trustworthy. They don't list trans fat, yet there are 8 instances of partially hydrogenated soybean oil in the ingredient list.

1,040 calories
Hungry-Man Classic Fried Chicken

The Best Supermarket

THESE IMPRESSIVE PANTRY-WORTHY PACKAGES WILL HELP YOU CUT

BEST FROZEN ENTRÉE

Marie Callender's Oven Baked Chicken

- 320 calories
- 12 g fat (3 g saturated)
- 990 mg sodium

This is exactly the well-rounded meal you should be looking for in a frozen entrée. The chicken gives it a load of lean protein, and the sides—potatoes and mixed vegetables—provide it with a source of complex carbohydrates and cancer-fighting phytonutrients. Keep a couple of these around so you don't resort to a bag of potato chips for dinner.

BEST FROZEN PIZZA

Kashi Sicilian Veggie Pizza
($^1/_3$ pizza)

- 220 calories
- 5 g fat (0.5 g saturated)
- 530 mg sodium

No other pizza maker in the country comes anywhere close to Kashi in terms of fiber- and protein-loaded pies. And Kashi goes one step further by avoiding high-fat ingredients like sausage and pepperoni. Instead, on this pie, you'll find a spread of cannellini beans and a layer of toppings such as eggplant, tomatoes, peppers, basil, and garlic. Add that to Kashi's whole-grain crust and you're looking at 5 grams of fiber and 11 grams of protein per serving.

BEST FROZEN SIDE

Cascadian Farms Wedge Cut Oven Fries (8 fries)

- 100 calories
- 3 g fat (0 g saturated)
- 10 mg sodium

Most home freezers in America house a bag of frozen fries, ready for last-minute meals on busy weeknights. Make these thick-cut, oven bound fries your standby spuds. Cascadian's recipe is impressively low in calories and light on oil. (To make sure they brown up nice and evenly, they've been tossed with a splash of apple juice.) The only better fry is one you cut from taters yourself.

BEST YOGURT

Fage Total 2%
(7 ounces)

- 130 calories
- 4 g fat (3 g saturated)
- 17 g protein
- 8 g sugars

You won't find a better low-calorie source of high-quality protein than this tasty Greek-style yogurt. And here's the kicker: Protein from milk is like protein from meat in that it contains all the essential amino acids your body needs to function. Stick to plain and sweeten it with fresh berries, banana slices, or a drizzle of honey at home. Once you've tried it, you'll never want your runny old yogurt again.

Foods in America

CALORIES AND MAXIMIZE NUTRITION

BEST FROZEN TREAT
Fudgsicle Original Fudge Bar (1 bar)

- *60 calories*
- *1.5 g fat (1 g saturated)*
- *9 g sugars*

Want to know why we love Fudgsicles? Two reasons: One, they're made from real milk, the way an ice-cream treat ought to be. And two, they're portioned just right, so that they satisfy your sweet tooth without busting your calorie bank. In fact, this is one treat that we deem safe enough to eat on a daily basis, so long as it's taking the place of your usual dessert. Nobody said eating had to be dull.

BEST FROZEN BREAKFAST
Jimmy Dean D-Lights Canadian Bacon, Egg White, and Cheese Honey Wheat Muffin (1 sandwich)

- *230 calories*
- *6 g fat (3 g saturated)*
- *790 mg sodium*

Every morning, thousands of cars across America cram into the fast-food lane to grab a breakfast that drivers can eat with one hand. Well, here's your excuse to skip the line. Jimmy's D-Light sandwich replaces the traditional sausage patty with Canadian bacon and drops the yolk from the eggs to cut down on saturated fat. Most important, it packs 15 grams of protein and 2 grams of fiber.

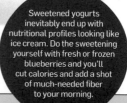

130 calories
Fage Total 2%

Sweetened yogurts inevitably end up with nutritional profiles looking like ice cream. Do the sweetening yourself with fresh or frozen blueberries and you'll cut calories and add a shot of much-needed fiber to your morning.

177

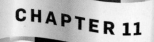

CHAPTER 11

The Best
(&Worst)
Snack
Foods

Eat This

Muir Glen Organic Garlic Cilantro Salsa

(2 Tbsp)

10 calories
0 g fat
130 mg sodium

MUIR GLEN *Organic*

USDA ORGANIC

MEDIUM

Garlic Cilantro Salsa

Save 80 calories!
Chronic dippers take notice! Snack savings add up quick.

Add a handful of Garden of Eatin' Black Bean Tortilla Chips and you'll have a near-perfect mid-afternoon snack: 150 calories, 6 grams of fiber, and a concentrated dose of tasty produce.

Save 7 g fat!
Fat-free food never tasted so good.

Not That!

Kraft Cheez Whiz Original Cheese Dip

90 calories
7 g fat (1.5 g satuated)
440 mg sodium

(2 Tbsp)

TOP SWAP!

These two dips represent the best and the worst of our industrial food system. One is made from 7 different vegetables and little else. The other is made from maltodextrin, sodium phosphate, and "natural flavor."

Even if you dip nothing but broccoli into your whiz, you'd still be better off with the chips and salsa.

BUTTON IS UP

KRAFT

Cheez Whiz

HEESE DIP

REFRIGERATE AFTER OPENING

"No word in the American lexicon has gotten as unfair a rap as the word

"snack."

Except maybe the word "banker." Many of us blame bankers for America's ongoing financial crisis, thanks to subprime lending practices and other money schemes so complicated that even John Grisham couldn't unravel their plots. And snacks are being blamed for America's obesity crisis, thanks to all the chocolaty sweets and greasy crunchables found swinging from every checkout counter in the country.

No wonder we're so angry at bankers and snack foods, those get-fat-fast schemers who want to create giant bubbles in the economy (or in your waistline) and then skip out just before the bubble—or the bathroom scale—bursts.

But just as there are plenty of bad bankers out there, there are plenty of good ones, too—regular men and women who help people invest their income, allow businesses to grow, and provide needed fuel for the economy. And the same goes for snacks. The good ones provide your body with all-day energy, keeping you alert and on top of your game and fending off attacks of hunger.

You need to snack. But at the same time, you need to beware of the nutritional Bernie Madoffs lurking in the supermarket aisles. Smart snacking is like smart money management—it keeps your account full and steady, and you never have to worry about caloric overload—or energy foreclosure.

So think of this chapter as your entry-level management school course, except in this case you're getting schooled in the art of operating a smart, lean, highly efficient business called your body.

Skittles:
Taste the rainbow of artificial food colorings, corn syrup, and hydrogenated oil.

47 grams of sugar
Skittles

The Worst Snack Foods in America

13 Kraft Cheez Whiz Original Cheese Dip (2 Tbsp)

- *90 calories*
- *7 g fat (1.5 g saturated)*
- *440 mg sodium*

The way most people dip, 2 tablespoons means 4 chips' worth of dip. And when have you ever stopped at 4 chips? That means these empty calories—all processed cheese goo spiked with nefarious food additives—add up quickly, as does that shocking sodium number. There are too many great dips (salsa, guac, hummus) to rely on the Whiz for flavor.

WORST CRACKER

12 Ritz (10 crackers)

- *160 calories*
- *9 g fat (2 g saturated)*
- *270 mg sodium*

The most famous name in crackers is also an easy way to get fat. Each cracker contains 2 grams of refined carbohydrates, nearly 1 gram of fat, and nary a scrap of fiber. Choose the Triscuit Original, which is about as unadulterated as wheat gets without chewing on chaff.

WORST CHIP

11 Gardetto's Special Request Roasted Garlic Rye Chips (½ cup)

- *160 calories*
- *10 g fat*
  (2 g saturated, 2.5 g trans)
- *40 mg sodium*

Gardetto extracts the worst part of its original snack mix and tries to serve it as a gourmet snack—a sneaky move that might have serious repercussions for even casual munchers. Each single serving exceeds the amount of trans fat deemed safe to consume daily by the American Heart Association.

WORST YOGURT

10 Yoplait Original 99% Fat Free Cherry Orchard

- *170 calories*
- *1.5 g fat (1 g saturated)*
- *27 g sugars*

There are a few yogurts with higher calorie counts (none worse than Stonyfield's 220-calorie Chocolate Underground), but it's the promise of a virtuous "99 percent fat-free" breakfast that makes this Yoplait cup so egregious. Who are they kidding? The

nutritional profile—with as much sugar as a pair of Twix bars and just 5 meager grams of protein—is closer to ice cream than to the healthy yogurt paradigm. If you're going to have a dairy breakfast, just make sure the protein offering is equal to or greater than the sugar content.

WORST POPCORN

9 Pop-Secret Kettle Corn (⅓ bag)

- *180 calories*
- *13 g fat*
  (3 g saturated, 6 g trans)
- *150 mg sodium*

The only "secret" here is that the company has no qualms about trans fat. Choose Orville Redenbacher's Movie Theater Butter for fewer calories and no trans fat.

WORST VENDING MACHINE SNACK

8 Austin Cheese Crackers with Cheddar Jack Cheese (1 package)

- *200 calories*
- *11 g (2 g saturated, 4.5 g trans)*
- *390 mg sodium*

The American Heart Association cautions consumers

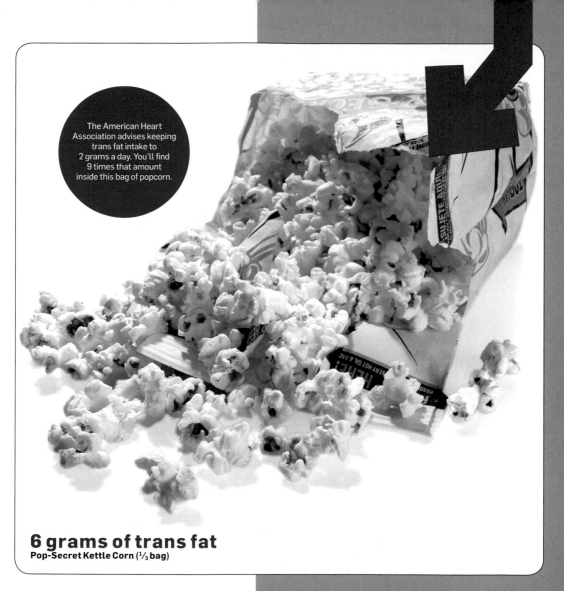

The American Heart Association advises keeping trans fat intake to 2 grams a day. You'll find 9 times that amount inside this bag of popcorn.

6 grams of trans fat
Pop-Secret Kettle Corn (⅓ bag)

The Worst Snack Foods in America

to cap their trans-fat intake at 1 percent of their total calories. For a 2,000-calorie diet, that's about 2 grams, the amount in 4 of these crackers. Care to keep your heart ticking longer than the shelf life of this package? We recommend leaving the Austins on the rack.

WORST CANDY

7 Skittles Original Fruit (1 package)

- 250 calories
- 2.5 g fat (2.5 g saturated)
- 47 g sugars

It's hard to imagine any candy being worse than this. Each colored bead is essentially sugar and corn syrup glued together with hydrogenated palm kernel oil.

WORST COOKIE

6 Oreo Cakesters (2 cookies)

- 250 calories
- 12 g fat (2.5 g saturated)
- 24 g sugars

Sugar, white flour, and oil—a timeless recipe for bad health. The Cakesters have more than twice as many calories as a Chewy Chips Ahoy!

WORST "HEALTHY" BAR

5 Kashi GoLean Chewy Oatmeal Raisin Cookie Bar (1 bar)

- 280 calories
- 5 g fat (3 g saturated)
- 33 g sugars

Despite all the bells and whistles surrounding this protein and fiber bar, its nutritional profile more closely resembles the Twix bar on this page than a legitimately nutritious snack. ("GoLean" in this case is more likely to mean, "Go lean against the wall until the sugar rush passes!") We love most of what Kashi has to offer, but this is just another example of why indiscriminate brand loyalty can come back to bite you.

WORST CANDY BAR

4 Twix (2-ounce package)

- 280 calories
- 14 g fat (11 g saturated)
- 27 g sugars

Twix takes the already-dubious candy-bar reputation and drags it through a murky pool of saturated fat. It would take 11 strips of

bacon to achieve that sort of heart-stopping potential, which makes this one potentially hazardous after-lunch snack.

WORST "HEALTHY" SNACK

3 Pop-Tarts Whole Grain Brown Sugar Cinnamon (2 pastries)

- 400 calories
- 12 g fat (4 g saturated)
- 24 g sugars

Don't think for a second that Kellogg's can fix Pop-Tarts by sprinkling a little whole wheat flour into the mix—not when that flour's held together with a glut of vegetable oil and stuffed with 7 different types of sugar.

WORST MUFFIN

2 Otis Spunkmeyer Banana Nut Muffin (1 muffin)

- 460 calories
- 22 g fat (3 g saturated)
- 32 g sugars

Despite popular belief, muffins are very rarely healthy. Case in point: The first ingredient in this muffin is sugar. The result is metabolic mayhem: Blood sugar climbs, the pancreas goes into overdrive, and the body is more likely to be storing sugar as fat. Think of muffins as cake to keep this snack of mostly empty calories in perspective.

1 Hostess Chocolate Pudding Pie

- *520 calories*
- *24 g fat*
  (14 g saturated, 1.5 g trans)
- *45 g sugars*

This is the type of snack you pick up at a gas station in a pinch and feel vaguely guilty about, not knowing that you just managed to ingest nearly three-quarters of a day's worth of saturated fat before your tank finished filling up. And considering these little packages of doom cost a buck or less across the country, the pudding pie qualifies as one of the cheapest sources of empty calories in America. The 2 best snacks to score at a gas station: fresh fruit (if they have it) and beef jerky.

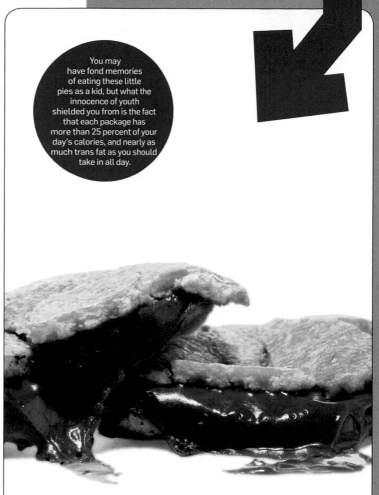

You may have fond memories of eating these little pies as a kid, but what the innocence of youth shielded you from is the fact that each package has more than 25 percent of your day's calories, and nearly as much trans fat as you should take in all day.

520 calories
Hostess Chocolate Pudding Pie

The Best Snacks in

THESE LITTLE BITES PACK HUGE BENEFITS. MAKE THEM A PART OF

BEST NUTS
Emerald Cocoa Roast Almonds, Dark Chocolate (¼ cup)

- 150 calories
- 13 g fat (1 g saturated)
- 25 mg sodium

They taste like candy, but these almonds contain almost no sugar. What they do contain, though, is a super dose of heart-healthy fats and fiber.

BEST HUNGER SQUASHER
Jack Link's Original Beef Jerky (1 ounce)

- 80 calories
- 1 g fat (0 g saturated)
- 590 mg sodium

Jerky is the world's easiest source of quick-and-convenient protein.

BEST TORTILLA CHIPS
Garden of Eatin' Black Bean Tortilla Chips (1 ounce)

- 140 calories
- 7 g fat (0.5 g saturated)
- 70 mg sodium

It's unheard of for chips to offer 4 grams of fiber. Credit the black beans these chips are made from.

BEST DIP
Wholly Guacamole Classic (2 Tbsp)

- 50 calories
- 4 g fat (0.5 g saturated)
- 75 mg sodium

This dip delivers all the heart-healthy monounsaturated fats guacamole should. Use it as a stand-in for mayo on sandwiches.

BEST SNACKING CHEESE
The Laughing Cow Mini Babybel Light Original (1 piece)

- 50 calories
- 3 g fat (1.5 g saturated)
- 160 mg sodium

Forget the puffs and doodles, this is real cheese made with low-fat milk. Nearly half of the calories come from protein.

BEST CRISP
True North Almond Crisps (about 15 crisps)

- 140 calories
- 7 g fat (0.5 g saturated)
- 240 mg sodium

Made from almonds, these chips pack more fiber and protein than potato or corn chips, plus a dose of vitamin E.

BEST PRETZEL
Snyder's of Hanover MultiGrain Olde Tyme Pretzel Twists (about 8 twists)

- 120 calories
- 2 g fat (0 g saturated)
- 170 mg sodium

Low in sodium and made from whole wheat flour, sesame seeds, and flax seeds.

BEST POPCORN
Orville Reden-bacher's Natural Buttery Salt & Cracked Pepper Popcorn (2 cups popped)

- 40 calories
- 2 g fat (1 g saturated)
- 160 mg sodium

High in fiber, low in dangerous fats and excess sodium.

America

YOUR DAILY ROUTINE

BEST TRULY HEALTHY BAR
Lärabar Jacalat Chocolate Coffee (1 bar)

- 190 calories
- 11 g fat (2 g saturated)
- 19 g sugars

No added sugar, just cocoa, nuts, dried fruit for sweetness, and coffee for a bonus buzz.

BEST CRACKER
Nabisco Triscuit Original (6 crackers)

- 120 calories
- 4.5 g fat (1 g saturated)
- 180 mg sodium

Made from whole wheat, oil, and salt. That's how they manage to serve up 3 grams of fiber and 3 grams of protein. Make these the cracker for all your snacking needs.

BEST POTATO CHIP
Popchips All Natural Barbecue (1 ounce)

- 120 calories
- 4 g fat
- 250 mg sodium

Popchips aren't baked or fried; they're placed in an enclosed environment and hit with high measures of heat and pressure until they puff up with air, leaving a perfectly crisp, oil-free potato chip. While the result would never qualify as a health food, it does contain 40 fewer calories and less than half the fat of traditional potato chips—our choice for genius packaged product of the year.

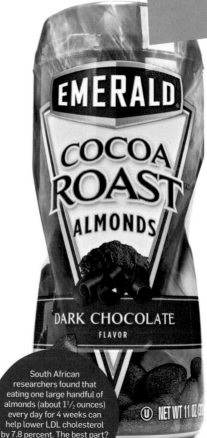

150 calories
Emerald Cocoa Roast Almonds

South African researchers found that eating one large handful of almonds (about 1½ ounces) every day for 4 weeks can help lower LDL cholesterol by 7.8 percent. The best part? These almonds taste like dessert.

The Vending Machine SURVIVAL GUIDE

You have a dollar in your pocket and a raging hunger in your belly. How do you snuff out the appetite without breaking the caloric bank? By using this blow-by-blow breakdown of the best and worst vending machine snacks.

BARS

Eat This
100 Grand
- 190 calories
- 8 g fat
  (5 g saturated)
- 22 g sugars

This is the safest candy bar we've come across. Make it your first choice.

Not That!
Snickers
- 280 calories
- 14 g fat
  (5 g saturated)
- 28 g sugars

The only thing Snickers satisfies are the requisites for a sugar crash.

Eat This
Take 5
- 210 calories
- 11 g fat
  (5 g saturated)
- 18 g sugars

Take 5 keeps the sugar in check by using crunchy pretzel instead of the standard nougat.

Not That!
Butterfinger
- 270 calories
- 11 g fat
  (6 g saturated)
- 28 g sugars

Switch to Take 5 and you'll save 60 calories per indulgence.

Eat This
Kit Kat Bar
- 210 calories
- 11 g fat
  (7 g saturated)
- 22 g sugars

Spread the love. Just because there are 4 pieces in a package doesn't mean you need to eat them all yourself.

Not That!
3 Musketeers
- 260 calories
- 8 g fat
  (5 g saturated)
- 40 g sugars

It's not the fat that does this bar in; it's the sugar. Forty grams is more than 2 Twinkies' worth—and it's nearly double the quantity you'll find in a Kit Kat.

Eat This
Nestlé Crunch Bar
- 220 calories
- 12 g fat
  (7 g saturated)
- 24 g sugars

The Crunch Bar is less dense than pure milk chocolate, which means less fat and sugar in each bite.

Not That!
Hershey's Milk Chocolate Bar
- 270 calories
- 16 g fat
  (10 g saturated)
- 31 g sugars

Bite-size pieces might work for s'mores, but eat a whole bar as a snack and you just sacrificed half a day of saturated fat.

CRUNCHY SNACKS

Eat This
Handi-Snacks Ritz Crackers 'n Cheez
- 100 calories
- 6 g fat
  (1.5 g saturated)
- 330 mg sodium

Perfect for mindless munchers. The self-contained vessel means you don't wind up looking down at a huge empty bag, wondering where all the food went.

Not That!
Doritos Nacho Cheese Crackers
- 210 calories
- 12 g fat
  (3 g saturated,
  3 g trans)
- 280 mg sodium

Be careful with individually packaged crackers; they're often swimming in trans fat. This package has a half gram per cracker.

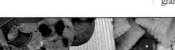

GOODIES

Eat This
Baked! Lays Potato Chips
· 110 calories
· 1.5 g fat
· 150 mg sodium

Baked! Lays are the best chips in the vending machine. The sodium's low and the saturated fat's nonexistent.

Not That!
Sun Chips Original
· 210 calories
· 10 g fat
  (1.5 g saturated)
· 180 mg sodium

New standards and healthier options have pushed Sun Chips out of the spotlight as the healthier alternative to potato chips. Plus, with its inflated serving size (1.5 ounces rather than 1 ounce), it has about twice as much damage potential as Baked! Lays.

Eat This
Planters Honey Roasted Peanuts
· 160 calories
· 13 g fat
  (2 g saturated)
· 110 mg sodium

This is the safest snack in the vending machine. It's loaded with protein, fiber, and heart-healthy monounsaturated fats.

Not That!
Corn Nuts Original
· 210 calories
· 8 g fat
  (1 g saturated)
· 310 mg sodium

Don't let the name trick you into thinking this snack is anything remotely similar to real nuts. It's just a blend of salted corn and partially hydrogenated oil.

Eat This
Rice Krispies Treat
· 150 calories
· 3.5 g fat
  (1 g saturated)
· 12 g sugars

The bulk of this bar is a fairly innocuous cereal, which keeps the damage to a minimum.

Not That!
Pop-Tarts Brown Sugar Cinnamon
· 400 calories
· 14 g fat
  (4.5 g saturated)
· 31 g sugars

A cookie-crust boat full of high-fructose corn syrup and partially hydrogenated oils: not an acceptable treat at any time of day.

Eat This
Mini Chips Ahoy!
· 170 calories
· 8 g fat
  (2.5 g saturated)
· 10 g sugars

This is hardly a nutritious snack, but its modest size makes certain that you won't overindulge. Plus, it still beats a chocolate bar any day.

Not That!
Famous Amos Chocolate Chip Cookies
· 280 calories
· 13 g fat
  (4 g saturated)
· 18 g sugars

What you want is a small snack, not a trough of cookies. Choose Famous Amos and you're stuck with the latter, and it will cost you more than 100 extra calories.

Eat This
Welch's Fruit Snacks, Mixed Fruit
· 195 calories
· 0 g fat
· 37.5 g sugars

These fruit snacks are made with real fruit and fortified with vitamins C, A, and E. It might not be as good as real fruit, but it's as close as you'll get at the vending machine.

Not That!
Original Fruit Skittles
· 250 calories
· 2.5 g fat
  (2.5 g saturated)
· 47 g sugars

Here's the base of every Skittle: sugar, corn syrup, and partially hydrogenated palm kernel oil. That's why the fat is completely saturated, and there's nearly as much sugar as 6 Dunkin' Donuts Chocolate Frosted Cake Donuts.

Eat This
Kraft Cinnamon Bagel-fuls
· 200 calories
· 4 g fat
  (2.5 g saturated)
· 190 mg sodium
· 8 g sugars

Surprisingly, not one of Kraft's bagel-and-cream-cheese fusions has more than 200 calories or 6 grams of fat, and the cinnamon in this one will keep your blood sugar from rising too quickly.

Not That!
Lance Glazed Honey Bun
· 320 calories
· 13 g fat
  (4 g saturated)
· 13 g sugars

The calories in this snack come from 3 sources: fat, sugar, and refined carbs.

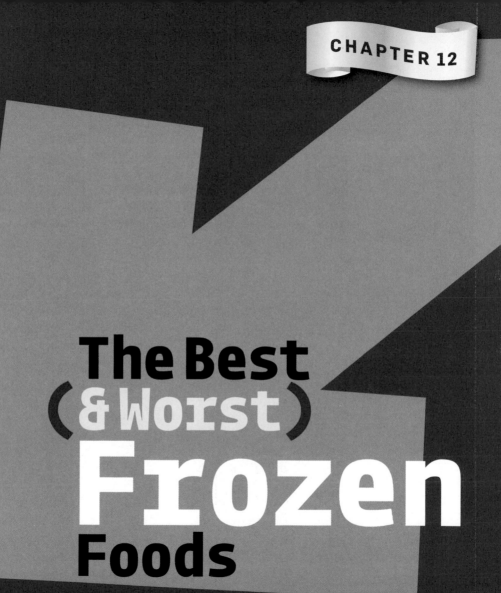

The Best
(&Worst)
Frozen
Foods

Eat This

Kashi Mexicali Black Bean Pizza

(⅓ pizza)

210 calories
7 g fat
(3 g saturated)
560 mg sodium

Trans fat free!
You'll find none of that cholesterol-raising junk in this pizza.

Save 630 calories!
Bake *this* pizza, not *that* one once a week and you'll cut 9 pounds out of your diet in a year.

Save 37 g fat!

194

DiGiorno For One Supreme Pizza

Garlic Bread Crust

840 calories
44 g fat
(16 g saturated,
3.5 g trans)
1,450 mg sodium

It's not just about cutting calories, it's about adding nutrition. Each Kashi pizza has 12 grams of fiber, 39 grams of protein, and plenty of produce.

Regardless of the crust you choose, DiGiorno's For One line is dominated by nutritional duds. Switch to the new Crispy Flatbread pizzas if you must have DiGiorno.

Urban legend

has it that if you're recently single and want to meet someone new, there are three places to hang out: the singles bars, the local museums, and the frozen-food aisle of the supermarket.

We can't help you with dating advice (your mom probably gives you enough of that already), and we haven't scoped out your local singles bar—yet. But we can tell you that the frozen-food aisle isn't the "meat market" it's cracked up to be (and let's face it, the lighting isn't exactly flattering, either). It's a far more democratic place, and all of us—not just the lonely ones—seek help in the freezer section: From August 2007 to August 2008, supermarkets sold more than $30 billion worth of frozen foods—and that doesn't even include all the chilled chow bought at Wal-Mart and other superstores.

Convenience is the obvious reason why the freezer aisle is so popular, but there are a lot of other reasons why you should make regular stops in the frozen-food section—even if you haven't seen a singles bar in 20 years. For example, frozen foods can be not only cheaper and more convenient but also healthier, especially when it comes to fruit and vegetables. One study found that vegetables such as green beans and spinach lose up to 75 percent of their vitamin C after being stored in the fridge for a week; same goes for ready-to-drink orange juice. But frozen foods don't suffer the same loss of superpowers. They're picked at the peak of ripeness, and they don't lose their edge once they're fast-frozen. And frozen foods are better for the environment as well, since they can be picked locally and stored in season, instead of trucked all the way from Chile. (Where do you think "fresh" strawberries come from in February?) The freezer also offers nutritional superstar

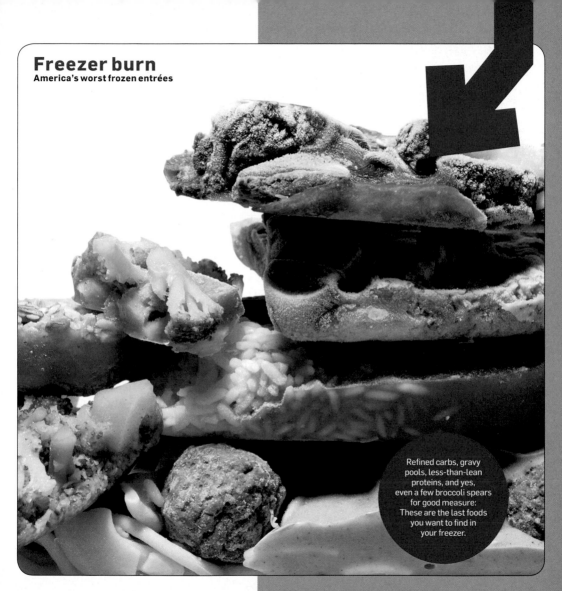

Freezer burn
America's worst frozen entrées

Refined carbs, gravy pools, less-than-lean proteins, and yes, even a few broccoli spears for good measure: These are the last foods you want to find in your freezer.

197

The Worst Frozen Foods in America

foods—like wild blue-berries—that simply can't be found fresh.

That said, all is not necessarily cool when it comes to the freezer section. A lot of food manufacturers see frozen foods as opportunities to conduct chemistry experiments—on your body. And because so many frozen meals have multiple components, the ingredients lists, especially the sodium content, can creep up and up, until the nutrition label reads like *Ulysses*. (Perhaps marketers are hoping that the boxes will be so cold you won't be able to hold them in your hands long enough to read the labels!)

Fortunately, we've braved the cold and uncovered what, exactly, is lurking behind the freezer door. Here are the frozen foods to embrace—and the ones to give the cold shoulder.

WORST MEAT SUBSTITUTE
15 Boca Meatless Chik'n Patties Original (1 patty)

- *160 calories*
- *6 g fat (1 g saturated)*
- *430 mg sodium*

A good meat substitute consists of little besides protein and seasoning. Boca's, on the other hand, earns more calories from fat than protein. Switch over to Quorn's and you'll cut out more than half the fat without sacrificing a single gram of protein.

Eat This Instead!
Quorn Naked Chik'n Cutlets (1 cutlet)
- *80 calories • 2.5 g fat (0.5 g saturated)*
- *420 mg sodium*

WORST FROZEN "HEALTHY" ENTRÉE
14 Healthy Choice Complete Selections Sweet & Sour Chicken (1 package)

- *400 calories*
- *10 g fat (1 g saturated)*
- *500 mg sodium*

Healthy Choice wants us to believe that they have quality standards that ensure their foods live up to their name, but this battered belly buster casts a dubious light on the company's commitment to nutritious frozen entrées. It hosts a load of fried chicken that's been battered in a syrup with as much sugar as you'll find in 3 Krispy Kreme original glazed doughnuts.

Eat This Instead!
Kashi Southwest Style Chicken (1 package)
- *240 calories • 5 g fat*
- *680 mg sodium*

WORST BREAKFAST SANDWICH
13 Jimmy Dean Sausage, Egg, and Cheese Croissant Sandwich (1 sandwich)

- *430 calories*
- *29 g fat*
  (9 g saturated, 3.5 g trans)
- *740 mg sodium*

Breakfast breads consistently carry a walloping dose of trans fat. Manufacturers claim it's hard to make biscuits and croissants without trans fat, but we always have the same response: If other companies can do it, then why can't you? By inviting sausage to the party, you end up with a one-two punch of trans and saturated fats.

Jimmy Dean D-Lights Turkey Sausage, Egg White & Cheese on a Whole Grain Muffin (1 sandwich)

- *260 calories • 7 g fat (3.5 g saturated)*
- *790 mg sodium*

WORST FROZEN SNACK

12 Don Miguel Beef & Cheese Empanadas
(5 small empanadas)

- *430 calories*
- *22 g fat (8 g saturated, 2 g trans)*
- *680 mg sodium*

The empanada is Latin America's answer to the calzone, and like its cousin from Italy, an empanada often tucks excessive quantities of calories and fat into its flaky sheath. All said, trans and saturated fats account for more than one-fifth of the calories in each little paunch-building pocket. Find a less risky snack.

Eat This Instead!
Lean Pockets Mexican Style Steak Fajita (1 pocket)

- *250 calories • 7 g fat (3.5 g saturated)*
- *670 mg sodium*

To the north, you'll find a starchy sea of refined carbohydrates. To the south, a murky, brackish tide comprising three-quarters of a day's saturated fat allotment. Together, they are the worst frozen beef entrée in America.

760 calories
Boston Market Swedish Meatballs

The Worst Frozen Foods in America

11 Toll House Ice Cream Chocolate Chip Cookie Sandwich (1 sandwich)

- *520 calories*
- *23 g fat (9 g saturated)*
- *44 g sugars*

If the nearly 11 teaspoons of sugar don't scare you away, then getting a quarter of your day's calories from an ice-cream novelty should. If you're going to take in this much fat and calories in one sitting, it'd better be dinner.

Eat This Instead!

Skinny Cow Low Fat Vanilla Ice Cream Sandwich (1 sandwich)

- *140 calories • 2 g fat (1 g saturated)*
- *15 g sugars*

WORST FROZEN PIE

10 Claim Jumper Chocolate Motherlode Cake (⅙ cake)

- *520 calories*
- *27 g fat (7 g saturated, 3 g trans)*
- *54 g sugars*

Premade pies and cakes are notorious for carrying outrageous amounts of trans fat, but none other than Claim Jumper's delivers more calories than 5 Quaker

Chewy Chocolate Chip granola bars in each slice. Either make cakes at home or seek out solid lines like Amy's.

Eat This Instead!

Amy's Organic Chocolate Cake (⅙ cake)

- *170 calories*
- *6 g fat (0 g saturated, 0 g trans)*
- *16 g sugars*

WORST FISH ENTRÉE

9 Claim Jumper Shrimp Scampi (1 meal)

- *550 calories*
- *30 g fat (13 g saturated, 3.5 g trans)*
- *1,130 mg sodium*

Scampi is a food industry code word for excessive amounts of butter and oil. In this case, a good portion of that oil is partially hydrogenated, blanketing a perfectly healthy plate of shrimp in a bath of trans fat. It's a great choice if you're looking for something to grease the door hinges, but not so great for greasing your palate.

Eat This Instead!

Weight Watchers Smart Ones Dragon Shrimp Lo Mein (1 package)

- *240 calories • 4 g fat (1 g saturated)*
- *690 mg sodium*

WORST FROZEN HANDHELD MEAL

8 Hot Pockets Four Meat & Cheese Calzone (1 calzone)

- *580 calories*
- *24 g fat (10 g saturated)*
- *1,660 mg sodium*

Hot Pockets tries to avoid responsibility for this caloric calamity by listing the serving size as half of a calzone, but honestly, who wants to split something as messy as this? And it's not even particularly huge to begin with. Hot Pockets pioneered the world of handheld microwave grub, but that doesn't mean other producers aren't offering better options. Seek out alternatives like this creation from Kashi or resign yourself to Lean Pockets.

Eat This Instead!

Kashi Turkey Fiesta Pocket Bread (1 piece)

- *270 calories • 6 g fat (1 g saturated)*
- *660 mg sodium*

7 Celentano Eggplant Parmigiana (1 package)

- 660 calories
- 44 g fat (10 g saturated)
- 960 mg sodium

This meatless meal has more fat than you'd find in a 12-ounce sirloin steak. Not exactly the type of health boon you bargained for if you gave up beef for Lent.

Eat This Instead!

Cedarlane Eggplant Parmesan (1 package)

- 320 calories • 16 g fat (6 g saturated)
- 780 mg sodium

WORST STIR-FRY

6 Bertolli Grilled Chicken Alfredo & Fettuccine Complete Skillet Meal for Two (½ package)

- 710 calories
- 42 g fat (22 g saturated)
- 1,370 mg sodium

A strip of bacon carries about a gram of saturated fat, which puts this skillet on par with 2 or 3 frying pans heaped full of smoked pork belly. In fact, the only thing this Meal for Two is good for is splitting with an enemy.

400 calories
Healthy Choice Sweet & Sour Chicken

Sometimes you need to focus less on the final calorie count and more on the quality of the calories. Here, 29 percent of them come directly from sugar—in the syrupy sweet and sour sauce and in the apple crisp. Not such a healthy choice after all.

The Worst Frozen Foods in America

Any other Bertolli bag would be an improvement, as would the impressive line of pastas and stir-fries from Birds Eye.

Eat This Instead!
Birds Eye Steamfresh Meals for Two Grilled Chicken in Roasted Garlic Sauce (¹/₂ bag)
· 340 calories · 13 g fat (5 g saturated)
· 880 mg sodium

WORST BEEF ENTRÉE
5 Boston Market Swedish Meatballs

· 760 calories
· 43 g fat
 (16 g saturated, 2 g trans)
· 1,290 mg sodium

Boston Market is in the business of selling comfort food, but all too often that savvy sales approach spells trouble for the consumer. The writing is on the box here: Fat-speckled meatballs, sour cream sauce, and egg noodles combine to bring a day's worth of trans fat to your dinner table. Meat loaf is no less comforting, but it is certainly a lot less fattening.

Eat This Instead!
Stouffer's Meatloaf
· 340 calories · 20 g fat (9 g saturated)
· 780 mg sodium

WORST PASTA ENTRÉE
4 Marie Callender's Fettuccini Alfredo & Garlic Bread

· 770 calories
· 46 g fat
 (16 g saturated, 1 g trans)
· 1,300 mg sodium

Here's some bad news for Alfredo fans: The base of this sauce is essentially pure fat. That makes it extremely unwise to eat it by the plateful. Red sauces will always trump white, but if you're determined to eat Alfredo, eat it in moderate portions and alongside something with true nutritional substance.

Eat This Instead!
Michelina's Budget Gourmet Lasagna Alfredo with Broccoli
· 300 calories · 12 g fat (6 g saturated)
· 560 mg sodium

WORST FROZEN PIZZA
3 DiGiorno For One Garlic Bread Crust Supreme Pizza

· 840 calories
· 44 g fat
 (16 g saturated, 3.5 g trans)
· 1,450 mg sodium

The bloated crust and the greasy toppings will saddle you with 60 percent of your day's sodium, 80 percent of your day's saturated fat, and nearly twice the amount of trans fat you should take in daily. Hands off!

Eat This Instead!
South Beach Diet Deluxe Pizza
· 340 calories · 11 g fat (4 g saturated)
· 650 mg sodium

WORST CHICKEN ENTRÉE
2 Hungry-Man Classic Fried Chicken

· 1,040 calories
· 59 g fat (13 g saturated)
· 1,610 mg sodium

Unless you're a professional marathoner, there's never a need to eat this much food in a sitting. Strangely enough, fried chicken in the world of frozen foods is usually a reasonable caloric investment, so don't settle for a package that packs half a day's worth of calories and nearly a full day's worth of fat. Want to save the easiest 730 calories of your life? Make this Swanson swap, which offers you the exact same meal in a more modest portion size.

Swanson Classics Boneless Fried Chicken with Mashed Potatoes and Corn

• *330 calories* • *17 g fat (3.5 g saturated)*
• *610 mg sodium*

WORST FROZEN FOOD IN AMERICA

1 **Stouffer's White Meat Chicken Pot Pie** (large)

• *1,160 calories*
• *66 g fat (26 g saturated)*
• *1,780 mg sodium*

The potpie is one of the world's worst dietary inventions to begin with, and the damage is all the more extreme when the pie seems as big as a child's head. Stouffer's tries to get away with it by falling back on the serving-size sleight of hand; that is, to list as 2 servings what every person with a fork will consume as 1. Nobody splits potpies, and eating this whole thing will fill your belly with more saturated fat than you should ever eat in an entire day.

Marie Callender's Oven Baked Chicken

• *320 calories* • *12 g fat (3 g saturated)*
• *990 mg sodium*

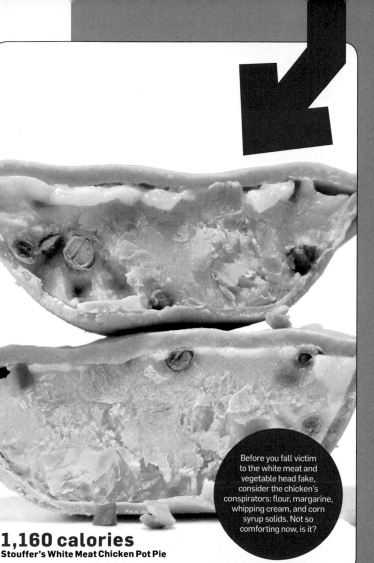

1,160 calories
Stouffer's White Meat Chicken Pot Pie

Before you fall victim to the white meat and vegetable head fake, consider the chicken's conspirators: flour, margarine, whipping cream, and corn syrup solids. Not so comforting now, is it?

The Best Frozen Foods

PACK YOUR ICE BOX WITH THESE FRIGID PHENOMS

BEST FROZEN BEEF ENTRÉE

Stouffer's Meatloaf

- 340 calories
- 20 g fat (9 g saturated)
- 780 mg sodium

Stouffer's line of frozen entrées run the nutritional gamut, from low-calorie, nutrient-dense dishes to full-fledged caloric catastrophes with nutritional stats that read like the Dow Jones Industrial Average. Thankfully, this beef entrée fits firmly into the former category, delivering 22 grams of protein and a dose of fiber for considerably fewer calories than Mom's famous meat loaf would saddle you with.

BEST FROZEN BREAKFAST

Jimmy Dean D-Lights Turkey Sausage Breakfast Bowl (1 package)

- 230 calories
- 7 g fat (3 g saturated)
- 730 mg sodium

Too bad not all of Jimmy Dean's meals are as good as the D-Lights line. As we've noted before, the regular pancake- and sausage-stuffed breakfast bowls comprise some of the worst morning meals in America. This surprising winner uses turkey sausage to keep the fat to a minimum, and with 23 grams of protein, it does a resounding job at shaking your metabolism from its slumber.

BEST FROZEN FUSION PIZZA

Kashi Mexicali Black Bean Pizza (⅓ pizza)

- 210 calories
- 7 g fat (3 g saturated)
- 560 mg sodium

Kashi's pizzas are hands down the best in the freezer. And oddly enough, this entire full-size pie has fewer calories than a single DiGiorno's For One Pizza, so even if you end up eating all of it, you're still saving calories. But low calories aren't the only boon; Kashi also squeezes in a load of belly-filling nutrients. Each serving here has 4 grams of fiber and 13 grams of protein.

BEST FROZEN APPETIZER

Green Giant Broccoli and Cheese Giant Bites (3 nuggets)

- 150 calories
- 5 g fat (1 g saturated)
- 530 mg sodium

The breaded outer crust makes these Bites look like nothing more than run-of-the-mill, deep-fried grease-bombs, but flip the package and you'll see otherwise. The main ingredient, instead of the usual white flour, is actually broccoli. That means the breading, oil, and cheese are all kept in their place: as flavor enhancers to something much more nutritional.

in America

BEST CHICKEN ENTRÉE

Ethnic Gourmet Lemongrass & Basil Chicken
(1 meal)

- *380 calories*
- *9 g fat (5 g saturated)*
- *310 mg sodium*

Most frozen foods rely on the same sad standbys to build flavor: sodium, sugar, and cheap oils. But the foundation of Southeast Asian–inspired dishes—whether Thai, Vietnamese, or Indian—relies on antioxidant-rich spices, fresh herbs, and bold, low-calorie condiments. As a result, they deliver big flavors with impressively low calorie, fat, and sugar counts. This one is our favorite.

BEST FROZEN TREAT

Skinny Cow French Vanilla Truffle Bars
(1 bar)

- *100 calories*
- *2 g fat (2 g saturated)*
- *12 g sugars*

By using skim milk in place of cream and going easy on the sugar, Skinny Cow manages to make some of the leanest ice-cream treats in the supermarket. Keep a box of these in your freezer to prevent you from reaching for something more dangerous. Just keep it to a single bar; they might be light, but they're still junk food.

You'll find plenty of diet entrées in the freezer section with fewer calories, but most are miniscule, incapable of satisfying even a meager appetite. Not so with Stouffer's meatloaf; this hearty dish delivers substance for a really reasonable caloric cost.

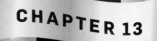

CHAPTER 13

The Best
(&Worst)
Drinks
in America

Eat This

Honest Tea Community Green Tea

34 calories
0 g fat
10 g sugars

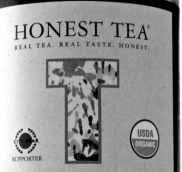

Cut 63 g sugars!
You'll save more added sugar than you should take in each day.

Save more than 250 calories!
If you drink tea once a day, this sippable swap translates into 26 pounds of body fat a year.

Burn fat!
The antioxidants found in green tea have been proven to increase metabolism.

HONEST TEA®
REAL TEA. REAL TASTE. HONEST.

USDA ORGANIC

SUPPORTER

COMMUNITY GREEN TEA
GREEN TEA WITH MALTESE ORANGE
16 FLUID OUNCES 473 mL

300 calories
0 g fat
73 g sugars

Not That!

TOP SWAP!

Arizona RX Energy Herbal Tonic

Any of tea's proven health benefits are drowned out by the sea of sugar awaiting inside this can.

The most egregious part of this can is the implication that this is somehow healthy for you. The name is at least half-true; by the time you finish with RX, you may need a prescription for insulin just to regulate your blood sugar.

SCENE I:
INTERIOR: A CROWDED, NOISY CHURCH BASEMENT.

SAM STANDS AT A PODIUM IN A BLUE COAT THAT IS FAR TOO SMALL TO COVER HIS FLABBY BELLY. HE SPORTS A RED-AND-WHITE-STRIPED TOP HAT AND WHITE BEARD. HE WAITS FOR THE ROOM TO QUIET.

SAM: Hi, everyone. My name's Uncle Sam, and I have a drinking problem.

CROWD: Hello, Sam.

SAM: Now, my drinking problem isn't *that* kind of drinking problem—the kind that typically inspires confession, rehab, and maybe an appearance on *The Surreal Life*. No, my drinking problem is very different indeed.

See, as a typical American, I just plain drink too much. Too much soda, too much juice, too many "enhanced" beverages, and way, way too many flavored coffees. In fact, as an average American, I consume so much bad stuff in liquid form that drinks now account for nearly 25 percent of my calories—about 450 calories every day, twice as much as I drank 30 years ago. That's the equivalent of tossing two slices of Domino's Sausage Pizza into a blender, pressing puree, and then slurping it up.

CROWD: Gasp!

SAM: And I'm doing this every single day. Is it any wonder that I'm 50 percent more obese than in the 1960s? [SAM GRABS HIS FLABBY BELLY AND GIVES IT A SHAKE] How is this possible? [TWO HANDS GO UP IN THE BACK OF THE ROOM]

DAVE AND MATT: Uncle Sam, it's not your fault! In fact, we doubt you're actually drinking more. In fact, so many Americans are struggling with their weight because beverage

Among the foods and beverages that are better for you than this calamitous cocktail: 19 Chicken McNuggets; 13 Beck's Premier Light Beers; 8 bowls of Froot Loops; 6 orders of Burger King Onion Rings; Wendy's Baconator.

890 calories
Red Lobster Traditional Lobsterita

The Worst Drinks in America

marketers are enlarging their serving sizes by adding cheap sugar substitutes, a variety of hard-to-pronounce chemicals, and tons of fats. It's the same thing they're doing to our food. **SAM:** Those bastards! **CROWD:** Boo! **DAVE AND MATT:** But we have great news! Those liquid calories are the easiest ones to cut out. And a recent study from Johns Hopkins University found that people who cut liquid calories from their diets lose more weight—and keep it off longer—than people who cut food calories. In fact, cutting those calories in half could mean you could drop almost 23½ pounds in just 1 year! And you could still eat exactly what you're eating now! **CROWD:** Hooray! **DAVE AND MATT:** All you need to know are the secrets of the drink industry. And, in fact, we have them right here...

WORST FUNCTIONAL BEVERAGE

20 Snapple Tropical Mango Antioxidant Water (20-ounce bottle)

- 150 calories
- 0 g fat
- 30 g sugars

Here's the thing about sugar: It has only one function, and that is to make you fat. Of course, bottlers of the so-called functional beverages try to hide this fact behind a flurry of healthy buzz-terms, such as antioxidants. Too bad 2 out of 3 antioxidants in this bottle are actually vitamins A and E, both of which are fat soluble, making them difficult to absorb in a fat-free beverage. If you want flavored water, just make sure it comes without calories. If it's more vitamins you seek, increase your fresh fruit intake or pop a multivitamin.

Drink This Instead!
Hint Mango Grapefruit (16-ounce bottle)
· 0 calories · 0 g fat · 0 g sugars

WORST KIDS' DRINK

19 SunnyD Smooth Style (16-ounce bottle)

- 260 calories
- 0 g fat
- 60 g sugars

It's not the most caloric beverage in the supermarket, but SunnyD irks us for more than just its caloric load. Here's a drink marketed toward children and displaying real fruit on the label, yet the contents of the bottle are actually 95 percent high-fructose corn syrup. That means aside from the added vitamin C, this is essentially a bottle of empty calories, which is the last thing a child needs. The emerging line of water-based beverages from Capri Sun and Minute Maid provide more real fruit juice and a tiny fraction of the sugar and calories.

Drink This Instead!
Capri Sun Tropical Fruit Roarin' Water (6.8-ounce pouch)
· 35 calories · 0 g fat · 9 g sugars

18 Rockstar Original

(16-ounce can)

- *280 calories*
- *0 g fat*
- *62 g sugars*

Americans spent $4.2 billion on high-octane elixirs in 2008. Even with dozens of brands found in the cooler, Rockstar stands out as the most sugar-loaded of the various and sundry energy drinks. Compared with its closest competitor, it has 20 extra calories, which is just enough to make it the worst possible choice for instant energy. And with research on the long-term effects of taurine and guarana still cloudy, you're better off getting your buzz from coffee, a proven source of antioxidants and other beneficial nutrients. But if you must grab a can, you can't get better than the low-carb concoction below.

Drink This Instead!

Monster Lo-Carb Energy (16-ounce can)

- *20 calories • 0 g fat • 6 g sugars*

62 grams of sugar
Rockstar Energy Drink

GINSENG

ROCKST★
ENERGY DRIN

Doub

16 fl/oz (473ml)

> Looking for a lift? You won't find it here. Sure, you'll reap the fleeting rewards of the temporary buzz, but the sugar crash will strike soon after, dragging you down lower than when you started. Want a worthwhile buzz? Try coffee. Black.

The Worst Drinks in America

17 Starbucks Coffee Frappuccino
(13.7-ounce bottle)

- *290 calories*
- *4.5 g fat (2.5 g saturated)*
- *46 g sugars*

Most people don't associate coffee with milk shakes—like loads of sugar, but that's exactly what's happening inside this bottle. Add one of these to your diet every morning and you'll add about 28 pounds of flab to your body in a year.

Drink This Instead!
Java Monster Lo-Ball Coffee + Energy (15-ounce can)
- *100 calories · 3 g fat (2 g saturated)*
- *8 g sugars*

WORST BOTTLED ICED TEA

16 Arizona RX Energy Herbal Tonic (20-ounce can)

- *300 calories*
- *0 g fat*
- *73 g sugar*

Proceed cautiously through the tea aisle; there are far too many bottlers using tea's good reputation to hawk their syrupy concoctions. Sure, this brew is made with green tea, but it's also made with a massive dose of high-fructose corn syrup. If you're hoping for green tea's metabolic boost, you'll be disappointed when your belly starts bulging instead of shrinking.

Drink This Instead!
Honest Tea Tropical Mate (16-ounce bottle)
- *34 calories · 0 g fat · 10 g sugars*

WORST BEER

15 Sierra Nevada Bigfoot Ale (12-ounce bottle)

- *304 calories*
- *32 g carbohydrates*
- *9.6% alcohol*

You know a beer is in trouble when it needs to invoke the image of an oversize mythical beast just to describe itself. Perhaps a better name would have been Jabba the Hut Ale. Beer gets most of its calories from the booze itself, and with nearly 10 percent alcohol in each bottle, this brew is likely to create a beer belly nearly as quickly as it creates a buzz.

Drink This Instead!
Guinness Draught (12-ounce bottle)
- *126 calories · 10 g carbohydrates*
- *4% alcohol*

WORST BOTTLED BEVERAGE

14 Sobe Liz Blizz
(20-ounce bottle)

- *310 calories*
- *1 g fat (0.5 g saturated)*
- *77 g sugars*

Don't be fooled by the natural motifs that adorn Sobe's bottles. Spin this one around and you'll see that it's made from water, sugar, skim milk, and cream. We've said it before and we'll say it again: Don't buy products with cartoon animals on the front.

Drink This Instead!
Sobe Lean Energy (20-ounce bottle)
- *13 calories · 0 g fat · 2.5 g sugars*

WORST SODA

13 Sunkist (20-ounce bottle)

- *320 calories*
- *84 g sugars*

All full-sugar sodas are evil, but they weren't all created equal. A 12-ounce can of Coke—the tooth-rotting standard—contains 140 calories and 39 grams of sugar. That same size can from Sunkist packs 190 calories and a staggering 52 grams of sugar. Tack on the extra 8 ounces in this orange monster and you begin to understand why soft drinks are often cited as one of the top contributors to obesity and diabetes in this country.

Drink This Instead!
Honest Ade Orange Mango (16.9-ounce bottle)

• *100 calories* • *24 g sugars*

WORST JUICE IMPOSTOR

12 Arizona Kiwi Strawberry (23.5-ounce can)

• *360 calories*
• *0 g fat*
• *84 g sugars*

If kiwi and strawberry are both fruits (and they are, we fact-checked it), then why does this can contain only 5 percent juice? Because it's made from watered-down high-fructose corn syrup—enough of it, in fact, to give this drink the sugar equivalent of 7 bowls of Froot Loops cereal. The most disturbing part of this beverage is that it normally costs just $0.99, making it the cheapest source of empty calories we've ever uncovered.

Drink This Instead!
Snapple Kiwi Pear Juice (17.5-ounce bottle)

• *33 calories* • *0 g fat* • *4.5 g sugars*

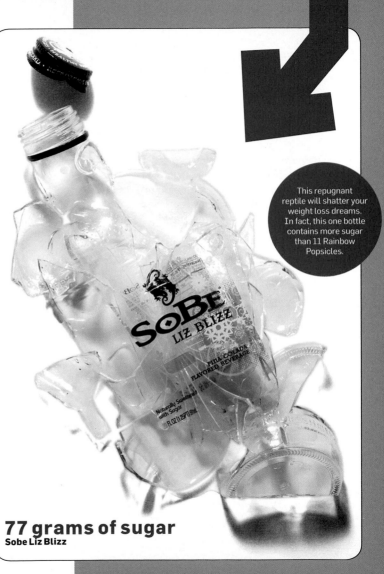

This repugnant reptile will shatter your weight loss dreams. In fact, this one bottle contains more sugar than 11 Rainbow Popsicles.

77 grams of sugar
Sobe Liz Blizz

The Worst Drinks in America

WORST CHOCOLATE MILK
11 Nesquik (16-ounce bottle)

· *400 calories*
· *10 g fat (6 g saturated)*
· *60 g sugars*

Nesquik seals its fate on our Worst List in two ways. The first is with the oversize dose of sugar; it's enough to give each 8-ounce serving as much sugar as a Snickers bar. The second problem is the bottle; it's twice the size of a normal serving of milk. Don't give up on the treat— studies show the balance of protein, fat, and carbs in chocolate milk makes a great postworkout recovery beverage. Just reach for the low-fat variety or drink the regular stuff in moderation.

Drink This Instead!
Organic Valley Lowfat Chocolate Milk (8-ounce carton)

· *160 calories · 2.5 g fat (1.5 g saturated)*
· *25 g sugars*

WORST BOTTLED SMOOTHIE
10 Naked Protein Zone Banana Chocolate (15.2-ounce bottle)

· *480 calories*
· *3 g fat (1 g saturated)*
· *32 g protein*
· *70 g sugars*

Naked makes fantastic smoothies, but this isn't one of them. The flood of protein can't justify the calorie counts, which will catapult your blood sugar and activate your body's fat-storing mechanism. Shave off a few by going out for a nice dinner. A 6-ounce sirloin steak has 60 percent more protein and 160 fewer calories.

Drink This Instead!
Bolthouse Farms Perfectly Protein Vanilla Chai Tea (15.2-ounce bottle)

· *300 calories · 5.5 g fat (2 g saturated)*
· *19 g protein · 40 g sugars*

The Truth about Diet Soda

When confronted with the growing tide of calories from sweetened beverages, the first response is, "Why not just drink diet soda?" Well, for a few reasons.

● **Just because diet soda is low in calories doesn't mean it can't lead to weight gain.**
It may have only 5 calories or less per serving, but emerging research suggests that consuming sugary-tasting beverages—even if they're artificially sweetened—may lead to a high preference for sweetness overall. That means sweeter (and more caloric) cereal, bread, dessert—everything.

● **Guzzling these drinks all day long forces out the healthy beverages you need.**
Diet soda is 100 percent nutrition free, and again, it's just as important to actively drink the good stuff as it is to avoid that bad stuff. So 1 diet soda a day is fine, but if you're downing 5 or 6 cans, that means you're limiting your intake of healthful beverages, particularly water and tea.

● **There remain some concerns over aspartame, the low-calorie chemical used to give diet sodas their flavor.**
Aspartame is 180 times sweeter than sugar, and some researchers claim to have linked it to brain tumors and lymphoma. The FDA maintains that the sweetener is safe, but reported side effects include dizziness, headaches, diarrhea, memory loss, and mood changes. Bottom line: Diet soda does you no good, and it might just be doing you wrong.

9 Sonic Route Large Lemon-Berry CreamSlush
(20 ounces)

- *630 calories*
- *15 g fat*
  (9 g saturated, 0.5 g trans)
- *99 g sugars*

To be fair, this belly blaster is more of a shake-slush hybrid: half sugar-saturated ice and half high-fat ice cream. Think it sounds tasty alongside a Sonic Cheeseburger and fries? Maybe so, but that's a meal that will cost you more than 1,500 calories.

Drink This Instead!
Small Strawberry Real Fruit Slush (14 ounces)

- *210 calories • 0 g fat • 52 g sugars*

WORST HOLIDAY COFFEE DRINK

8 Starbucks Venti 2% Peppermint White Chocolate Mocha
(20 ounces)

- *660 calories*
- *22 g fat (15 g saturated)*
- *95 g sugars*

Between the candies and the casseroles, we already have plenty of temptations to deal

760 calories
Starbucks Salted Caramel Hot Chocolate

For the caloric cost of this towering hot chocolate, you could slurp down 6 mugs of Swiss Miss and still have calories to spare.

with during the holidays. We certainly don't need Starbucks' surreptitious sugar overload thrown into the mix. The name implies indulgence, sure, but the fact that this cup holds more sugar than 9 Krispy Kreme original glazed doughnuts is pretty appalling. Settle for a candy cane in your coffee or find a different drink.

Drink This Instead!
Grande Skinny Cinnamon Dolce Latte (16 ounces)
· *130 calories · 0 g fat · 17 g sugars*

WORST HOT CHOCOLATE

7 Starbucks Venti 2% Salted Caramel Signature Hot Chocolate (20 ounces)

· *760 calories*
· *37 g fat (22 g saturated)*
· *85 g sugars*
· *380 mg sodium*

Since when did hot chocolate require salt and caramel to meet the expectations of consumers? Seems a bit gratuitous, no? Thanks to Starbucks' monstrous creation, the classic winter comfort beverage is now sullied with more than a full day's worth of saturated fat and as much

sugar as nearly 4 Hershey's chocolate bars.

Drink This Instead!
Grande Nonfat Vanilla Crème (16 ounces)
· *270 calories*
· *7 g fat (4.5 g saturated)*
· *38 g sugars*

WORST COCKTAIL

6 Red Lobster Traditional Lobsterita
· *890 calories*
· *0 g fat*
· *183 g carbohydrates*

Lobsterita means a lobster tank–size glass filled with booze and high-fructose corn syrup. You'd have to drink 4 regular on-the-rocks margaritas to outdo the massive calorie load. Pair that with a dinner and you might be pushing a full day's calories in one meal. If you want to get drunk, take a shot. If you want to enjoy a cocktail, make sure it doesn't start with a bottle of mix—your body and your taste buds will thank you.

Drink This Instead!
Malibu Hurricane
· *200 calories · 0 g fat*
· *36 g carbohydrates*

WORST FLOAT

5 Baskin-Robbins Large Ice Cream Soda with Vanilla Ice Cream Float (32 ounces)

· *960 calories*
· *40 g fat*
  (25 g saturated, 1.5 g trans)
· *136 g sugars*

If you're going to have a float, it's best to limit yourself to one small scoop of ice cream and a reasonable pour of soda, yet Baskin-Robbins' smallest portion is 32 ounces! Unfortunately, if the ice cream mogul doesn't begin offering smaller sizes, your options are limited. Either split a small float or cut the soda out of the equation.

Eat This Instead!
Vanilla Ice Cream Scoop (4 ounces)
· *260 calories*
· *16 g fat (10 g saturated, 0.5 g trans)*
· *26 g sugars*

The *Eat This, Not That!* Drink Decoder

All-Natural Disaster
7UP

The Claim:
"All natural flavors"

The Truth:
The FDA doesn't have a definition for this claim. Case in point: 7UP now boasts that it's made with 100 percent natural ingredients. That's because they've switched from carbonated water to filtered water, from citric acid to natural citric acid, and from calcium disodium EDT to natural potassium citrate. Got it? Here's the kicker: The soft drink is still sweetened with high-fructose corn syrup, which can't be made without the help of a centrifuge.

The Better Option:
A healthy choice, like seltzer with a squeeze of lemon or lime.

When it comes to beverage labels, things aren't always as they seem. Use this decoder to separate fact from fiction before sipping.

Got Milk?
Yoo-Hoo

The Claim:
"Chocolate drink"

The Truth:
Ever notice the conspicuous absence of milk in the title of this popular drink? The first ingredient in this kid favorite is water; the second, high-fructose corn syrup. In fact, nonfat dry milk does not appear until the 9th ingredient, 3 slots below partially hydrogenated soybean oil. As a result, Yoo-Hoo offers less than half the calcium and vitamin D provided by the real thing.

The Better Option:
For a kid in need of nutrition, real chocolate milk will always be the better choice. Organic Valley Chocolate Lowfat Milk comes in 8-ounce cartons for automatic portion control.

A Not-So-Juicy Cocktail
Ocean Spray Cran-Raspberry

The Claim:
"Juice drink"

The Truth:
Words like "juice drink" and "juice cocktail" are industry euphemisms for a huge dose of sugar water. In this case, the product is also adorned with a cluster of other claims that attempt to hide this simple fact. (Most of Ocean Spray's juice products suffer from a serious lack of juice; this particular one, with just 18 percent juice, is one of the worst offenders.) Ocean Spray, to be sure, is not the only juice purveyor guilty of this sleight of hand: Dozens of manufacturers, including Welch's, Minute Maid, and SunnyD, perpetrate similar nutritional injustices.

The Better Option:
Every juice that hits your lips should be 100 percent juice. Period.

100 Percent Misleading
Tropicana Pure 100% Juice Pomegranate Blueberry

The Claim:
"100% juice pomegranate blueberry"

The Truth:
Drinks may be labeled 100 percent pure juice, but that doesn't mean they're made exclusively with the advertised juice. Pomegranate and blueberry get top billing here, even though the ingredient list reveals that pear, apple, and grape juices are among the first 4 ingredients. These juices are used because they're cheap to produce and because they're very sweet—likely to keep you coming back for more. Labels loaded with of-the-moment superfoods like acai and pomegranate are especially susceptible to this type of trickery.

The Better Option:
To avoid the huge sugar surge, pick single-fruit juices. POM and R.W. Knudsen both make smart choices.

The Worst Drinks in America

WORST ICE BLENDED COFFEE DRINK

4 Così Gigante Double OH! Arctic (23 ounces)

- *1,210 calories*
- *19 g fat*
- *259 g carbohydrates*

How does Così's coffee creation reach such abysmal heights? By dropping a giant Oreo cookie into the blender with a flood of chocolate syrup and then sticking another Oreo on top. The only thing stronger than the massive caffeine jolt will be the sugar crash to follow. "Blended coffee drinks" is a troubled genre in need of a name change; we think "caffeinated milk shakes" is a more apt description.

Drink This Instead!
Grande Latte (15 ounces)
- *210 calories • 7 g fat*
- *21 g carbohydrates*

WORST MILK SHAKE

3 Cold Stone Creamery Gotta Have It PB&C Shake

- *2,010 calories*
- *131 g fat (68 g saturated)*
- *153 g sugars*

The PB&C is intended to denote peanut butter and chocolate, but the more accurate translation might be potbellies and cardiovascular disease. After all, this one drink does pack more calories than a dozen ice cream sandwiches and more saturated fat than nearly 20 large orders of McDonald's French fries. And what's even more depressing is that no shake on Cold Stone's menu, not even the small sizes, falls below 1,000 calories. Choose a small ice cream and use the 1,640 calories for something with at least a trace of nutritional value.

Eat This Instead!
Peanut Butter Ice Cream Like It Size
- *370 calories*
- *24 g fat (13 g saturated, 0.5 g trans)*
- *28 g sugars*

WORST SMOOTHIE

2 Smoothie King's The Hulk, Strawberry (40 ounces)

- *2,088 calories*
- *70 g fat (32 g saturated)*
- *240 g sugars*

To be fair, this smoothie is designed to help people gain weight. The problem is that we live in a nation in which two-thirds of us are overweight, and the number of professional bodybuilders doesn't constitute a significant demographic. Plus, if you really want to put on some pounds, just eat 9 Odwalla Super Protein bars. That's how many it would take to match this caloric load.

Drink This Instead!
The Shredder, Strawberry (20 ounces)
- *356 calories • 1 g fat • 41 g sugars*

1 Baskin-Robbins Large Chocolate Oreo Shake

- *2,600 calories*
- *135 g fat*
  (59 g saturated fat,
  2.5 g trans fat)
- *263 g sugars*
- *1,700 mg sodium*

Is this the worst drink on the planet? All signs point to yes. First off, it has an ingredient list that reads like an O-chem final. Those 70-plus ingredients conspire to pack this shake with more sugar than 29 Fudgsicles, as much fat as a stick and a half of butter, and more calories than 48 actual Oreos. Oh, it also has 3 days' worth of saturated fat and, most bizarre of all, as much salt as you'll find in 9 bags of Lay's Classic potato chips. Need more proof? Let's hope not.

Drink This Instead!
Small Chocolate Chip Shake
- *540 calories*
- *21 g fat (14 g saturated, 0.5 g trans)*
- *72 g sugars*

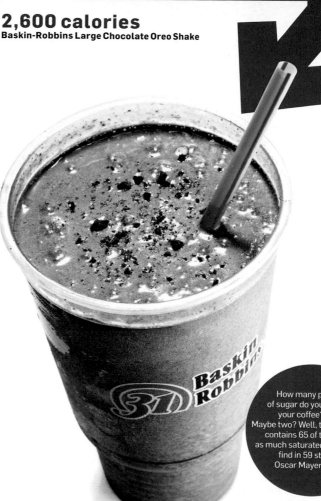

2,600 calories
Baskin-Robbins Large Chocolate Oreo Shake

How many packets of sugar do you like with your coffee? One? Maybe two? Well, this one shake contains 65 of them, plus as much saturated fat as you'd find in 59 strips of Oscar Mayer bacon.

The Best Drinks in Am

CUT YOUR LIQUID CALORIES IN HALF AND YOUR BODY WILL REJOICE.

BEST COFFEE DRINK

Tall Starbucks Skinny Vanilla Latte + Protein (12 ounces)

- *120 calories*
- *0 g fat*
- *15 g protein*
- *12 g sugars*

Despite its large selection of hypersweetened beverages, Starbucks does make an effort to provide healthy options. Nothing beats plain coffee, of course, but among the more flavored selections, this is the best we've seen. Because it's made with sugar-free syrup and nonfat milk, the Skinny Latte has always been one of the safest options on the menu, but if you ask for protein, it gets even better.

BEST ICE BLENDED COFFEE DRINK

Smoothie King Skinny Coffee Smoothie Mocha (20 ounces)

- *160 calories*
- *2 g fat*
- *17 g protein*
- *13 g sugars*

A Smoothie King coffee drink? That's right; the blended beverage purveyor took the lessons it learned making healthy smoothies (leaving the lessons they learned from their more problematic products thankfully behind) and applied them to the mocha; the result is a lightly sweetened coffee-and-milk concoction with a healthy dose of protein. Think of it as a small meal that tastes like a big treat.

BEST BOTTLED JUICE

Odwalla Farms 100% Pure Pressed Carrot Juice (15.2 ounces)

- *133 calories*
- *0 g fat*
- *24.5 g sugars*

Poor carrot juice. It's so often passed by as busy shoppers rush to buy apple and grape juices by the jug, and all the while it sits there, nutritionally superior, lower in calories, and equally delicious. Don't believe it? Give it a taste test. The natural sugars are concentrated in the juice, so you'll feel like you're drinking a smoothie while you casually sip down a week's worth of vitamin A.

BEST BOTTLED TEA

Honest Tea Community Green Tea (16 ounces)

- *34 calories*
- *0 g fat*
- *10 g sugars*

Honest Tea came out as the catechin winner in a *Men's Health* analysis of multiple green teas. And this one has exactly what you want: metabolism-boosting and cancer-fighting antioxidants packaged in a bottle with a mere 10 grams of organic cane sugar. The rest of the flavor comes from the essence of Maltese orange. Drink this one to your health.

erica

THESE DRINKS WILL HELP

BEST ALL-FRUIT SMOOTHIE

Jamba Juice Peach Perfection
(16 ounces)

- *230 calories*
- *0 g fat*
- *46 g sugars*

Smoothies lose their luster as a health food when they come in giant cups laced with added sugars (and don't be fooled by sugar euphemisms: honey, evaporated cane juice, and turbinado all count). Keep it small and keep it all 100 percent fruit, like this really solid Jamba offering, and you can afford to suck a couple down a week.

BEST BEER

Guinness Draught
(12-ounce bottle)

- *126 calories*
- *10 g carbohydrates*

Yes, there are beers out there with fewer calories (both Beck's and Miller make 64-calorie bottles), but you'll never find a beer with a better flavor-to-calorie ratio than the pride of Dublin.

Studies show strategic sipping is the most effective way to lose weight—whether you're a kid or an adult.

35 calories
Capri Sun Roarin' Waters

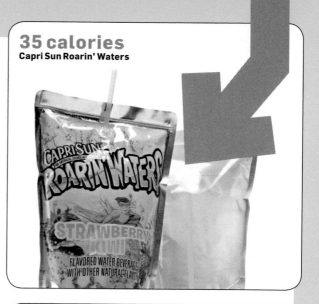

120 calories
Tall Starbucks Skinny Latte

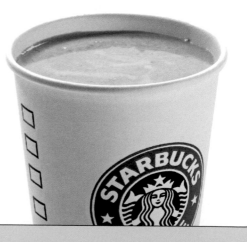

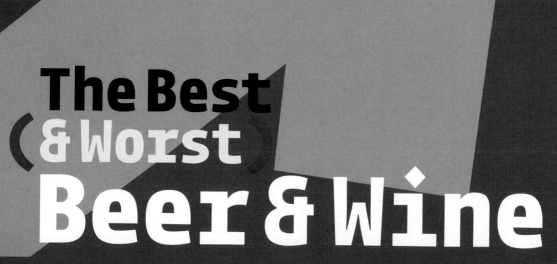

CHAPTER 14

The Best
(& Worst)
Beer & Wine

Beer and wine
have a lot of magical effects on the body,
both positive and negative.

On the downside, alcohol can make you sloppy, indiscriminate, and as blabbery as Joe Biden on sodium pentothal. Plus, combining mugs and shots is scientifically proven to increase your risk of mug shots—just ask Lindsay Lohan and Mel Gibson.

On the positive side, a lot of research on red wine (and some on beer and white wine) indicates that one drink a day can help protect against stroke, coronary artery disease, dementia, and more. Indeed, some studies suggest that drinking in moderation can actually help deflate a beer belly: In a recent study of 8,000 people, Texas Tech University researchers determined that those who downed a daily drink were 54 percent less likely to have a weight problem than teetotalers. Between one and two drinks a day resulted in a 41 percent risk reduction. But that's where the trend ends. Consumption of three or more daily drinks increases your risk of obesity, says the study.

And therein lies the rub. If you can limit yourself to one or two a day, then you can get the health benefits without too many extra calories—if you choose wisely. Here's a rundown of what, exactly, you're really getting each time you reach for a cold one.

The Best (& Worst) Beer in America

(all per 12 ounces)

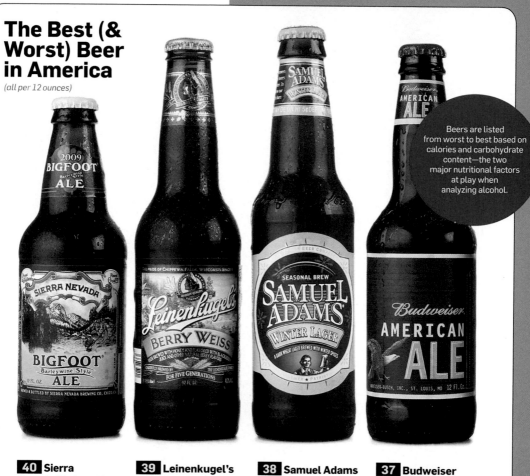

Beers are listed from worst to best based on calories and carbohydrate content—the two major nutritional factors at play when analyzing alcohol.

40 Sierra Nevada Bigfoot Ale
- *330 calories*
- *32 g carbohydrates*
- *9.6% alcohol*

39 Leinenkugel's Berry Weiss
- *207 calories*
- *28 g carbohydrates*
- *4.7% alcohol*

38 Samuel Adams Winter Lager
- *200 calories*
- *14 g carbohydrates*
- *5.8% alcohol*

37 Budweiser American Ale
- *182 calories*
- *18 g carbohydrates*
- *5.3% alcohol*

The Best (&Worst) Beer in America

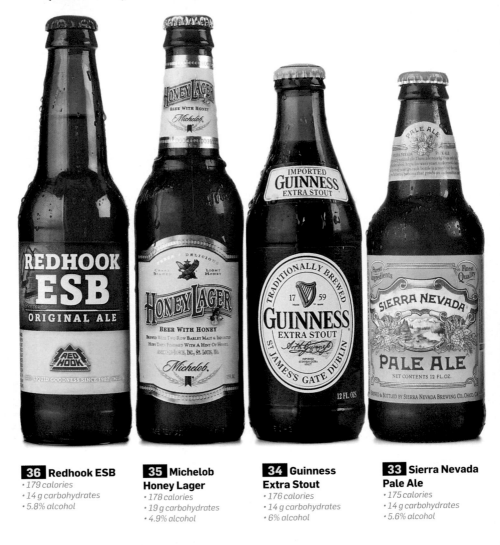

36 **Redhook ESB**
- 179 calories
- 14 g carbohydrates
- 5.8% alcohol

35 **Michelob Honey Lager**
- 178 calories
- 19 g carbohydrates
- 4.9% alcohol

34 **Guinness Extra Stout**
- 176 calories
- 14 g carbohydrates
- 6% alcohol

33 **Sierra Nevada Pale Ale**
- 175 calories
- 14 g carbohydrates
- 5.6% alcohol

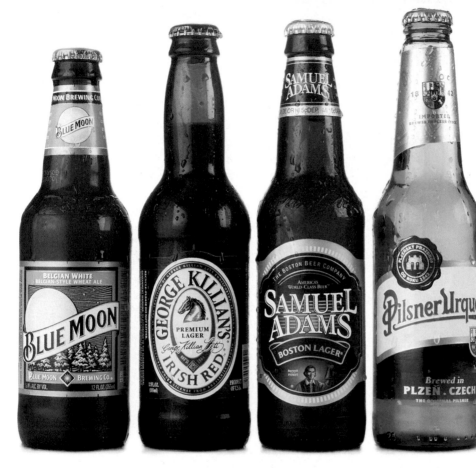

32 **Blue Moon Belgian White**
- *164 calories*
- *13 g carbohydrates*
- *5.4% alcohol*

31 **George Killian's Irish Red**
- *162 calories*
- *15 g carbohydrates*
- *5% alcohol*

30 **Samuel Adams Boston Lager**
- *160 calories*
- *18 g carbohydrates*
- *4.8% alcohol*

29 **Pilsner Urquell**
- *156 calories*
- *16 g carbohydrates*
- *4.4% alcohol*

The Best (&Worst) Beer in America

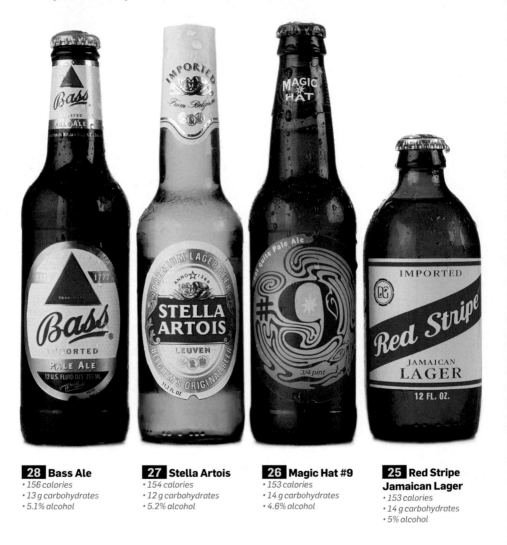

28 Bass Ale
- *156 calories*
- *13 g carbohydrates*
- *5.1% alcohol*

27 Stella Artois
- *154 calories*
- *12 g carbohydrates*
- *5.2% alcohol*

26 Magic Hat #9
- *153 calories*
- *14 g carbohydrates*
- *4.6% alcohol*

25 Red Stripe Jamaican Lager
- *153 calories*
- *14 g carbohydrates*
- *5% alcohol*

Mix This, Not That! Best and Worst Mixers

The sidecar. The Singapore sling. The Harvey Wallbanger. The cocktail lounge is a potpourri of mysterious concoctions with magic powers. Be it vodka, gin, or whiskey, a shot of the hard stuff will cost you about 110 calories, but what else, exactly, is in those witches' brews? Here's a rundown of the most common mixers. (Nutritional info for eye of newt not available.)

Drink This
Sauza Margarita Mix
(4 ounces)
· 93 calories
· 0 g fat
· 24 g sugars

The goal with mixers is to keep the sugar count as low as possible. While you'd be better off making margaritas with fresh lime, this will work in a pinch.

Not That!
1800 The Ultimate Margarita Mix
(4 ounces)
· 170 calories
· 0 g fat
· 39 g sugars

Ounce for ounce, this mix is three times sweeter than most soda. An 8-ounce margarita made with this will pack on 400 calories.

Drink This
Jose Cuervo Strawberry Margarita Mix
(4 ounces)
· 100 calories
· 0 g fat
· 24 g sugars

Add rum and you've just turned it into a daiquiri, and you've saved a load of sugar calories in the process.

Not That!
Mr & Mrs T Strawberry Daiquiri-Margarita Mix
(4 ounces)
· 180 calories
· 0 g fat
· 44 g sugars

There's no nutrition in all these calories, just a lot of high-fructose corn syrup.

Drink This
V8 Spicy Hot
(4 ounces)
· 25 calories
· 0 g fat
· 4 g sugars
· 310 mg sodium

Low in sugar and high in nutrients, a Bloody Mary is one of the world's healthiest cocktails. By using V8, you'll cut down on the only real drawback—the salt.

Not That!
Master of Mixes Bloody Mary Mixer Smooth & Spicy
(4 ounces)
· 50 calories
· 0 g fat
· 11 g sugars
· 910 mg sodium

This mix has as much sodium as 2 full cups of salted peanuts.

Drink This
Canada Dry Club Soda
(8 ounces)
· 0 calories
· 0 g fat
· 0 g sugars

Club soda and its cousin seltzer water are nothing more than carbonated water, which makes them the safest mixers at the party.

Not That!
Canada Dry Tonic Water
(8 ounces)
· 90 calories
· 0 g fat
· 23 g sugars

This tonic water is made from carbonated water, high-fructose corn syrup, and flavoring— basically a glorified soft drink.

Drink This
Reed's Premium Ginger Brew
(8 ounces)
· 100 calories
· 0 g fat
· 22 g sugars

Ginger has many known health benefits; just don't fall for the imitation ales that include no actual ginger on their ingredient list, unlike this one. Still, there's plenty of sugar, so use sparingly.

Not That!
Sprite Lemon-Lime Soda
(8 ounces)
· 100 calories
· 0 g fat
· 26 g sugars

Don't succumb to the misconception that Sprite is a "healthier" soda. It has just as many calories as nearly every other major type of soda.

Drink This
R.W. Knudsen Pineapple Coconut 100% Juice
(4 ounces)
· 85 calories
· 0.5 g fat
· 18.5 g sugars

This is the best piña colada stand-in you'll find. It's 100 percent juice and contains no added sweeteners.

Not That!
Master of Mixes Piña Colada Mixer
(4 ounces)
· 210 calories
· 1.5 g fat
· 50 g sugars

This typical piña colada mix contains only 24 percent actual juice. The rest of the calories are from high-fructose corn syrup and sugar.

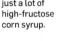

The Best (&Worst) Beer in America

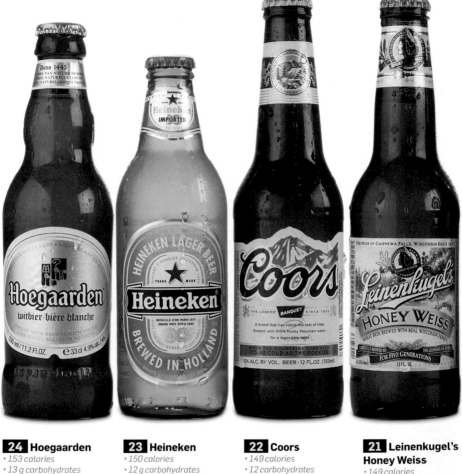

24 **Hoegaarden**
- *153 calories*
- *13 g carbohydrates*
- *4.9% alcohol*

23 **Heineken**
- *150 calories*
- *12 g carbohydrates*
- *5% alcohol*

22 **Coors**
- *149 calories*
- *12 carbohydrates*
- *4.9% alcohol*

21 **Leinenkugel's Honey Weiss**
- *149 calories*
- *12 g carbohydrates*
- *4.9% alcohol*

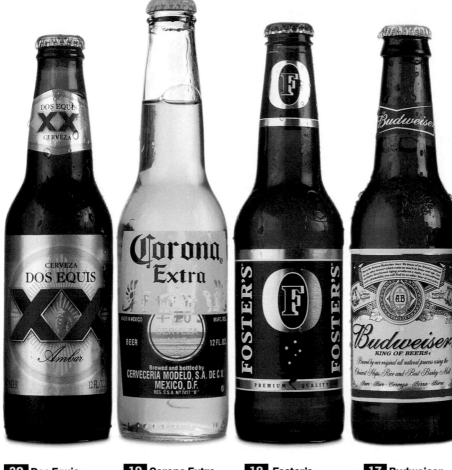

20 Dos Equis
- *149 calories*
- *12 g carbohydrates*
- *4.9% alcohol*

19 Corona Extra
- *148 calories*
- *14 g carbohydrates*
- *4.6% alcohol*

18 Foster's
- *145 calories*
- *11 g carbohydrates*
- *5% alcohol*

17 Budweiser
- *145 calories*
- *11 g carbohydrates*
- *5% alcohol*

The Best (&Worst) Beer in America

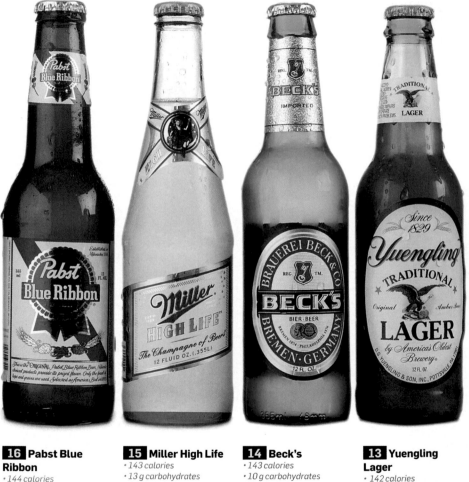

16 Pabst Blue Ribbon
- *144 calories*
- *13 g carbohydrates*
- *5% alcohol*

15 Miller High Life
- *143 calories*
- *13 g carbohydrates*
- *4.7% alcohol*

14 Beck's
- *143 calories*
- *10 g carbohydrates*
- *5% alcohol*

13 Yuengling Lager
- *142 calories*
- *12 g carbohydrates*
- *4.6% alcohol*

Best (& Worst) Bar Foods

They call it "belly-ing up to the bar" for a reason: Over time, nothing can pack on extra pounds like stopping by the pub for a daily dose of the dog that bit ya. It's not that your regular pint or pinot is so perilous. Often, it's the food you eat with the booze that really threatens your waistline.

Here's why: Your body sees booze as a toxin and puts a priority on burning off those alcohol-related calories. So the fat deposits from the nachos and the sliders sit in your gut as your metabolism focuses on that last pint. But proper noshing not only cuts calories, it's also known to prevent the dreaded potbelly hangover. (That's the kind that hangs over your belt.) Here's how.

WORST SEAFOOD DISH

Fish 'n' Chips

- 1,080 calories
- 49 g fat
  (9 g saturated)
- 1,650 mg sodium
- 117 g carbohydrates

Don't be distracted by the cutesy name: fish 'n' chips are just deep-fried fish and French fries. If you're going to bother with seafood, choose peel-and-eat shrimp, which come with all the health-boosting omega-3s and -6s, and none of the artery-clogging deep-fried fats.

Eat This Instead!

Peel-and-Eat Shrimp (12 large shrimp with 2 tablespoons cocktail sauce)

- 165 calories
- <1 g fat
- 480 mg sodium

WORST APPETIZER

Nachos with the Works (cheese, beans, ground beef, salsa, and sour cream)

- 623 calories
- 37 g fat
  (15 g saturated)
- 1,822 mg sodium
- 57 g carbohydrates

These stats apply to just 9 fully loaded nacho chips. Chances are, though, that you aren't going to stop there. For a similar taste at only a fraction the caloric load, choose a simple cup of chili con carne. You'll pass on the carbo-loaded chips and fat-blasted cheese and dips, and you'll keep all the belly-filling, protein-packed meat.

Eat This Instead!

Chili con Carne (1 cup)

- 298 calories
- 13 g fat (4 g saturated)
- 1,043 mg sodium
- 28 g carbohydrates

WORST FRIED SIDE

Jalapeño Poppers (4)

- 720 calories
- 48 g fat
  (21 g saturated)
- 1,440 mg sodium
- 45 g carbohydrates

The peppers are rendered a helpless vessel for a glut of cream cheese and a deep-fried bread-crumb batter. Pop just 4 poppers and you've consumed your daily allowance of saturated fat and as many calories as you should eat during dinner. Calamari is really the only fried dish you'll find at a bar with any substance. Yes, the calamari soak up their share of oil, but at least they bring otherwise-lean protein to your bar binge.

Eat This Instead!

Fried Calamari (1 cup)

- 300 calories
- 13 g fat (5 g saturated)
- 17 g carbohydrates

WORST CHICKEN DISH

Chicken Fingers (4) with Ranch Dressing

- 750 calories
- 48 g fat
  (11 g saturated)
- 1,970 mg sodium

Neither of these is a model of sound nutrition, but nothing you eat at the bar really is. Buffalo wings have the advantage of escaping the breading that fingers invariably receive, which acts as an oil sponge in the deep fryer. But if you like to cool off your wings with blue cheese, the margin between these two chicken standbys narrows by 100 calories.

Eat This Instead!

Buffalo Wings (6) with BBQ Sauce

- 390 calories
- 24 g fat (8 g saturated)
- 900 mg sodium

The Best (&Worst) Beer in America

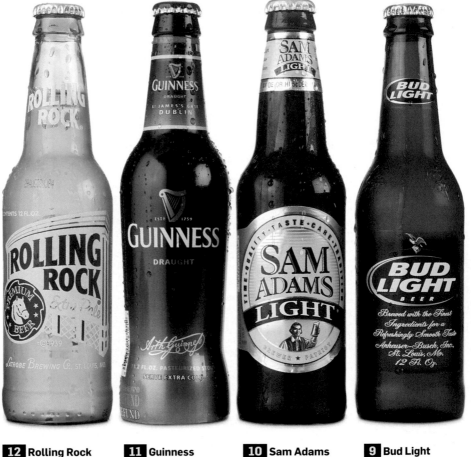

12 Rolling Rock Premium
- 132 calories
- 10 g carbohydrates
- 4.5% alcohol

11 Guinness Draught
- 126 calories
- 10 g carbohydrates
- 4% alcohol

10 Sam Adams Light
- 119 calories
- 10 g carbohydrates
- 4% alcohol

9 Bud Light
- 110 calories
- 7 g carbohydrates
- 4.2% alcohol

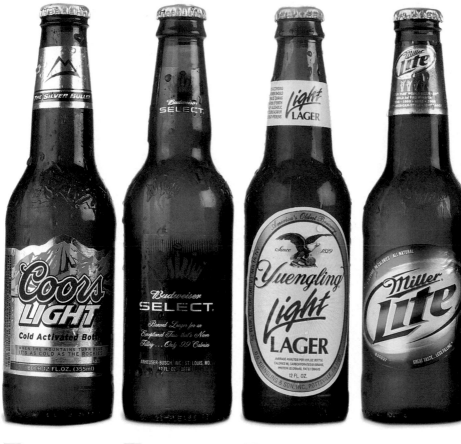

8 **Coors Light**
- *104 calories*
- *5 g carbohydrates*
- *4.2% alcohol*

7 **Budweiser Select**
- *99 calories*
- *3 g carbohydrates*
- *4.3% alcohol*

6 **Yuengling Lager Light**
- *99 calories*
- *9 g carbohydrates*
- *3.8% alcohol*

5 **Miller Lite**
- *96 calories*
- *3 g carbohydrates*
- *4.2% alcohol*

The Best (&Worst) Beer in America

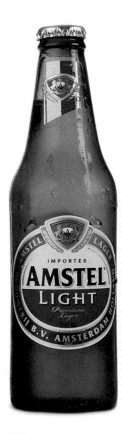

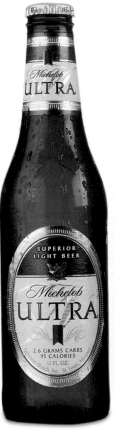

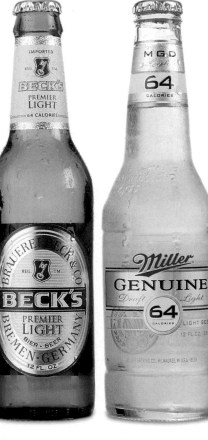

4 Amstel Light
- 95 calories
- 6 g carbohydrates
- 3.5% alcohol

3 Michelob Ultra
- 95 calories
- 3 g carbohydrates
- 4.2% alcohol

2 Beck's Premier Light
- 64 calories
- 4 g carbohydrates
- 3.8% alcohol

1 MGD 64
- 64 calories
- 2 g carbohydrates
- 2.8% alcohol

The World's Healthiest Grapes

A fine merlot is like . . . medicine. That's because, like all red wines, it contains resveratrol, an antioxidant that can help ward off everything from cancer to heart attacks. But not every varietal packs the same disease-fighting potency. Researchers at the University of Southern Mississippi tested 11 reds and discovered these 8 wine-cellar standouts.

Pinot Noir California	5.01
Beaujolais France	3.55
Cabernet Sauvignon and Merlot Chile	1.56
Zinfandel California	1.38
Cabernet Sauvignon California	0.99
Sauvignon Blanc California	≤ 0.02
Chardonnay California	≤ 0.02
Dry Sherry California	≤ 0.01

Resveratrol in milligrams per liter

Buy This, Not That!

LESSONS ON HOW TO NAVIGATE A WINE STORE

Treat your local wine cellar like a barbershop. Stay loyal to one store and befriend a clerk who knows about the wines you like. Once he or she understands your tastes, your options will become endless. Here are a few other dos and don'ts.

DON'T: Buy the label

There's a saying in the wine industry: "Put critters on the label, sell cases." Labels are designed by marketing companies who know how to trick you into buying juice that doesn't pack the thunder. Playful labels and cartoons are major warning signs. Be wary of red or yellow labels, which are designed to stand out.

DO: Double-check the ratings card

Often, wine shops post ratings for the wrong year. How much can the quality of wine vary from year to year? A ton. Most 2000 California cabernets are just average wines, for example, but the 2001 vintage is exceptional.

DON'T: Choose from a display near the counter

Chances are, they're trying to unload wines that didn't sell as well as expected or are aging quickly. Either way, these won't be among the best bottles in the store.

Ultimate Wine Decoder

Stymied by the staggering array of vino? Focus on finding a wine with an intensity that suits your palate and your dinner plans—less intense wines for, say, Thai and sushi and more intense for heavy meats. Calories and carbohydrates don't differ much among most major grape varietals, but we've provided counts for 5-ounce pours (courtesy of the USDA) for your reference.

Flavor Intensity
1 (low intensity) to 10 (high intensity)

Sauvignon Blanc: 1.5
· 119 calories
· 3 g carbohydrates

New World (recent producers): New Zealand
Old World (original sources): Loire, France

Pinot Grigio/ Pinot Gris: 2.0
· 122 calories
· 3 g carbohydrates

New World: Oregon
Old World: Italy

Riesling: 2.5
· 118 calories
· 6 g carbohydrates

New World: Australia
Old World: Germany

Chardonnay: 5.0
· 120 calories
· 4 g carbohydrates

New World: California
Old World: Burgundy

Pinot Noir: 5.5
· 121 calories
· 3 g carbohydrates

New World: Central Otago, New Zealand
Old World: Burgundy

Merlot: 6.5
· 122 calories
· 4 g carbohydrates

New World: Argentina
Old World: Pomerol, France

Red Zinfandel: 7.5
· 129 calories
· 4 g carbohydrates

New World: California
Old World: Italy

Syrah: 8.5
· 122 calories
· 4 g carbohydrates

New World: Australia; California
Old World: Rhône, France

Cabernet Sauvignon: 9.0
· 127 calories
· 4 g carbohydrates

New World: California
Old World: Bordeaux

CHAPTER 15

The Best (& Worst) Foods for Any Symptom

Psssst! C'mere.

You feelin' a little down? Wanna pick-me-up? You wanna feel no pain? You want a little somethin' that will take away those bad feelings, make you happier? Give you more energy? Boost your sex drive? Put a little topspin on your brain, get you thinkin' sharper and smarter all day and into the night? Then I got what you need, right here, under my coat.

What I got here is . . . I got food.

No, for real. Food can be the right cure for all your ills. And it's cheaper and more effective than seeing the doctor, or popping a bunch of pills, or calling up your no-good cousin, the one with the shady connections. You don't need pharmaceuticals to battle depression, ease anxiety, fend off aches and pains, or pick you up when you're beat. Simply altering your diet will do the same thing, much more safely, cheaply, and effectively.

See, our bodies and how we feel inside them are nothing more than a reflection of the various chemicals that flow through our system on a daily basis. And when those chemicals are the healthy kind you get from the right mix of fruits and vegetables, proteins and fats, you'll feel healthier, more energetic, and happier than you have in years.

Unfortunately, most Americans are suffering from two separate but related maladies: We're overmedicated and undernourished. When something goes awry with the way our bodies function, our first instinct is to head to the pharmacy. But food is—or should be—our first line of defense, a way to both stop symptoms when they arise and protect ourselves long-term from their reappearance. Healthy fats and high-octane nutrients have been shown to perform little miracles across the medical spectrum—fighting off disease, guarding against memory loss, beating back inflammation, and boosting both our mood and our brain power. Next time you're feeling low, don't call Doctor Feelgood. Call Chef Feelgood.

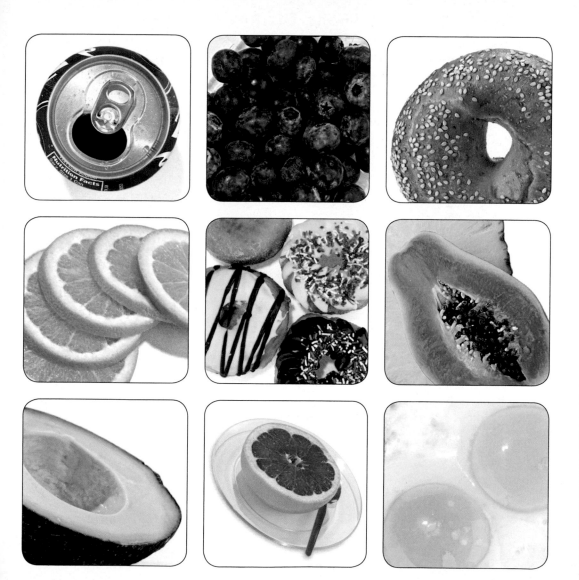

The Best and Worst Foods for
When You're Stressed

Modern life is a big, boiling cauldron of anxiety stew, and we get a heaping helping every day. Whether you're talking to your boss about a promotion, talking to your spouse about the credit card bills, or talking to your kids about that chocolate stain on the new couch, stress is lurking around every corner. So calm yourself quick with these natural nerve settlers.

Eat This

1 cup of plain yogurt with 2 tablespoons mixed nuts

Scientists in Slovakia gave people either 3 grams each of two amino acids (lysine and arginine) or a placebo and asked them to deliver a speech. Blood measurements of stress hormones revealed that the amino acid—fortified speakers were half as anxious during and after the speech as those who took the placebo. Yogurt is one of the best food sources of lysine; nuts pack tons of arginine.

Red bell peppers

Researchers at the University of Alabama fed rats 200 milligrams of vitamin C twice a day and found that it nearly stopped the secretion of stress hormones. Add raw slices of red peppers to salads and sandwiches; calorie for calorie, no food gives you more vitamin C.

Peppermint tea

One study found that peppermint kept drivers more alert and less anxious while they were on the road. One reason for this might be because it helps you breathe easier. An acid in peppermint encourages your cells to produce a substance called prostacyclin, which keeps your airways propped open.

A handful of sesame seeds

Stress hormones can deplete your body's supply of magnesium, reducing your stress-coping abilities and increasing your risk of developing high blood pressure. Sesame seeds are packed with this essential mineral.

Not That!
A can of soda

A study from the *American Journal of Public Health* found that people who drink 2½ cans of soda daily are three times more likely to be depressed and anxious, compared with those who drink less.

The Best and Worst Foods to
Improve Your Mood

Watch enough TV advertising and you begin to think the only answer to a bad mood is a bottle of pills. Wrong! Your next meal can have as dramatic an impact on your mood as your next prescription refill. So the next time you have a gnawing feeling that something's amiss, try gnawing on one of these.

 Eat This

An arugula or spinach salad

Leafy greens—arugula, chard, spinach—are rich sources of B vitamins, which are part of the assembly line that manufactures feel-good hormones such as serotonin, dopamine, and norepinephrine. In fact, according to a study published in the *Journal of Neuroscience Nursing*, a lack of B_6 can cause nervousness, irritability, and even depression.

A tuna roll or a fillet of grilled salmon

A study in Finland found that people who eat more fish are 31 percent less likely to suffer from depression. And skip sweet, simple carbs (like the rice with your sushi)—the inevitable sugar crash can deepen depression.

Canola oil

Canola oil is one of the cheapest sources of omega-3 fats and one of the easiest to incorporate into your diet. When consumed, these fats concentrate in your brain and help elevate your mood. Make a canola oil vinaigrette or use a little to sauté vegetables.

Dark chocolate

Research shows that dark chocolate can improve heart health, lower blood pressure, reduce LDL cholesterol, and increase the flow of blood to the brain. It also boosts serotonin and endorphin levels, which are associated with improved mood and greater concentration. Look for chocolate that is 60 percent cocoa or higher.

 Not That!
White chocolate

White chocolate isn't technically chocolate, since it contains no cocoa solids. That means it also lacks the ability to stimulate the euphoria-inducing chemicals that real chocolate does, especially serotonin.

The Best and Worst Foods to
Make You Look and Feel Slim

Whether you're trying to revert to prom-era size for your high school reunion or recovering from a season of holiday bingeing, you want to get rid of the extra pounds (and that sluggish feeling) in a hurry. So don't tailor your clothes; tailor your meals.

Eat This
Grilled chicken breast

The protein in lean meat and poultry fills you up and speeds metabolism, which cuts your cravings while easing off the pounds. High-protein diets also help to build muscle and attack extra belly fat.

Grapefruit

A grapefruit a day in addition to your regular meals can speed weight loss. The fruit's acidity slows digestion, helping you feel fuller longer. And the vitamin C—packed grapefruit works to lower cholesterol and decrease risk of stroke, heart disease, and some types of cancer.

A small scoop of tuna salad

A study at the University of Oxford in England found that eating salmon and tuna can speed up the movement of food from your stomach to your intestines, which leaves your stomach calmer and quells bloating. Credit the omega-3 fatty acids found in the fish, which stimulate hormones that regulate food intake, body weight, and metabolism.

Not That!
Canned soup and salty snacks

Sodium binges can lead to water retention, which makes your stomach feel like a beach ball. Avoid inflation by skipping salty foods like salted nuts and potato chips. And resist your cravings for Chinese takeout and Mexican food, two of the most salt-laden cuisines.

Broccoli and cauliflower

Over the long term, you should be eating all the broccoli and cauliflower your heart desires; but if you plan on hopping into a swimsuit tomorrow, just know that both vegetables (along with all cruciferous vegetables) contain the compound raffinose, which has been shown to cause prolonged bloating.

The Best and Worst Foods to
Increase Energy

In Spanish culture, the siesta is a midday nap that replenishes the body's energy and prepares it for an evening of hard work and hard partying. Sadly, explaining a 3 P.M. snooze in such terms to your boss probably won't go very far. Instead, use this arsenal of foods to power through the midday slump.

Eat This

A handful of trail mix

Raisins provide potassium, which your body uses to convert sugar into energy. Nuts stock your body with magnesium, which is important in metabolism, nerve function, and muscle function. When magnesium levels are low, your body produces more lactic acid—the same fatigue-inducing substance that you feel at the end of a long workout.

A bowl of cereal

Cereal is an excellent source of thiamin and riboflavin. Both vitamins help your body use energy efficiently, so you won't be nodding off mid-PowerPoint.

High-protein salad with vinaigrette

The oil in the dressing will help slow down digestion of protein and carbs in the salad, stabilizing blood-sugar levels and keeping energy levels high. Build your salad on a bed of romaine or spinach for an added boost in riboflavin and add chicken and a hard-boiled egg for energizing protein.

Not That!

Espresso-based drinks

Sure, the caffeine will perk you up, but with anywhere from 25 grams (latte) to 74 grams (white chocolate mocha) of sugar in your Starbucks or local coffee shop drink of choice, the spike in blood sugar will ultimately send you crashing. Blended frozen drinks are even more sugar-saturated. Stick to brewed coffee or Americanos.

Pancakes and bagels

MIT researchers analyzed blood samples from a group of people who had eaten either a high-protein or a high-carbohydrate breakfast. Two hours after eating, the carb eaters had tryptophan levels four times higher than those of the people who had eaten protein. The higher your tryptophan level, the more likely you are to feel tired and sluggish.

247

The Best and Worst Foods for
Your Metabolism

Who doesn't want a little help from this natural fat-burning engine? These foods will get the pistons pumping.

Eat This

Green tea

Catechins, the powerful antioxidants found in green tea, are known to increase metabolism. A study by Japanese researchers found that participants who consumed 690 milligrams of catechins from green tea daily had significantly lower body mass indexes and smaller waist measurements than those in a control group.

Steak and eggs

A British study found that people who increased the percentage of protein-based calories in their diets burned 71 more calories a day (that's 7.4 pounds a year). Jump-start your metabolism as soon as you wake up with a protein-rich breakfast of scrambled eggs and end your day with 4 to 6 ounces of high-quality protein like lean beef, chicken, or fish.

Not That!

Nothing

That's right; there's no better way to grind your metabolism to a halt than skipping a meal. When your body goes without food, it switches into survival mode, storing calories rather than burning them. Breakfast is most important, since your body is still in shutdown mode and your metabolism needs a jump start. In a perfect nutritional world, we would all eat six small, 300-calorie meals a day, but failing that, a couple of 200-calorie snacks strategically taken throughout the day will have to do.

Low-fat fruit-flavored yogurt

Pay less attention to fat and more attention to sugar when picking meals and snacks. Foods high in sugar and simple, refined carbohydrates cause your blood sugar to elevate, which in turn signals to your body to store fat, rather than burn it. Be particularly mindful of hidden sources of added sugar: low-fat yogurt, "healthy" cereal, juice, and more.

The Best and Worst Foods for
Shut-Eye

Nothing makes it harder to fall asleep than knowing how important it is to fall asleep. So when the pressure's on, try chowing on one of these snacks before bedtime to ensure some serious shut-eye.

Eat This

Nonfat popcorn

Pop a bag half an hour before bedtime: The carbs will induce your body to create serotonin, a neurochemical that makes you feel relaxed. Skip the butter—fat will slow the process of boosting serotonin levels.

Oatmeal with sliced banana and walnuts

Sleep is inspired by the hormone melatonin, but stress or excitement can disrupt melatonin's release. Bring your brain back down to earth by whipping up a bowl of instant oatmeal and topping it with a sliced banana and crushed walnuts, both of which are rich in melatonin.

A pile of sesame seeds

Sesame seeds are one of the best natural sources of tryptophan, the sleep-inducing amino acid responsible for all of those post-Thanksgiving turkey comas.

Not That!

A glass of warm milk

Forget what your mom told you: This popular remedy for sleeplessness could be making matters worse. The protein in milk boosts alertness. Plus, unless it's skim, the fat in milk slows down digestion and makes sleep more fitful.

The Best and Worst Foods for
When You're Sick

The first line of defense in the war on your well-being isn't found in the pharmacy—it's in the aisles of the supermarket. Warm up your cold, send the flu flying, and bolster your immune system with these foods.

Eat This

Ginseng

In a Canadian study, people who took 400 milligrams of ginseng a day had 25 percent fewer colds than those popping a placebo. Ginseng helps kill invading viruses by increasing the body's production of key immune cells. You can find ginseng supplements at most pharmacies or brew up a cup of ginseng tea.

Green tea

EGCG, a chemical compound that is potent in green tea, has been shown to stop the adenovirus (one of the bugs responsible for colds) from replicating. Start pumping green tea into your system at the first sign of a cold and you should be able to stave off worse symptoms. The best brand to brew? Go with Tetley; it was the most effective brand in studies.

Oranges

The zinc and vitamin C in oranges won't prevent the onslaught of a cold, but they might decrease the severity and duration of your symptoms. One orange provides more than 100 percent of your daily recommended intake of vitamin C.

Olive oil and avocados

Foods rich in healthy fats, such as olive oil and avocados, help reduce inflammation, a catalyst for migraines. One study found that the anti-inflammatory compounds in olive oil suppress the same pain pathway as ibuprofen.

Not That!

Caffeinated beverages and energy drinks

Excessive caffeine screws with your sleep schedule and suppresses functions of key immune agents. And insufficient sleep opens the door to colds, upper respiratory infections, and other ills. What's more, caffeine can dehydrate you, and hydration is vital during illness: Fluids not only transport nutrients to the illness site but also dispose of toxins.

The Best and Worst Foods to
Boost Libido

The idea of an aphrodisiac has been around since early man pulled the first oyster from the ocean. But not all passion foods are quite so expensive—and they don't need to be eaten raw. Unleash these mood foods to boost arousal and sexual stamina.

Eat This

Dark chocolate

The cocoa in chocolate contains methylxanthines, stimulants that increase your body's sensitivity. Chocolate also contains phenylethylamine, a chemical that can give you a slight natural high. And Italian researchers found that women who eat chocolate often have a higher sex drive than those who don't. Make sure your chocolate has at least 60 percent cocoa.

6-ounce sirloin steak

Protein has been shown to naturally boost levels of dopamine and norepinephrine, two chemicals in the brain that heighten sensitivity during sex. Your steak is also packed with zinc—a mineral that boosts libido by reducing production of a hormone called prolactin, which may interfere with arousal.

Vanilla ice cream

Ice cream has high levels of calcium and phosphorus, two minerals that build your muscles' energy reserves and boost your libido. All that calcium—200 milligrams in the typical bowl—can also make you more sexually charged, since the muscles that control sexual response need calcium in order to contract properly.

Not That!

Oysters

Okay, they won't exactly inhibit your bedroom behavior, but these legendary "aphrodisiacs" have never been proven to actually boost libido. While zinc, abundant in oysters of all shapes and sizes, is linked to male fertility, the connections to actual arousal have never been borne out in clinical research.

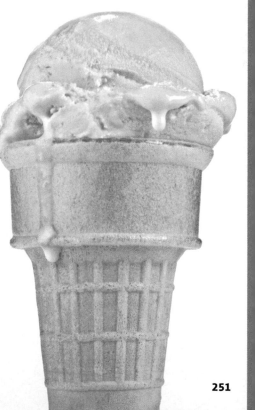

The Best and Worst Foods for
Fertility

It's one of life's great ironies that couples who spend their teens and 20s trying to avoid getting pregnant often find themselves in their 30s and 40s doing just the opposite. While the miracle of conception depends on many factors, you can tweak the odds in your favor through a careful diet.

 Eat This

Brazil nuts
Cigarette smoke, air pollution, and other toxins in the air can damage sperm, altering the DNA inside the cells and possibly increasing your child's risk of birth defects. Your best bet? Call in the Brazilians. Brazil nuts are a top source of selenium, a mineral that boosts sperm health while also helping the little buggers swim faster.

Liver
It might not sound sexy, but ounce for ounce there are few better sources of fertility-boosting vitamin A than liver. Studies show that men who get plenty of A each day have higher sperm counts and perform better sexually than men who don't. Can't stomach the liver? Try a salad made with red leaf lettuce and shredded carrots.

Frozen peaches
University of Texas researchers found that men who consumed at least 200 milligrams of vitamin C a day had higher sperm counts than men who took in less. Vitamin C also keeps sperm from clumping, meaning they'll have a better chance of finding their target. Keep a bag of frozen peach slices—they have more C than fresh ones do—in your freezer to dump into smoothies or add to your morning cereal. A single cup has more than twice your daily vitamin C requirement.

Not That!

Doughnuts and fries
Researchers from Harvard found that women who took in 2 percent of their calories from trans fat had a 70 percent greater risk of infertility than those who skipped trans fat altogether. Avoid fast-food and chain restaurants that still fry in trans-fatty oil and skip packaged foods like cookies and pastries with partially hydrogenated oils on the ingredient list.

The Best Foods for
Working Out

The right postworkout meals help build lean muscle, repair your body, and ensure gains long after you've done your last rep.

Eat This

PB&J or pasta

The perfect post—weight training repast has about 400 calories, with 20 to 30 grams of protein (to build new muscle) and 50 to 65 grams of carbohydrates (to repair old muscle). Peanut butter and jelly sandwiches or a small bowl of pasta with meat sauce fits that formula.

Pork tenderloin

Lean meats are a great low-calorie source of protein, and scientists at McMaster University in Hamilton, Ontario, found that eating more protein may reduce the fat around your midsection. People who ate 20 more grams of protein every day than the group average had 6 percent lower waist-to-hip ratios.

Pineapple and papaya

Both of these tropical fruits are loaded with bromelain and papain, enzymes that not only help break down proteins for digestion but also have anti-inflammatory properties to speed up your postworkout recovery.

8 ounces of chocolate milk

The best sports drink may come from a cow. British researchers found that milk does a better job than water or sports drinks at rehydrating the body after exercise. Why? To begin with, milk has more electrolytes and potassium. The addition of chocolate gives milk the perfect balance of carbs, protein, and fat for speedy muscle recovery.

Coffee

University of Georgia scientists revealed that taking a caffeine supplement (equal to two cups of coffee) after exercise reduces muscle soreness more than pain relievers can. Caffeine blocks a chemical that activates pain receptors.

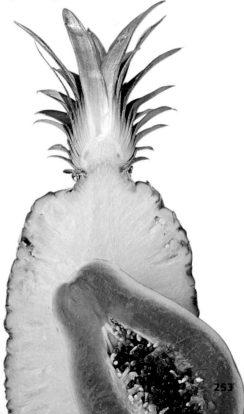

253

The Best and Worst Foods for
Your Brain

Believe it or not, that wrinkled old sponge in your noodle is actually an energy-starved engine responsible for guzzling down about 20 percent of your body's fuel. If you want to keep the spark plugs firing properly, you've got to make sure you're pumping in the right nosh. Stock up on these foods and you'll be better prepared to face any cognitive challenge, from the morning ideas meeting with the boss to the evening cocktail party with the coworkers.

Long-Term Memory

Eat This
Blueberries
Antioxidants in blueberries help protect the brain from free-radical damage, which could decrease your risk of Alzheimer's and Parkinson's diseases and improve cognitive processing. Wild blueberries, if you can find them—check the freezer section—have even more brain-boosting antioxidants than the cultivated variety.

Not That!
Fresh fruit out of season
Here's a cool tip: If the berries are out of season, you're better off buying them frozen. The freezer holds in nutrients longer, and it also ensures that your berries were picked ripe at peak antioxidant capacity. Out-of-season fruit, on the other hand, is picked too soon and allowed to "ripen" on a truck.

Short-Term Memory

Drink This
Coffee
Fresh-brewed joe is the ultimate brain fuel. Caffeine has been shown to retard the aging process and enhance short-term memory performance. In one study, British researchers found that people consuming the caffeine equivalent of one cup of coffee experienced improved attention and problem-solving skills.

Not That!
Energy drinks and Venti lattes
Like a politician whose smile is just a little too eager, caffeine has a dark side, too. Too much of it can make you jittery, anxious, and unsure of yourself. It can also derail your sleep schedule, meaning that extra cup of coffee today can blunt your cognitive powers tomorrow. Nobody performs at peak when groggy (except maybe Lil Wayne).

Extra Brainpower

Eat This
Salmon or mackerel
The omega-3 fatty acids found in fish are one of the primary building blocks of brain tissue, so they're essential to boosting brainpower. Salmon is also rich in niacin, which

wards off Alzheimer's disease and slows the rate of cognitive decline.

▶ Not That!
Full-fat ice cream

Not all fats are created equal, and about 60 percent of those found in ice cream are saturated, which is the kind that raises blood cholesterol. Over time, this cholesterol can clog blood vessels and prevent the flow of nutrients and blood to the brain.

Focus

▶ Drink This
A cup of peppermint tea

Researchers in Cincinnati found that it took a mere whiff of peppermint to increase subjects' concentration and performance on tedious tasks, and a professor in West Virginia claimed that he used the magical herb to improve athletes' performance.

▶ Not That!
Candy

Sugary foods incite sudden surges of glucose that result in energetic highs and lows. Unfortunately, the lows outlast the highs, as do the possible headaches and lack of concentration. And if you're wolfing down candy with the hopes of prolonging the rush, your problem might soon turn into one of midsection girth.

Sharper Senses

▶ Eat This
1 tablespoon of ground flaxseed daily

Flax is the best source of alpha-linolenic acid (or ALA)—a healthy fat that improves the workings of the cerebral cortex, the area of the brain that processes sensory information, including that of pleasure. To meet your quota, sprinkle flaxseed on salads or mix it into a smoothie or shake.

▶ Not That!
Alcohol

This one's obvious, but worth mentioning anyway. While a drink or two can increase arousal signals, more than a few drinks will actually depress your nervous system. This will dull sensations and make you tired, not sharp—in your brain or throughout your body.

The 10 Best Foods for

BEST SUN BLOCKERS: COOKED TOMATOES
Lycopene, the phytochemical that makes tomatoes red, helps eliminate skin-aging free radicals caused by ultraviolet rays. Cooking tomatoes helps concentrate their lycopene levels, so tomato sauce, tomato paste, and even ketchup pack on the protection. So does a hunk of lycopene-rich watermelon.

BEST WRINKLE FIGHTERS: SWEET POTATOES
They're loaded with vitamin C, which smoothes out wrinkles by stimulating the production of collagen. A recent study in the *American Journal of Clinical Nutrition* found that volunteers who consumed 4 milligrams of C (about half a small sweet potato) daily for 3 years decreased the appearance of wrinkles by 11 percent. Try papaya and carrot, too.

BEST WRINKLE FIGHTERS: FLAXSEEDS
These little seeds offer a payload of omega-3 fatty acids, which erase spots and iron out fine lines. The British *Journal of Nutrition* reported that participants in one study who downed about half a teaspoon of o-3s in 6 weeks experienced significantly less irritation and redness, along with better-hydrated skin. Beyond flax, salmon is an omega king.

BEST NATURAL MOISTURIZER: SAFFLOWER OIL
The omega-6 fatty acids found in safflower oil can be the ultima moisturizer for people who suffer f dry, flaky, or itchy skin. They kee cell walls supple, allowing water better penetrate the epidermis. Scientists have found that this o may even help people who suffe from severe conditions such as eczema.

BEST SUN BLOCKERS: ALMONDS
Almonds are stuffed with vitamin E, which helps defend against sun damage. Volunteers who consumed 14 milligrams of the vitamin per day (about 20 almonds) and then were exposed to UV light burned less than those who took none. And because vitamin E is an antioxidant, it also works to keep your arteries free of dangerous free radicals.

Your Skin

BEST BLEMISH BANISHER: CARROTS

Think of carrots as orange wonder wands—good for the eyeballs and good for clearing up breakouts. No magic here, though, just plenty of vitamin A, which prevents overproduction of cells in the skin's outer layer. That means fewer dead cells to combine with sebum and clog pores. Plus, vitamin A reduces the development of skin-cancer cells.

BEST CANCER DEFENDERS: SPINACH

In a study published in the *International Journal of Cancer*, people who ate the most leafy greens had half as many skin tumors over 11 years as those who ate the least. The folate in these veggies, which helps maintain and repair DNA, may reduce the likelihood of cancer-cell growth.

BEST SKIN TIGHTENER: TUNA IN A CAN

Your favorite deli sandwich has a little secret: selenium. This nutrient helps preserve elastin, a protein that keeps your skin smooth and tight. The antioxidant is also believed to buffer against the sun (it stops free radicals created by UV exposure from damaging cells).

BEST CANCER DEFENDERS: GREEN TEA

Green tea releases catechin, an antioxidant with proven anti-inflammatory and anticancer properties. Research found that drinking 2 to 6 cups a day not only helps prevent skin cancer but might also reverse the effects of sun damage by neutralizing the changes that appear in sun-exposed skin. (The tea's antioxidants degrade as it cools, so drink it while it's hot.)

BEST SUN BLOCKERS: DARK CHOCOLATE

Flavonols, the antioxidants in dark chocolate, reduce roughness in the skin and provide sun protection. In a study from the *Journal of Nutrition*, women who drank cocoa fortified with a chocolate bar's worth of flavonols had better skin texture and stronger resistance to UV rays than those who drank significantly fewer flavonols.

15 Foods That Cure

BEST BLOOD SUGAR STABILIZER: RASPBERRIES
Raspberries contain anthocyanins, which boost insulin production and lower blood sugar levels, providing a strong defense against diabetes.

BEST SKIN SAVER: CARROTS
National Cancer Institute researchers found that people with the highest intake of carotenoids—pigments that occur naturally in carrots—were six times less likely to develop skin cancer than those with the lowest intakes.

BEST HEART PROTECTOR: SALMON
A diet of heart-healthy fats, like those found in salmon and olive oil, raises good HDL cholesterol levels. And salmon contains a huge dose of omega-3 fatty acids, which can ward off heart disease.

BEST BREAST CANCER BEATER: WHOLE-GRAIN CEREAL
Women getting at least 30 grams of fiber daily are half as likely to develop breast cancer, according to research. A bowl of Fiber One with blueberries will get you halfway there.

BEST COLON CANCER GUARD: GREEN OR WHITE TEA
Drinking just one cup of tea a day may cut your risk of colon cancer in half. Antioxidants in the tea, called catechins, inhibit the growth of cancer cells, found researchers at Oregon State.

BEST BONE PROTECTOR: SHRIMP
Shrimp is high in vitamin B_{12}, which aids bone density, is crucial in the generation of new cells, and is a good source of vitamin D, an essential ingredient for bone strength.

BEST VISION DEFENDER: SPINACH OR ROMAINE LETTUCE

The National Institutes of Health found that people who consume the most lutein—found in leafy greens—are 43 percent less likely to develop macular degeneration.

BEST ANTI-AGING ELIXIR: RED WINE

Oxidative stress plays a major role in aging, and an antioxidant in red wine called resveratrol may help extend life by neutralizing disease-causing free radicals. Pop a Pinot Noir: It packs the most resveratrol per glass.

BEST LUNG CANCER FIGHTER: GRAPEFRUIT

A grapefruit a day can reduce your risk of developing lung cancer by up to 50 percent. Grapefruit contains naringin, which may help lower levels of cancer-causing enzymes.

BEST PROSTATE PROTECTOR: GARLIC

Compounds in garlic have been shown to reduce risk of prostate cancer by up to 50 percent.

BEST CAVITY KILLER: MONTEREY JACK CHEESE

Researchers found that eating less than a quarter ounce of Jack, Cheddar, Gouda, or mozzarella cheese will boost pH levels to protect your pearly whites from cavities.

BEST HAIR REJUVENATOR: BEEF

Iron in the meat stimulates hair turnover and replenishment. Beef is also rich in zinc, which helps guard against hair loss.

BEST CHOLESTEROL REDUCER: OLIVE OIL

Antioxidants found in olives have been shown both to raise HDL (good) cholesterol and lower LDL (bad) cholesterol, making olive oil a doubly potent protector against cardiovascular disease.

BEST BLOOD PRESSURE REDUCER: BAKED POTATO

Besides the obvious factors—obesity, high salt intake—diets containing too little potassium are the primary cause of hypertension. Fight back with a baked potato.

BEST BRAIN BOOSTER: COFFEE

Beyond boosting alertness for up to 90 minutes, that morning cup is the number-one source of antioxidants in the American diet and can help decrease your risk of developing Alzheimer's disease by as much as 60 percent.

CHAPTER 16

The Best (& Worst) Foods for Your Blood Pressure

Eat This

Red Lobster Wood Grilled Sole

with Fresh Asparagus

590 mg sodium
305 calories
6.5 g fat
(2 g saturated)
11 g carbohydrates

More omega-3s!
Fight high cholesterol with these healthy fats.

Save 595 calories!
Plus nearly a full day's worth of saturated fat.

Save 2,900 mg sodium!
You'll eliminate the same amount of salt as you'd find in 105 saltine crackers!

Not That!

3,490 mg sodium
900 calories
41 g fat
(17 g saturated)
82 g carbohydrates

Olive Garden Grilled Shrimp Caprese

Red Lobster has plenty of salt licks, too. But their line of simple grilled and broiled fish provides some of the finest fare you'll find in a chain restaurant.

Not even seafood is safe in the hands of most chain restaurants. Tack on 2 breadsticks and the garden salad that comes with this meal and you'll take in 1,550 calories and 6,180 milligrams of sodium—nearly 3 days' worth!

Few things in world history have done as much good, and caused as much damage, as the simple mineral salt.

On the upside, salt made modern civilization possible, allowing ancient man to preserve food so that he could concentrate on more important things, like curing ulcers with leeches and creating the subprime mortgage crisis. But while salt has long been used to make food more easily available, it can also be used to cause starvation— "salting the land" meant poisoning crops with salt so your enemies couldn't grow grains and produce. In fact, salt was once so precious and

powerful, some scholars believe the word "salary" comes from the Latin *salarium,* which was how Roman soldiers were paid. I believe it means "thanks for killing the natives, here's some money, go buy salt."

Today, salt is cheaper than dirt. (Literally— just go to a gardening store and you'll see.) But salt isn't done causing its damage. When you eat out at most restaurants, from the highest of the high-end to the cheapest and fastest of the drive-thrus, you're all but guaranteed to

take in more than your recommended daily intake for sodium— about 2,300 milligrams of sodium, max. But salt is so cheap and, let's face it, makes so many foods taste delicious, that it's in nearly everything. In fact, the average American takes in about 3,300 milligrams of sodium every single day!

And it's not because of what comes out of our saltshakers. According to Monell Chemical Senses Center researchers, 77 percent of that sodium intake comes from processed-food

6,540 mg sodium
On the Border Firecracker
Stuffed Jalapeños

Tex-Mex cooks are never shy with the salt, but this dish breaks even their reckless boundaries. Each little cheese-stuffed popper contains more than 1,000 milligrams of sodium.

purveyors. Their motivation: Pile on the salt so we don't miss natural flavors and fresh ingredients.

Why is that a problem? With ever-expanding portion sizes, supersalty foods are displacing fresh fruits and vegetables, which are rich in potassium. And a 1:1 ratio of dietary salt to potassium is critical for your health. Studies show that a high-sodium, low-potassium diet is linked to a host of maladies, including high blood pressure, stroke, osteoporosis, and exercise-induced asthma.

To protect your heart, your bones, your muscles, and your taste buds, we scoured takeout menus and supermarket shelves to expose the top 14 saltiest foods in America. No need to take the information with a grain of salt. These dishes provide plenty.

SALTIEST PACKAGED SIDE

14 Rice-A-Roni Rice Pilaf
(1 cup prepared with margarine)

- *1,200 mg sodium*
- *310 calories*
- *9 g fat*
  (1.5 g saturated, 1.5 g trans)

Sodium equivalent:
6½ small bags of Lay's Classic potato chips

The San Francisco treat is more like a nutritional Alcatraz, imprisoning your hopes for a decent day of eating. The most alarming part here is the serving size: If just a cup of this stuff packs more than 50 percent of your day's recommended sodium intake, this certainly qualifies the pilaf as being one of the most salt-dense foods in the supermarket.

Eat This Instead!
Rice-A-Roni Whole Grain Chicken & Herb Classico (1 cup prepared)
- *760 mg sodium • 260 calories*
- *8 g fat (1 g saturated)*

SALTIEST SUPERMARKET LUNCH

13 Hormel Chili 98% Fat Free Turkey
with Beans (1 can)

- *2,500 mg sodium*
- *420 calories*
- *6 g fat (2 g saturated)*

Sodium equivalent:
206 Rold Gold Pretzel Sticks

Think you're doing yourself a favor by seeking out the low-fat option? Think again. This chili can is just another example of the classic bait and switch, a tactic where food producers replace fat with salt and/or sugar. To underscore just how bad this bowl of red really is, a whole tray of seemingly treacherous mac and cheese spiked with chili will save you more than 1,500 milligrams of sodium. Next time, ignore the front label and go straight for the back, where the only information you need resides.

Eat This Instead!
Hormel Chili Meals Chili 'n Mac (1 tray)
- *980 mg sodium • 270 calories*
- *7 g fat (3 g saturated)*

2,550 mg sodium
Dairy Queen Chili Cheese Fries

This is DQ's real Blizzard. You can almost feel your blood pressure rise just looking at this catastrophe. Too bad it's listed as a side, gobbling up an entire day's worth of sodium and half a day of calories before you move on to your burger.

The Worst Foods for Your Blood Pressure

12 Dairy Queen Chili Cheese Fries

- 2,550 mg sodium
- 1,240 calories
- 71 g fat
  (28 g saturated, 0.5 g trans)

Sodium equivalent:
15 strips of bacon

This one's a no-brainer: chili, cheese, fried potatoes. But even a savvy eater couldn't possibly anticipate how bad these 3 ingredients could be when combined by one heavy-handed fast-food company. Stick with classic ketchup and recapture nearly a day's worth of sodium and 930 calories.

Eat This Instead!
French Fries (regular)
- 640 mg sodium • 310 calories
- 13 g fat (2 g saturated)

SALTIEST KIDS' MEAL

11 Romano's Macaroni Grill Chicken Fingerias and Fries

- 3,080 mg sodium
- 960 calories
- 58 g fat (10.5 g saturated)

Sodium equivalent: 20 Chicken McNuggets and 3 large orders of McDonald's French Fries

The dearth of healthy, well-balanced meal options for kids at chain restaurants is a serious issue in this country. You can't fault a restaurant for offering chicken fingers and fries—it's easily one of the most popular kids' meals out there—but you can fault it for stuffing that perennial favorite with nearly 1,000 calories, a full day's worth of fat, and more than a day's worth of sodium. Until restaurants take more responsibility for their youngest customers, parents need to do whatever possible to lead their kids to smarter choices on the menu.

Eat This Instead!
Mona Lisa's Cheese Masterpizza
- 940 mg sodium • 480 calories
- 14 g fat (8 g saturated)

SALTIEST "HEALTHY" MEAL

10 Olive Garden Grilled Shrimp Caprese

- 3,490 mg sodium
- 900 calories
- 41 g fat (17 g saturated)
- 82 g carbohydrates

Sodium equivalent: 20 individual canisters of Pringles Originals

Grilled shrimp on its own makes for one of the healthiest sources of protein on the planet, but when corrupted by the imaginations of the corporate cooks at Olive Garden, the result is considerably bleaker. The melted mozzarella and the garlic butter sauce are to blame for the high sodium numbers. Stick with the sea, but choose grilled salmon, instead of a platter that's soaked in salty sauce.

Eat This Instead!
Herb-Grilled Salmon
- 760 mg sodium • 510 calories
- 26 g fat (6 g saturated)
- 5 g carbohydrates

SALTIEST BURGER

9 Chili's Southern Smokehouse Bacon Big Mouth Burger

- 4,200 mg sodium
- 1,650 calories
- 108 g fat (36 g saturated)

Sodium equivalent: A pound of salted peanuts

Where there's smoke, there's salt, at least when left in the hands of the restaurant industry. Here, smoky thick-cut bacon combines with

Only one bowl of pasta at Macaroni Grill has less than 1,000 milligrams of sodium—the Capellini Tre Pomodoro. You're better off personalizing your pasta. We like whole wheat penne with broccoli, grilled chicken, and spicy tomato sauce.

4,900 mg sodium
Romano's Macaroni Grill Spaghetti and Meatballs

The Worst Foods for Your Blood Pressure

smoked Cheddar and an ancho chile barbecue sauce to smother this huge patty and buttered bun with nearly 2 days' worth of salt. We can't argue that any of the burgers at Chili's are actually "good" for you, but switching to the Oldtimer will cut nearly three-quarters of the sodium and 64 grams of fat.

Eat This Instead!
Oldtimer
- *1,310 mg sodium • 821 calories*
- *44 g fat (12 g saturated)*

SALTIEST SALAD
8 Chili's Boneless Buffalo Chicken Salad
- *4,380 mg sodium*
- *1,070 calories*
- *78 g fat (15 g saturated)*
- *46 g carbohydrates*

Sodium equivalent: 43 cups of Pop-Secret Homestyle Popcorn

What's scary about this salad is that it sounds relatively harmless. That's the case for almost all the leafy fare you'll find at Chili's—

most salads that aren't labeled as a "side" tack on at least a day's worth of sodium and an average of 1,000 calories. Choose the house garden salad or side Caesar and a reasonable main dish for a much smarter, healthier order.

Eat This Instead!
Side Salad Caesar
- *550 mg sodium • 350 calories*
- *31 g fat (6 g saturated)*
- *13 g carbohydrates*

The *Eat This, Not That!* Guide to HIGH BLOOD PRESSURE

What it is: Think of your circulatory system as the Erie Canal—a series of locks and gates that move blood to where it's needed. Without them, blood would simply succumb to gravity and be pulled down to the lower parts of your body and extremities (bad news for your brain and, uh, lots of other important things!). Simply put, blood pressure is the pressure of the blood against the walls of the arteries, and it's the result of both the force of the heart pumping blood into the arteries and the force of the arteries resisting the blood flow.

It's expressed in two numbers (example: 115/75 mmHg). **The top number** in the fraction is your systolic blood pressure—the measurement of the heart beating. **The bottom number** is your diastolic blood pressure—the heart's relaxation rate between beats.

The system works incredibly well—until you start sabotaging it with weight gain and unhealthy habits. How?

❶ All that new fatty padding needs blood, too, and your heart has to pump extra hard to get it there.

❷ Eating high-sodium foods leads your body to retain water (so it can attempt to dilute all that excess salt), which increases blood volume.
❸ The fatty meals you've been eating are lining your arteries with plaque—that means your vessels are narrower, so pressure has to increase to squeeze the same amount of blood through a smaller space.
❹ Letting stress get to you makes your brain release fight-or-flight hormones, which also lead to your heart pumping harder.

These factors and more drive your blood pressure into

dangerous territory. Anything between 120/80 and 139/89 is considered "prehypertension," meaning that if you don't take steps to improve your lifestyle now, you've written yourself a prescription for high blood pressure in the future. That's a level of 140/90 or higher—a dangerous condition that makes the heart and arteries work too hard, increasing your risk for heart disease, stroke, and other health problems.
What you can do: Once you've reached hypertensive blood pressure levels, drug therapy is usually a must. But

7 Red Lobster Admiral's Feast

- *4,662 mg sodium*
- *1,506 calories*
- *93 g fat (9 g saturated)*

Sodium equivalent: 7 medium orders of Burger King Onion Rings

The Admiral is piloting a sinking ship if this is the vessel he's steering. It's a sea of dreaded beige, with 4 different varieties of deep-fried seafood filling out the plate. Add on the Caesar and the fries that come with the meal and you're looking at more than 6,000 milligrams of seafood before you. Red Lobster is filled with low-calorie options, but sodium's definitely an enduring issue here, so choose wisely. Grilled fish and vegetables is a great place to start.

Eat This Instead!

Wood Grilled Sole with Fresh Asparagus

- *590 mg sodium • 305 calories*
- *7.5 g fat (2.5 g saturated)*

6 Arby's Sausage Gravy Biscuit

- *4,699 mg sodium*
- *1,040 calories*
- *60 g fat*
  (22 g saturated, 2 g trans)

Sodium equivalent:
13 large orders of McDonald's French fries

This is absolutely one of the worst ways you could start your day. Make a date with this and you'll have consumed 2 full days' worth of

whether your numbers are healthy, prehypertensive, or even full-blown hypertensive, you can still make some healthy changes to reduce your risk of the health problems associated with high blood pressure. **Eat less sodium.** If you do nothing else, make this one change. Eat absolutely no more than 2,300 milligrams of sodium each day and aim for 1,500 or less. This can be tough if your meals are based around chain restaurants and canned or frozen foods, so read nutrition facts carefully and center your meals around lean meats flavored with spices rather than salt, lots of fresh vegetables and fruits, and whole grains. Avoid cold cuts, cans, and jars. **Eat more potassium.** Potassium helps remove extra salt from the circulatory system, which helps dilate blood vessels, making blood flow more easily. Great sources include bananas, sweet potatoes, spinach, raisins, and tomatoes. **Make your last call earlier.** Heavy alcohol consumption can dramatically increase blood pressure, but having one or two drinks per day can decrease it slightly.

Other Picks

Tea: Flavonoids help relax blood vessels and thin blood, reducing clotting.
Black currant jelly: The antioxidant quercetin may help prevent buildup of free radicals that allow plaque to penetrate artery walls.
Fresh berries: Blackberries, strawberries, and blueberries contain salicylic acid, an anti-inflammatory known to fight heart disease.
Tuna: The omega-3 fats help strengthen the heart and lower blood pressure. Just make sure it's not mayo-heavy tuna salad.

Olive and sesame seed oils: Use them for cooking instead of corn or vegetable oil. The monounsaturated fats have been found to lower blood pressure dramatically.

Other Passes

Licorice: It's been found to spike blood pressure.
Condiments: Mustard, ketchup, soy sauce, and teriyaki sauce are all major sources of sodium.
Prepackaged dinners: Processed meals can carry up to 5,000 milligrams of sodium per serving. Take the extra time to cook for yourself.

sodium before the noon hour. The key to maintaining a reasonable blood pressure for most folks is to take in at least the equivalent amount of sodium and potassium throughout your day. (A 1:1 ratio is seen as ideal.) The problem with this biscuit is that you're consuming a heart-stopping level of sodium and almost no potassium. Throw in an abundance of calories and trans fat and you may have been better off sleeping in.

Eat This Instead!
Bacon and Egg Croissant
· 651 mg sodium · 337 calories
· 22 g fat (10 g saturated)

SALTIEST PASTA
5 Romano's Macaroni Grill Spaghetti and Meatballs with Meat Sauce (dinner)
· 4,900 mg sodium
· 1,810 calories
· 118 g fat (54 g saturated)

Sodium equivalent: 8½ cups of Chex Mix Original

The only thing more unappetizing than the sky-high sodium levels here is the fact that a single bowl of pasta can pack as much saturated fat as 54 strips of bacon. Unfortunately, when ordering pasta out, options that contain any kind of meat or seafood usually come with an unnaturally large dose of calories, fat, and sodium. Save those dishes for the stove at home and stick to the tomato-based capellini next time you find yourself at Macaroni Grill.

Eat This Instead!
Capellini Tre Pomodoro
· 990 mg sodium · 640 calories
· 25 g fat (3 g saturated)

SALTIEST SANDWICH
4 Blimpie Turkey and Bacon 12" Super Stacked
· 5,244 mg sodium
· 1,165 calories
· 48 g fat (21 g saturated)

Sodium equivalent: 28 strips of bacon

Deli meats are typically injected with salt solutions to lend them more moisture and flavor, but in the case of this turkey terror, it lends

The Sodium Spectrum
10 OF THE BIGGEST SOURCES OF SALT IN OUR DIETS

Soy sauce (about 3 tablespoons):
2,818 mg sodium

Teriyaki sauce (about 3 tablespoons):
1,916 mg sodium

Canned anchovies (about 12 anchovies):
1,834 mg sodium

Capers (about 5 tablespoons):
1,482 mg sodium

Cooked turkey bacon (about 3 slices):
1,142 mg sodium

Salami (about 6 thin slices):
1,130 mg sodium

Microwaved pork bacon (about 4 slices):
1,036 mg sodium

Ramen noodles (½ package):
1,001 mg sodium

Smoked salmon (about 3 thin slices):
1,000 mg sodium

Shredded Parmesan (about 10 tablespoons):
850 mg sodium

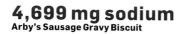

4,699 mg sodium
Arby's Sausage Gravy Biscuit

The name should be a dead giveaway: Sausage and gravy are two of the saltiest foods on the planet. Poured lavishly over a biscuit, they'll wipe out 2 full days' worth of sodium in one morning meal.

The Worst Foods for Your Blood Pressure

the consumer nearly 2½ days' worth of sodium intake. A word to the wise: If you're watching your salt intake, processed meat, processed cheese, and bacon will never serve you well. This is one of the few times that tuna is actually the smart sandwich selection.

Eat This Instead!
Tuna 6" Regular
· 776 mg sodium · 483 calories
· 21 g fat (3 g saturated)

SALTIEST APPETIZER
3 On the Border Firecracker Stuffed Jalapeños with Chili con Queso

· 6,540 mg sodium
· 1950 calories
· 134 g fat (36 g saturated)

*Sodium equivalent:
1,453 Pepperidge Farms Cheddar Goldfish*

Appetizers are the most problematic area of most chain-restaurant menus. That's because they're disproportionately reliant on the type of cheesy, greasy ingredients that catch hungry diners' eyes when they're most vulnerable—right when they sit down. Seek out lean

protein options like grilled shrimp skewers or ahi tuna when available; if not, simple is best—like chips and salsa.

Eat This Instead!
Chips and Salsa
· 440 mg sodium · 430 calories
· 22 g fat (3.5 g saturated)

SALTIEST ENTRÉE
2 Chili's Buffalo Chicken Fajitas with condiments and 4 flour tortillas

· 6,846 mg sodium
· 1,782 calories
· 108 g fat (29 g saturated)

Sodium equivalent: 68 cups of Pop-Secret Homestyle Popcorn

After Chinese food, Tex-Mex may be the saltiest cuisine on the planet, dedicated as it is to shredded cheese, refried beans, and massive tortillas. Even if you split this dish 3 ways, you'd still consume an entire day's allotment of sodium. Your best bet at Chili's is to avoid the Tex-Mex treatment and opt for more basic fare, like their Classic Sirloin.

Eat This Instead!
Chili's Classic Sirloin
· 990 mg sodium · 540 calories
· 50 g fat (18 g saturated)

THE SALTIEST FOOD IN AMERICA
1 P.F. Chang's Hot and Sour Soup Bowl

· 6,878 mg sodium
· 534 calories
· 20 g fat (4 g saturated)

*Sodium equivalent:
208 saltine crackers*

P.F. Chang's has published their nutrition facts for years sans sodium counts, which was cause for concern and—as it turns out—justified suspicion. Chinese food runs high on the sodium spectrum because of its reliance on viscous stir-fry sauces and salt-laden condiments like soy sauce. But this is an unfathomable amount of salt to pack into one 534-calorie bowl of soup. Unless you stick to vegetable sides and small servings of a select few entrées (Orange Peel Beef, Lemon Scallops), you're all but guaranteed to absorb 1 or more days' worth of sodium in a single sitting at P.F. Chang's.

Eat This Instead!
Sichuan-Style Asparagus
· 263 mg sodium · 213 calories
· 11 g fat (2 g saturated)

Consider this: Your calorie and sodium allotments are nearly identical numbers (both around 2,300). But for every calorie found in this soup, you'll be taking in 12.8 milligrams of sodium.

6,878 mg sodium
P.F. Chang's Hot and Sour Soup Bowl

The Best Foods for Yo

STRIP THE SODIUM FROM YOUR DIET WITH THESE SOLID STANDBYS

BEST FISH
Red Lobster Wood Grilled Sole
with Fresh Asparagus

- *590 mg sodium*
- *305 calories*
- *6.5 g fat*
  (2 g saturated)

Not only is this one of the dishes least likely to boost your blood pressure, it's also one of the finest entrées you'll find at a chain restaurant anywhere in America. The list of benefits is long: lean protein, heart-healthy omega-3s, the diverse nutrient package from asparagus, and impressively low calorie and sodium numbers.

BEST SANDWICH
Così Tuscan Pesto Chicken Sandwich

- *452 mg sodium*
- *510 calories*
- *18 g fat*

Most sandwiches crash right through the 1,000-milligram sodium ceiling, often packing more than an entire day's worth of sodium in one hand-held vessel. Così rebuts with this impressive offering, which not only goes easy on the salt but also offers up a dose of blood pressure–lowering monounsaturated fats in the pesto's olive oil base.

BEST BURGER
Five Guys Little Hamburger
with lettuce, tomato, onion, and sautéed mushrooms

- *487 mg sodium*
- *513 calories*
- *26 g fat*
  (11.5 g saturated)

Five Guys' greatest strength is also its most troubling weakness—its build-your-own-burger menu option. Avoid the allure of bacon, cheese, and mayo and go straight for the veggies. Here, onions offer quercetin, an antioxidant that can help protect your arteries, and mushrooms and tomatoes both pack major potassium, which helps remove excess salt from your circulatory system.

BEST MEXICAN
Baja Fresh Grilled Mahi Mahi Tacos (2)

- *600 mg sodium*
- *460 calories*
- *18 g fat (3 g saturated)*

These 2 tacos buck the trend of Mexican food being disproportionately prone to sodium spikes, which is reason enough to make our best list. But throw in the heart-strengthening, blood pressure–lowering benefits of mahi mahi's omega-3s and you have a true Hall of Famer on (or in) your hands.

ur Blood Pressure

Honest Tea
Green Dragon

- *20 mg sodium*
- *63 calories*
- *0 g fat*
- *10 g sugars*

The flavonoids found prominently in green tea aid in relaxing blood vessels, which allows for unrestricted blood flow from your heart to the rest of your body. *Men's Health* sent a variety of teas to an independent lab to test the concentrations of antioxidants in each, and this bottle came back the clear winner. Drink up.

Pesto trounces mayo and most other condiments as a sandwich spread for plenty of reasons: monounsaturated fat from olive oil and pine nuts, antioxidants from basil, and the cholesterol-lowering impact of fresh garlic.

452 mg sodium
Così Tuscan Pesto Chicken Sandwich

CHAPTER 17

The Best
(&Worst)
Foods for Your
Cholesterol

Eat This

Uno Chicago Grill Lemon Basil Salmon

with Steamed Broccoli

0 g trans fat
510 calories
39 g fat (5 g saturated)
1,030 mg sodium

This meal may have more calories, but it's packed full of vital nutrients and belly-filling protein.

More omega-3s!
Salmon is one of the best sources of these heart-healthy fats.

Save 7 g trans fat!
Considering you're only supposed to take in 2 grams a day, this is no small swap.

Not That!

Long John Silver's Breaded Clam Strips

7 g trans fat
320 calories
19 g fat (4.5 g saturated)
1,190 mg sodium

Add an order of regular fries and a soft drink and you'll have a 750-calorie meal with 10 grams of trans fat.

The restaurant industry began to shift away from frying in partially hydrogenated oil 10 years ago. Now, Long John Silver's is one of the few places left clinging to their trans-fatty fare.

POP QUIZ:
Define "Trans Fat."

☐ A mid-1960s Pontiac muscle car known for its luxurious curves
☐ A large, cross-dressing pool player from Minnesota
☐ A form of fat not found in nature but found in many convenience
foods and proven to increase your risk for heart disease

I suppose if Minnesota Fats did drive a Pontiac, his sweet ride would be known as Trans Fats. But the real trans fat—or, more accurately, trans-fatty acids—is a form of dietary flab invented in the beginning of the 20th century by food marketers looking for a cheaper, easier way to keep baked goods fluffy and moist while they sat for days or weeks on the supermarket shelf. On your grocery shelf, you'll find it under names like "shortening" or "par-

tially hydrogenated oil." In your local restaurant . . . well, you won't find it listed at all, because restaurants in most parts of the country aren't required to reveal it.

That's why we're here. While nutritionists and researchers may disagree about how certain foods and fats affect our overall cholesterol levels, one universal truth that everyone can agree on is that trans fat is an ultimate evil lurking in our food chain, proven

time and again to lower healthy HDL cholesterol, raise artery-clogging LDL cholesterol, and put us at increased risk for cardiovascular disease. Several studies have found a correlation between trans fat and type 2 diabetes; a French study found a connection between trans fat and breast cancer; and a 2003 study found a connection to Alzheimer's disease. All of which explains why the National Academy of Sciences recommends

5 grams trans fat
Boston Markets Classic
Chicken Salad Sandwich

With its multigrain roll and pile of fresh produce, this sandwich looks downright healthy. But the seemingly simple sub has a 5-inch ingredient list and more trans fat than you should consume in 2 days.

that people limit their intake of the harmful fat to no more than 1 percent of daily energy intake (about 2 grams tops, although zero sounds better to us). But even that's a compromise, since the Academy acknowledges that there's no "safe" amount. In fact, this artificial fat is so hazardous to our bodies that in 2007 the New York City Department of Health banned its use in restaurants.

Which of course led to the destruction of all the city's restaurants and caused New York to drop into the sea. Oh no,

wait . . . that didn't happen. In fact, the effect on New York's restaurants—including its fast-food joints—was pretty much zilch. That's because there are plenty of suitable, and much healthier, options out there and plenty of industry titans are using them. But to this day, many chain restaurants and food manufacturers in most parts of the country are still clinging to hydrogenated oils and shortening, and putting you, the consumer, in danger as a result.

Indeed, some chains are actually claiming to

be free of the harmful stuff when, in fact, they're still rolling around in it. Because the FDA allows the food industry to list trans fat content as "0 grams" per serving as long as it's less than 0.5 gram, restaurants can basically lie about serving trans fat-free food. Take KFC for example. They openly brag about having no trans fat, but "partially hydrogenated" oils show up 62 times on their menu's ingredient lists!

What's so unfair about this ongoing disregard for our health is that many fats are actually

Restaurants That Don't List Trans-Fat Content, as of May 2009

A number of restaurants didn't appear on our list, not because they don't have trans fat but only because they refuse to share their trans-fat content. It could be that one of these sneaky companies has items on its menu that are far worse than anything listed here—and, in fact, until they divulge their numbers, we're going to assume the worst. They've got to be hiding those numbers for a reason, right? Here's a list of the restaurants we checked out that didn't list trans-fat content. Order from their menus and drive-thru windows at your own risk.

- Applebee's
- Chevys Fresh Mex
- Chili's
- Chuck E. Cheese
- Così
- Hardee's
- IHOP
- Jimmy John's
- Olive Garden
- On the Border
- Outback Steakhouse
- P.F. Chang's
- Smoothie King
- T.G.I. Friday's

good for us—having a positive impact on our cholesterol profiles while also helping us stay fuller longer. Monounsaturated fats, like those found in olive and canola oils and healthy foods like avocados and nuts, can be used to make most any food better for us.

So in this chapter, you'll learn which foods out there can really set you up for heart disease and other health issues in the future and which carry healthier fats that can help you live a longer, leaner life. *Eat This, Not That!* researchers scoured nutrition tables from more than 60 chain fast-food and sit-down restaurants across the country in search of the trans-fattiest dishes. You'll be shocked by what we found. Protect your heart—avoid these ticker-harming fat blasts at all costs.

TRANS-FATTIEST SALAD

11 Jack in the Box Chicken Club Salad with Crispy Chicken Strips, Bacon Ranch Dressing, and Gourmet Croutons

- 4.5 g trans fat
- 840 calories
- 58 g fat (15 g saturated)
- 1,980 mg sodium

You know you deserve the dubious distinction of Trans-Fattiest Restaurant in America when even your salads come layered with more than 2 days' worth of the stuff. It all really comes down to one major factor: frying oil. Jack's is one of the last chain restaurants in the country to still be frying in partially hydrogenated oil, which means anything that touches the fryer will emerge soaking in trans fat. Until they do what nearly everyone else has already done and switch over to a trans-fat-free oil, stay away from the beige food.

Eat This Instead!
Asian Chicken Salad with Grilled Chicken
- 160 calories
- 1.5 g fat (0 g saturated, 0 g trans)
- 380 mg sodium

TRANS-FATTIEST MEXICAN FOOD

10 Baja Fresh Charbroiled Steak Nachos

- 4.5 g trans fat
- 2,120 calories
- 118 g fat (44 g saturated)
- 2,990 mg sodium

All Baja Fresh nachos come served with heaping piles of Jack and Cheddar cheeses, beans, guac, pico de gallo, your choice of meat, and a complete overload of trans fat. Even if you share this plate of nachos 4 ways, you'll each still consume more than your daily allowance of trans fat and more than 500 calories—that's as much as a reasonable sandwich should offer. And whoever heard of having a sandwich before your meal?

Eat This Instead!
Grilled Mahi Mahi Tacos (2)
- 460 calories
- 18 g fat (3 g saturated, 0 g trans)
- 600 mg sodium

The Worst Foods for Your Cholesterol in America

TRANS-FATTIEST SOUP

9 **Schlotzky's Wisconsin Cheese Soup Bowl**

- *5 g trans fat*
- *460 calories*
- *33 g fat (14 g saturated)*
- *1,821 mg sodium*

Schlotzky's Web site proudly claims "our soups are made with the highest quality ingredients and freshly cooked every day for optimum flavor." In the Bizzaro World of fast-food marketing, "high quality" translates into nearly a day's worth of sodium and twice your daily limit of trans fat. This dish has the dubious distinction of being one of the only soups we've ever seen with a significant trans-fat load. Even if you switched from the oversize bowl to a cup, you'd still take in 4 grams of the stuff. Our suspicion is that a decidedly low-quality cheese is to blame. Cheese has fat, of course, but only the cheap imitation stuff contains partially hydrogenated oil.

Eat This Instead!

Hearty Vegetable Beef Soup Cup

- *109 calories • 5 g fat
  (2 g saturated, 0 g trans)*
- *1,029 mg sodium*

TRANS-FATTIEST SANDWICH

8 **Boston Market Classic Chicken Salad Sandwich**

- *5 g trans fat*
- *800 calories*
- *41 g fat (7 g saturated)*
- *1,900 mg sodium*

The *Eat This, Not That!* Guide to HIGH CHOLESTEROL

What it is: Unless you've been living under a rock for the last few years, you know that the word "cholesterol" itself shouldn't inspire panic. In fact, it's as natural to our bodies as blood itself—we use cholesterol to form cell membranes, create hormones, and perform all sorts of important bodily procedures. We even make it ourselves—about 1,000 milligrams of it—every day. Some foods contain cholesterol, like egg yolks, meats, and whole-milk dairy, but most of it is made by the body.

Once you start chowing down on too much trans fat, though, your body starts churning out more cholesterol than you can use. Some of it is removed via the liver, but some of it sets up shop along the walls of your arteries, working with other substances to form plaque. This stuff narrows the space blood has to move through the arteries, forcing up your blood pressure, but it also can break off and form clots that cause strokes, paralysis, and death.

Two types of lipoproteins, molecules that carry cholesterol and other substances through the blood, determine your cholesterol levels.

HDL cholesterol, or good ("helpful") cholesterol, takes excess cholesterol to the liver, where it's passed from the body. It may also remove excess cholesterol from plaque, slowing its growth. High levels of HDL seem to protect against heart attack, and low levels indicate a greater risk of heart attack and, possibly, stroke.

LDL cholesterol, or bad ("lazy") cholesterol, rather than carrying excess cholesterol to your liver, simply deposits it in the blood, leading it to build up in your arteries. High levels mean an increased risk of heart disease, while lower levels reflect a lower risk.

Unfortunately, part of your risk of high cholesterol is out of your control. Some types of the condition run in the family, and your balance of HDL and LDL can strongly depend on your age and sex. For example, young men tend to have lower levels of HDL than women. Both sexes see higher levels of LDL as they age. Young women have lower levels of LDL, but after age 55, they see higher levels of LDL than men.

Chicken and tuna salad sandwiches might not be the models of health some purport them to be, but even we were surprised to see how bad this Boston Market sandwich really is. Where do they possibly find the room to cram 2½ days' worth of trans fat into chicken, mayonnaise, lettuce, and bread? The answer lies somewhere in the murky ingredient list, which, as with too many of their dishes, runs at more than 40 items long. Boston Market has a swath of solid entrées—from rotisserie chicken to slices of sirloin—and healthy sides on their menu. Get a sandwich stacked with lean white meat, minus the trans fat, with Boston Market's line of open-faced sandwiches.

Eat This Instead!
Rotisserie Turkey Open-Faced Sandwich
- *330 calories • 6 g fat (1.5 g saturated, 0 g trans)*
- *1,480 mg sodium*

7 Pop-Secret Kettle Corn (4 cups popped)

- *6 g trans fat*
- *180 calories*
- *13 g fat (3 g saturated)*
- *150 mg sodium*

The only secret here is that the popcorn purveyor uses partially hydrogenated oil to pop their kernels, turning a reasonable snack into a nutritional nightmare of heart-wrenching proportions. This

However, you have almost complete control over 2 huge factors in cholesterol health: diet and exercise.

What you can do: First and foremost, you must start watching trans-fat intake. This fearsome fat has been found to raise LDL more than anything else you eat (including cholesterol itself!). This may seem simple—just read the nutrition facts, right?—but the FDA allows manufacturers to claim that foods have "0 grams of trans fat" when 1 serving of the product contains less than 0.5 gram of trans fat. That number looks small, but it adds up quickly, and the American Heart Association says you shouldn't eat more than 2 grams per day. The only way to be sure is to check the ingredients list for any mention of "partially hydrogenated" oils—they're the source of all things trans fatty.

You also must exercise and watch your weight. A sedentary lifestyle leads to weight gain, which is associated with increased LDL and decreased HDL. And if you smoke, cut it out immediately—cigarette smoking is one of the biggest risk factors of heart disease, and it's been shown to lower HDL cholesterol.

Finally, drink water—tons of it. A Loma Linda University study found that drinking 5 or more glasses of water a day could help you lower your risk of heart disease by 50 to 60 percent—the same drop you get from cutting out cigarettes, lowering LDL, exercising, or losing weight.

Other Picks
- **Alcohol:** Drinking 1 or 2 alcoholic beverages per day is associated with a lower risk of heart disease.
- **Grapefruit:** Eating 1 each day can lower your total cholesterol and LDL levels by 8 and 11 percent, respectively.
- **Cranberry juice:** Drinking 3 glasses of cranberry juice daily can raise HDL levels by 10 percent. Just watch the sugar content and make sure you're getting at least 27 percent juice (it's often diluted).

Other Passes
- **Butter and margarine:** No matter which you pick, you'll end up with either saturated fat or trans fat. Better to go with Benecol spread, which contains a plant substance that inhibits cholesterol absorption; it can actually lower your LDL cholesterol.
- **Carbohydrate-rich snacks:** Replace them with nuts and you could decrease your risk of heart disease by 30 percent.

The Worst Foods for Your Cholesterol in America

box has 3 bags of popcorn, which means every time you buy it, you're bringing 54 grams of dangerous trans fat into your house. There's not an easier—or more important—swap to make.

Eat This Instead!
Orville Redenbacher's Smart Pop! Kettle Korn
- *130 calories*
- *2.5 g fat (0.5 g saturated, 0 g trans)*
- *370 mg sodium*

TRANS-FATTIEST COLD TREAT
6 Dairy Queen Chocolate Xtreme Blizzard (large)

- *6.5 g trans fat*
- *1,440 calories*
- *67 g fat (33 g saturated)*
- *165 g sugars*

Not a single Blizzard, shake, or malt at Dairy Queen comes without trans fat—which is ridiculous, because most other ice cream and smoothie places manage to leave it out of their products. This Chocolate Xtreme Blizzard is terrifying on every nutritional level: It's the sugar equivalent of 6 packs of peanut M&Ms, the caloric equivalent of nearly 6 McDonald's hamburgers, and more than three

times your daily limit of trans fat. Seek out relative safety in DQ's line of soft serve sundaes.

Eat This Instead!
Hot Fudge Sundae (small)
- *300 calories*
- *10 g fat (7 g saturated, 0 g trans)*
- *37 g sugars*

TRANS-FATTIEST SEAFOOD
5 Long John Silver's Breaded Clam Strips

- *7 g trans fat*
- *320 calories*
- *19 g fat (4.5 g saturated)*
- *1,190 mg sodium*

The word that should have set you off was "breaded"—it implies fried in oils, and in this case, those oils are packed with heart-harming trans fat. Who wants to order fried seafood through a squawk box anyway? Luckily, Long John also serves up a number of dishes that will boost good cholesterol, none better than the simple grilled fillet of salmon.

Eat This Instead!
Grilled Pacific Salmon
- *150 calories*
- *5 g fat (1 g saturated, 0 g trans)*
- *440 mg sodium*

TRANS-FATTIEST BURGER
4 Denny's Double Cheeseburger

- *7 g trans fat*
- *1,540 calories*
- *116 g fat (52 g saturated)*
- *3,880 mg sodium*

There's nothing redeeming about this atrocious cheeseburger—stacked between 2 buns is nearly three times your daily limit of trans fat, three-quarters of the calories you should consume in 1 day, and the sodium equivalent of 118 saltine crackers. Oh, and did we mention the 59 bacon strips' worth of saturated fat? Aside from the Fit Fare Boca, you're not going to find a reasonable burger on the Denny's menu, so it's either this or a grilled chicken sandwich.

Eat This Instead!
Top Sirloin Steak & Shrimp Skewers with Mixed Vegetables
- *370 calories*
- *12 g fat (3.5 g saturated, 0 g trans)*
- *820 mg sodium*

13 grams trans fat
Bob Evans NSA Apple Pie

Drop that fork! If you're watching your cholesterol or care about your heart health in general, pass on the pie. Piecrust traditionally gets its characteristic flakiness from shortening, which is why 4 slices out of 5 are likely to be crammed with trans fat.

The Worst Foods for Your Cholesterol in America

3 Bob Evans Stacked & Stuffed Caramel Banana Pecan Hotcakes

- *9 g trans fat*
- *1,543 calories*
- *77 g fat (26 g saturated)*
- *109 g sugars*
- *2,259 mg sodium*

These problematic pancakes keep popping up on our worst lists for a reason: They have more calories, sugar, carbs, sodium, and fat than nearly any other breakfast in America. Add to that list 4½ days' worth of trans fat and you begin to wonder why Bob Evans doesn't make you sign a waiver before applying the syrup. When ordering from Bob's breakfast menu, stick with items labeled "Fit from the Farm"—aside from scrambled eggs or a plain bowl of oatmeal, they're the only healthy breakfast foods Bob Evans offers.

Eat This Instead!
Fit from the Farm Breakfast with a Parfait
- *371 calories*
- *12 g fat (3 g saturated, 0 g trans)*
- *707 mg sodium*

2 Bob Evans NSA Apple Pie

- *13 g trans fat*
- *491 calories*
- *30 g fat (5 g saturated)*
- *19 g sugars*

It feels like just looking at Bob Evans's dessert menu will raise your LDL. More than 75 percent of the sweet stuff contains trans fat, with a full 7 desserts containing 7 grams or more of the troublesome lipid. Clearly Bob's bakers haven't found a way to make piecrust without shortening, despite the fact that the rest of the world figured it out long ago (here's a tip, guys: good old-fashioned butter). Until they get a grip on their penchant for partially hydrogenated fats, your only viable option for a meal capper is a simple, unadorned scoop of vanilla ice cream—the à la mode minus the pie.

Eat This Instead!
Vanilla Ice Cream
- *116 calories*
- *6 g fat (4 g saturated, 0 g trans)*
- *11 g sugars*

1 Jack in the Box Bacon Cheddar Potato Wedges

- *13 g trans fat*
- *760 calories*
- *52 g fat (16 g saturated)*
- *960 mg sodium*

It's no surprise this side dish is bursting with fat and calories—it's a plate of fried potatoes topped with bacon and melted cheese. To be fair, Bob Evans also offers 2 items with 13 grams of heart-hammering trans fat (Slow Roasted Chicken Pot Pie and the NSA Apple Pie)—but Jack's is so thoroughly swaddled in the junk that they truly have earned the bottom slot, and the troubling title of Trans-Fattiest Restaurant in America. The good news is that not all of Jack's items are filled with the bad stuff—a smarter appetizer or side dish would be the Grilled Chicken Pita Snack.

Eat This Instead!
Grilled Chicken Pita Snack
- *310 calories*
- *13 g fat (3 g saturated, 0 g trans)*
- *640 mg sodium*

13 grams trans fat
Jack in the Box
Bacon Cheddar Potato Wedges

No fried food on Jack's menu escapes the harsh bath in partially hydrogenated oil. Until they make the switch to trans fat free frying oil, skip all strips, fries, rings, nuggets, and, of course, wedges.

America's Best Foods

PROTECT YOUR TICKER WITH THESE HEART-HEALTHY FOODS

BEST BREAKFAST
Starbucks Perfect Oatmeal
with Nut Medley

- 240 calories
- 11 g fat
  (1.5 g saturated)
- 0 mg sodium

As that old Quaker guy has pointed out so many times on TV, research has shown a bowl of oatmeal every morning for breakfast can help reduce bad cholesterol levels. Add to that a dose of heart-healthy fats from the nut mix Starbucks throws in with their oatmeal and you have an incredible start to your day.

BEST LUNCH
Baja Fresh Grilled Mahi Mahi Tacos (2)

- 460 calories
- 18 g fat (3 g saturated)
- 600 mg sodium

Those 18 grams of fat come almost entirely from the one-two punch of heart-healthy, cholesterol-lowering omega-3 fats found in the fish and the generous serving of sliced avocado used to crown each taco. You'd be hard pressed to find a better ratio of flavor to nutrition anywhere in the restaurant world.

BEST SNACK
Wholly Guacamole Classic (2 Tbsp)

- 50 calories
- 4 g fat
  (0.5 g saturated)
- 75 mg sodium

Too many supermarket "guacamoles" are made with miniscule amounts of avocado—in some cases, less than 2 percent of that great green fruit. But Wholly Guacamole is as simple, unadorned, and avocado-packed as you could ever hope for, making this a dip rich in those HDL-spiking monounsaturated fats. Try a few tablespoons as a great sub for mayo on your next turkey sandwich.

BEST DINNER
Uno Chicago Grill Lemon Basil Salmon
with Steamed Broccoli

- 510 calories
- 39 g fat (5 g saturated)
- 1,030 mg sodium

That fat count may look high—and it is—but it's almost entirely good fat. That's because when it comes to cancer-fighting, inflammation-reducing, heart-strengthening omega-3 fatty acids, salmon is king, packing more of the stuff than nearly any other food found in nature. Team it up with a side of steamed broccoli and you and your heart will be happier than ever.

for Your Cholesterol

Whether you take yours at Starbucks or at home at the kitchen table, oatmeal is the best weapon you have for fighting high cholesterol in the breakfast hour.

240 calories
Starbucks Perfect Oatmeal

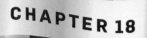

CHAPTER 18

The Best
(&Worst)
Foods for Your
Blood
Sugar

Eat This

Vivanno Banana Chocolate

Nonfat Milk

28 g sugars
250 calories
2 g fat (0.5 g saturated)

Blended drinks from coffee shops are usually atrocious, but the Starbucks Vivanno line bucks the trend.

VIVANNO™
nourishing blends

Save 500 calories!

Save 92 grams of sugar!
And do it all while slurping up chocolate.

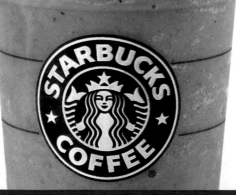

120 g sugars
750 calories
15 g fat (9 g saturated)

Not That!

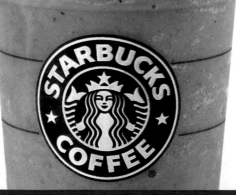

Starbucks Strawberries and Crème Frappuccino

Blended Crème with Whipped Cream

TOP SWAP!

Don't be fooled: This drink has more in common with milk shakes than it does with coffee or real fruit.

Sweetened drinks terrorize our blood sugar levels because they have no fiber or protein to slow down digestion. The Vivanno does more than cut out most of the sugar; it offers 21 grams of protein and 6 grams of fiber to slow down the sugar absorption.

A fully grown male deer.

The carbon body of a 2007 Shelby Mustang Funny Car. Tom Cruise. And all the sugar and other sweeteners you, the average American, will eat this year. What do they all have in common? They all weigh approximately 140 pounds.

Life is sweet, all right—so sweet that each of us will eat the sugar equivalent of 3,628 Reese's Peanut Butter Cups in the next 12 months.

Impossible, right? Sure, you like a piece of birthday cake now and again, and you're not above raiding the kids' Halloween stash or Christmas stockings or even stealing a serving of ice cream once a week or so. But 140 pounds of the sweet stuff? How can that be?

In this chapter, we'll show you that sugar doesn't lurk just in standard fare like cupcakes and brownies. Even if you keep your desserts to a minimum, you'll still be downing untold pounds' worth of sweetener—the equivalent of 460 calories of sugar every single day! Sugar is so much a part of our daily food intake because food marketers, eager to appeal to the sweet-toothed little kid in all of us, have found a way to add it to every food they can get their hands on—from ketchup to corn dogs to barbecued ribs, bread, and even pasta sauce. It's cheap, and it works.

The evidence? One in 5 health care dollars in America is spent caring for someone with diabetes, the disease most closely associated with an increased intake of sugar.

Sweeteners are so inexpensive because the US government subsidizes large industrial farms whose main crops include corn, which is easily converted into the ubiquitous sweetener

Blood sugar roller coasters aren't confined to desserts. Savory food in this country often comes with staggering deposits of sugar, as with these ribs, which pack more of the sweet stuff than 6 Klondike Bars.

110 grams of sugars
Uno Chicago Grill Baby Back Ribs

The Worst Foods for Your Blood Sugar

high-fructose corn syrup (HFCS). Consider this: A single US dollar buys 75 calories' worth of fresh broccoli, but thanks to our government's "help," that same dollar buys 1,815 calories'—empty calories—worth of sweetener. As a result, taxpayers like you and me take a double hit: We pay on the front end to have farmers grow surpluses of corn, which then get converted into food additives that create billions of dollars' worth of medical expenses on the back end.

To help you avoid the impact of stealth sugars that run rampant through our food supply, we've sifted through all the nutritional data to name the 18 biggest sugar bombs in America. Keep them from blowing up in your neighborhood.

MOST SUGAR-PACKED CANNED PRODUCT

18 Del Monte Peach Chunks in Heavy Syrup

- 23 g sugars
- 100 calories
- 0 g fat (0 g saturated)

*Sugar equivalent:
2 bowls of Frosted Flakes!*

Unlike most of the food in this chapter, these peaches aren't bona fide junk food; they are, after all, still fruit. But why manufacturers feel the need to can, package, and bottle nature's candy with excess sugar is a question we will never stop asking. In this case, the viscous sugar solution clings to the fruit like syrup to a pancake, soaking every bite with utterly unnecessary calories. Looking for cheap sources of fruit to have on hand at any time? Opt for the frozen stuff—it's picked at the height of season and flash frozen on the spot, keeping costs low and nutrients high.

Eat This Instead!
Dole Frozen Sliced Peaches (¾ cup)
- 9 g sugars • 500 calories • 0 g fat

MOST SUGAR-PACKED CEREAL

17 Quaker Natural Granola Oats & Honey & Raisins (1 cup)

- 30 g sugars
- 420 calories
- 12 g fat (7 g saturated)
- 6 g fiber

*Sugar equivalent:
3 Original Fudgsicle Pops!*

Like eating dessert for breakfast? Because that's basically what granola is. Sure, there's a splash of fiber, but it's completely diluted by a tidal wave of sugar. In fact, sugar accounts for more than a third of the calories in this bowl, and unfortunately, Quaker's is the rule, not the exception. The only acceptable use for granola is to crumble a small handful into plain yogurt. Save your bowls for a cereal more wholesome.

Eat This Instead!
Post Shredded Wheat (1 cup)
- 0 g sugars • 170 calories
- 1 g fat • 6 g fiber

MOST SUGAR-PACKED SIDE

16 Boston Market Cinnamon Apples

- 42 g sugars
- 210 calories
- 3 g fat

Sugar equivalent: 9 Oreos!

We're not apple-bashing here, but consider the numbers: A medium- to large-size apple contains about 18 grams of sugar. A candy apple, which is shrink-wrapped in pure sugar, contains about 38 grams of sugar. So even if Boston Market's side includes an entire apple, it's still encumbered with more sugar than 2 full apples or 1 carny-made indulgence. This dish is more fitting as a dessert than a side.

Eat This Instead!

Garlic Spinach
- 1 g sugars • 130 calories
- 9 g fat (6 g saturated)

23 grams of sugars
Del Monte Peach Chunks in Heavy Syrup

Most—96 percent, in fact—of the calories come from sugar, and only some of those are from the actual fruit. Anything canned in syrup has no place in your home. Frozen fruit is always the better buy.

Del Monte
Quality

PULL TOP LID

Peach Chunks
YELLOW CLING PEACHES IN HEAVY SYRUP

The Worst Foods for Your Blood Sugar

MOST SUGAR-PACKED SANDWICH

15 Subway Footlong Sweet Onion Chicken Teriyaki on Honey Oat Bread

- 44 g sugars
- 840 calories
- 11 g fat (2 g saturated)
- 2,340 mg sodium

Sugar equivalent: 5 Rice Krispies Treats!

Subway's menu board loudly reminds you that this creation is one of their sandwiches with "6 grams of fat or less." What it doesn't tell you is that the fat-free sweet onion sauce is like maple syrup in disguise, ratcheting up the calories and infusing your sandwich with the type of sugar counts you expect to find in a banana split—not in a supposedly wholesome sandwich. Trading fat for sugar is a losing strategy in the war on your waistline and well-being.

Eat This Instead!
6" Oven Roasted Chicken Breast on 9-Grain

- 9 g sugars • 310 calories
- 5 g fat (1.5 g saturated)
- 830 mg sodium

MOST SUGAR-PACKED CANDY

14 Skittles Original Fruit (1 package)

- 47 g sugars
- 250 calories
- 2.5 g fat (2.5 g saturated)

Sugar equivalent: 4 bowls of Froot Loops cereal!

Here's a reason to opt for the self-checkout instead of waiting for a cashier: You're more likely to make impulse buys while you wait for the disaffected teen to bag your dinner. And if the object of your impulse just happens to be a bag of Skittles, you'll have put a serious strain on your pancreas. Behind the rainbow motif of this bag lies a small bead of candy that consists of essentially 3 things: saturated fat, an amalgam of artificial colors, and sugar, which alone provides 75 percent of the calories in this bag.

Eat This Instead!
Jolly Ranchers (3 pieces)

- 11 g sugars • 70 calories • 0 g fat

The Truth about Artificial Sweeteners

While there is a robust debate among scientists about the potential dangers of alternative sweeteners, research is still too new to make any final judgments. With little evidence to support cancer-causing claims made by those who oppose aspartame and its ilk—and a supermarket's worth of research clearly documenting the ill effects of sugar—we see no clear reason to cut out artificial sweeteners entirely, if it means decreasing sugar in your diet. That being said, not all alternative sweeteners are created equal, and it's best to avoid excessively sweetened foods, artificial or not. When possible, shoot for natural ingredients and a short ingredients list.

Sugar Alcohols Limit	Saccharin Avoid	Sucralose Safe	Aspartame Limit	Acesulfame Potassium Limit
WHAT IS IT?				
A group of alcohols such as lactilol, sorbitol, and mannitol that provide roughly 25 percent fewer calories than sugar	A chemically complex zero-calorie sweetener	A zero-calorie sugar derivative made by joining chlorine particles to sugar molecules	A low-calorie artificial sweetener made by joining two amino acids with an alcohol	A zero-calorie sweetener that often appears with sucralose or aspartame to create a flavor closer to sugar
HOW SWEET IS IT?				
They vary from one alcohol to another, but generally they're slightly less sweet than sugar.	300 times sweeter than sugar	600 times sweeter than sugar	180 times sweeter than sugar	200 times sweeter than sugar
POTENTIAL DANGERS				
Sugar alcohols are applauded for not causing tooth decay and for providing a smaller impact on blood sugar. Because they are not well digested, however, sugar alcohols may cause intestinal discomfort, gas, and diarrhea. Some people also report carb cravings after ingesting too much of these sweeteners.	Between 1977 and 2000, the FDA mandated that saccharin-containing products carry a label warning consumers about the risk of cancer, due largely to the development of bladder tumors in saccharin-consuming rats. Saccharin still isn't in the clear. One recent study funded by Purdue and the National Institutes of Health showed that rats with a saccharin-rich diet gained more weight than those with high-sugar diets.	After reviewing more than 110 animal and human studies, the FDA decided in 1999 to approve sucralose for use in all foods. Sucralose opponents argue that the amount of human research is inadequate, but even groups like the Center for Science in the Public Interest have deemed it safe.	Some researchers claim to have linked aspartame to brain tumors and lymphoma, but the FDA insists that the sweetener is safe for humans. A list of complaints submitted to the Department of Health and Human Services includes headaches, dizziness, diarrhea, memory loss, and mood changes. The Center for Science in the Public Interest states that children should avoid drinks sweetened with aspartame.	In 2003, the FDA approved it for everything except meat and poultry. Although the FDA does not recognize the sweetener as a carcinogen, some experts disagree. They point to flawed tests as the basis for the FDA's acceptance of the additive. Large doses have been shown to cause problems in the thyroid glands of rats, rabbits, and dogs.
FOUND IN				
Smuckers Sugar Free Breakfast Syrup, Wrigley's Gum, **Jell-O Sugar Free cups**	**Sweet'N Low**	Splenda, Minute Maid Fruit Falls, **Dannon Light & Fit**	NutraSweet, Equal, **Diet Coke**, Sugar Free Popsicle	PowerAde Zero, Coke Zero, Breyers No Sugar Added Vanilla Ice Cream, **Hershey's Syrup Lite**

The Worst Foods for Your Blood Sugar

13 Odwalla PomaGrand Pomegranate Limeade

- *54 g sugars*
- *240 calories*
- *0 g fat*

Sugar equivalent: 4¹/₂ Reese's Peanut Butter Cups!

To most of Odwalla's bottled beverages, we offer nothing but praise, but this one's an exception. It lacks the nutritional punch provided by some of the thicker smoothies, but what's worse is that it's bogged down with a glut of evaporated cane juice, which is, of course, one of sugar's many euphemisms. Make it a rule to never drink a smoothie (or for that matter, anything) with added sugar. Choose the Dannon smoothie instead. It's calcium-rich yogurt flavored with berries and fortified with vitamins D, E, and B.

Drink This Instead!
Dannon Light & Fit Mixed Berry with Pomegranate
- *12 g sugars • 70 calories • 0 g fat*

12 Dairy Queen Corn Dog

- *55 g sugars*
- *460 calories*
- *19 g fat*
  (5 g saturated, 0.5 g trans)

Sugar equivalent: 4 scoops of Edy's Slow Churned Rich and Creamy Fudge Tracks ice cream!

When you eat a corn dog, you're generally aware of the fact that you're consuming a good deal of fat and a few refined carbs. If that corn dog happens to be from DQ, though, you'd probably be surprised to learn that there's also a towering ice cream cone's worth of sugar blended into the batter. To compare, a corn dog from Sonic has only 4 grams of sugar. That must be why Sonic's corn dog also has less than half as many calories. Apparently DQ got their "eats" and "treats" recipes mixed up.

Eat This Instead!
All-Beef Chili Dog
- *5 g sugars • 290 calories*
- *17 g fat (6 g saturated)*

11 Oscar Mayer Maxed Out Turkey & Cheddar Cracker Combo Lunchables

- *61 g sugars*
- *680 calories*
- *22 g fat (9 g saturated)*
- *1,440 mg sodium*

Sugar equivalent: 10 Dunkin' Donuts jelly-filled doughnuts!

The Maxed Out line is the worst of the lackluster Lunchables, with a back label that reads like a chemistry textbook. By cramming dessert and a supersweet drink into the box, Oscar manages to saddle this already-troubled package with more added sugar than your child should take in all day.

Eat This Instead!
Oscar Mayer Cracker Stackers Lean Ham & Cheddar
- *6 g sugars • 340 calories*
- *19 g fat (9 g saturated)*
- *1,110 mg sodium*

`10` Sobe Lizard Lava

- *75 g sugars*
- *310 calories*
- *1 g fat (0 g saturated)*

*Sugar equivalent:
11 Rainbow Popsicles!*

Sobe could use a marketing campaign just to explain to us exactly what "Lizard Lava" is. Process of elimination tells us it's not juice, tea, coffee, or soda, which leads us to the conclusion that it's a Frankenbeverage bred from an orgy of artificial colors, flavors, and an outrageous amount of sugar. It's not that we mind innovative new products, but when that innovation amounts to little more than a bottle of liquid sugar, we're compelled to point out that this is no lizard—it's a dinosaur.

Drink This Instead!
Sobe Lean Blackberry Currant
- *2 g sugars • 15 calories • 0 g fat*

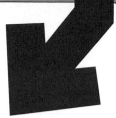

30 grams of sugars
Quaker Natural Granola Oats & Honey & Raisins

Thought the sweetest cereal in America would be one with a leprechaun or a rabbit on the box? Think again. Honey and brown sugar team up to cover these clusters with more sugar than you'd find in 3 Krispy Kreme original glazed doughnuts.

The Worst Foods for Your Blood Sugar

MOST SUGAR-PACKED "HEALTHY" BREAKFAST

9 Au Bon Pain Strawberry Yogurt with Blueberries (large)

- *80 g sugars*
- *470 calories*
- *4 g fat (3 g saturated)*

Sugar equivalent: 3 packs of Peanut M&M's!

Do you think there's any chance that strawberries and blueberries account for the 80 grams of sugar in this yogurt? Not unless Au Bon Pain managed to squeeze in about 9 cups of fruit. No, the real culprit here is the assault of added sweeteners: high-fructose corn syrup, corn syrup, and sugar. Some might call this an insult to natural flavors of fruit and yogurt. We would agree. Au Bon Pain redeems itself by being one the first companies savvy enough to turn the superfood quinoa (aka oatmeal on steroids) into a healthy breakfast staple.

Eat This Instead!
Cinnamon Walnut Quinoa (2 ounces)
- *2 g sugars • 90 calories • 6 g fat*

MOST SUGAR-PACKED ICE CREAM

8 Cold Stone Creamery Nutter Butter Ice Cream, Gotta Have It size (large)

- *84 g sugars*
- *940 calories*
- *59 g fat (30 g saturated, 1 g trans)*

Sugar equivalent: 21 Nutter Butter Cookies!

Companies often break from the standard small/medium/large serving size monikers, but renaming an oversize vessel of sugar and fat "Gotta Have It" is a grossly unfair marketing ploy. In this case,

The *Eat This, Not That!* Guide to HIGH BLOOD SUGAR

What it is: Like many things, a small amount of sugar isn't bad. Your body uses it for energy, and it knows how to handle it—your digestive system turns the food you eat into glucose and sends it into the bloodstream. When it hits your pancreas, you start producing insulin, which directs the glucose into your cells, where it helps you perform all the basic things you need to do.

But bad health habits, particularly eating too many high glycemic index foods, flood your body with glucose and overwhelm your pancreas. Your insulin loses its ability to direct glucose properly to cells, and you develop what's called insulin resistance. Eventually, the pancreas gets so tired that it slows down the amount of insulin it produces, giving you less than you need—that's type 2 diabetes. Glucose begins to build up in the blood, overflow into the urine, and pass out of the body without your cells even having the chance to use it in the right way.

Not surprisingly, you'll start to lose energy, and your body will start to essentially shut down. You'll be exhausted and extremely thirsty; you may suddenly lose weight; you'll likely get sick more often; and if you injure yourself, it'll take an unusual amount of time to heal. At the same time, the extra sugar in your blood will begin to damage your blood vessels and nerves, leading to blindness, impotence, numbness, and heart damage.

Scared yet? We'll give you a second to take a deep breath. **The good news:** Type 2 diabetes is largely preventable, and the right diet and exercise can even reverse some of its ill effects.

What you can do: Start by slimming down. About 80 percent of people with type 2 diabetes are overweight, which makes sense, consid-

Gotta Have It translates into nearly a pound of ice cream, 25 percent of which is pure sugar. Unless it's from natural sources (e.g., fruits), you should never consume that much sugar in an entire day, let alone a single dessert. But to make matters worse, Cold Stone has loaded this massive cup with the saturated fat equivalent of 30 strips of bacon. You'll definitely want to downsize.

Eat This Instead!
Egg Nog Ice Cream, Like It size (small)
· 21 g sugars · 260 calories
· 15 g fat (10 g saturated)

MOST SUGAR-PACKED "JUICE"

7 Au Bon Pain Homestyle Lemonade (large)

· 104 g sugars
· 460 calories
· 0 g fat

Sugar equivalent: 26 Nabisco Newtons Fruit Crisp Mixed Berry Individual Bars!

Fruit juice too often teems with sugar, and lemonade is the worst offender. In most cases, it seems inaccurate to even call it juice, as it almost always contains more sugar than fruit. In fact, any juice product with "ade" attached to it should be cause for immediate suspicion. Case in point: Au Bon Pain's Homestyle Lemonade, which contains more sugar than it does either water or lemon. The problem is that Au Bon Pain's drink menu is riddled with shocking sugar overloads. Either stick with water or settle for a small glass of real 100 percent juice.

Drink This Instead!
Small Orange Juice (1 cup)
· 26 g sugars · 110 calories · 0 g fat

---

ering that poor eating habits lead to both weight gain and diabetes. So get plenty of exercise and good sleep, but make sure you focus on your diet as well. And when you consider that "glucose-intolerant" is another term for "diabetic," it's clear what you need to cut down on: glucose-rich foods like bread, rice, pasta, and potatoes. But that doesn't mean you should starve yourself—in fact, you should make sure you eat until you feel satisfied, since letting your blood sugar drop too low can often

lead to carb binges.

Get to know the glycemic index, a measure of how quickly the carbs in a food are converted to glucose and released into the blood. People who eat foods with the lowest glycemic index are much less likely to develop diabetes than those who eat high glycemic index foods. Track your diet at glycemicindex.com.

Other Picks

Lean proteins: Center your meals around chicken breast, pork tenderloin, flank steak, and fish to stay satisfied and cut down on carbs.
Vegetables: Eat several servings of leafy green vegetables each day.
Whole grains: Soluble fiber can decrease your risk of heart disease and diabetes.
Apples: People who eat apples frequently can cut their risk of diabetes by nearly a third.
Raspberries: Raspberries contain anthocyanins, which boost insulin production and lower blood sugar levels, providing a strong defense against diabetes.

Other Passes

Solid fats: Since diabetes increases your risk of heart disease, a heart-healthy diet is important here, too.
Juice: Even 100 percent juice can send your blood sugar for a ride. Keep it to no more than 8 ounces a day.
"Multigrain" anything: You're looking for whole grains. Multigrain is a fancy way of saying "a whole lotta grains," even though they may be processed and stripped of their nutrients.

The Worst Foods for Your Blood Sugar

6 Bob Evans Stacked and Stuffed Caramel Banana Pecan Hotcakes

- *109 g sugars*
- *1,543 calories*
- *77 g fat*
  (26 g saturated, 9 g trans)

Sugar equivalent: 9 bowls of Cap'n Crunch!

We've deemed this mess the Worst Pancake Breakfast in America, the Trans-Fattiest Breakfast in America, and the Most Sugar-Packed Breakfast in America. Somehow, we doubt Bob will hang the plaques on his restaurant wall, but if he hopes to keep his clientele healthy, he'll consider banishing this dish from the menu. The combined force of cream cheese, caramel, and whipped cream blasts your beltline with 75 percent of your day's calories—a quarter of those from sugar.

Eat This Instead!
3 Scrambled Egg Lites with 2 slices of bacon and fresh fruit
- *19 g sugars • 502 calories*
- *19 g fat (7 g saturated)*

5 Uno Chicago Grill Baby Back Ribs

- *110 g sugars*
- *1,320 calories*
- *90 g fat (30 g saturated)*

Sugar equivalent: 11 Pillsbury Strawberry Toaster Strudels!

An overabundance of sugar represents a discouraging trend with today's barbecue sauces, and no food makes that more clear than restaurant-style ribs. Uno's version is slicked up with more sugar than you'll find in an oversize banana split, and we have a suspicion that Chili's Honey-Chipotle Baby Back Ribs are even worse (they don't release sugar counts). Either way, it's clearly time to start thinking of ribs as an appetizer to be split among friends instead of a meal for one. Your body's less likely to rebel if you limit yourself to 2 or 3 at a time.

Eat This Instead!
Sirloin (8 ounces)
- *0 g sugars • 400 calories*
- *14 g fat (5 g saturated)*

4 Starbucks Strawberries and Crème Frappuccino Blended Crème with Whipped Cream (24 ounces)

- *120 g sugars*
- *750 calories*
- *15 g fat (9 g saturated)*

Sugar equivalent: 9 scoops of Breyers All Natural Extra Creamy Vanilla Ice Cream!

Don't be fooled by the coffeehouse hoopla: This sugar-spiked pink beverage is a milk shake in drag. It allows you to suck the caloric equivalent of a Whopper with Cheese through a straw without actually absorbing any redeemable nutrients. If it's fruity and blended you seek, sip on something from the Vivanno line; this one packs real fruit, 21 grams of protein, and 6 grams of blood sugar—stabilizing fiber.

Drink This Instead!
Banana Chocolate Vivanno Nonfat (16 ounces)
- *28 g sugars • 250 calories*
- *2 g fat (0.5 g saturated)*

It's bad enough that these ubiquitous boxes are stuffed full of processed cheese and meat, but Kraft feels the need to throw fuel on the fire by including candy and Kool-Aid. No wonder kids love them so much.

61 grams of sugars
Oscar Mayer Maxed Out Turkey & Cheddar Lunchables

We dare you to try to count the number of ingredients used in this packaged lunch. We lost count after 50.

The Worst Foods for Your Blood Sugar

MOST SUGAR-PACKED SUNDAE

3 Baskin-Robbins York Peppermint Pattie Brownie Sundae

- 183 g sugars
- 1,610 calories
- 80 g fat
  (32 g saturated, 1 g trans)

Sugar equivalent: 14 Breyers Oreo Ice Cream Sandwiches!

Even if you split it 4 ways, this sundae would still pack 400 calories and the sugar equivalent of 2 packs of Peanut M&M's. It's disappointing that 2 of the 3 worst items on this list are from Baskin-Robbins. But as long as they keep dreaming up new ways to contribute to our nation's expanded waistlines and elevated insulin levels, we'll keep calling them out for it.

Eat This Instead!

Mint Chocolate Chip Ice Cream (4 ounces) in a Cake Cone
- 26 g sugars • 295 calories
- 16 g fat (10 g saturated)

MOST SUGAR-PACKED SMOOTHIE

2 Smoothie King Grape Expectations II (40 ounces)

- 250 g sugars
- 1,096 calories
- 0 g fat

Sugar equivalent: Eleven 100 Grand candy bars!

Smoothies are made from fruit, and fruit is a natural source of sugar. That much we understand. But what puzzles us is why smoothie makers feel the need to douse a naturally sweetened beverage with copious amounts of added sugars. Luckily, Smoothie King offers a way out of this downward diabetic spiral: Ask them to make your smoothie "skinny." That means they'll leave out the added sugars and just give you real fruit.

Drink This Instead!

Smoothie King Grape Expectations Skinny (20 ounces)
- 67 g sugars • 298 calories • 0 g fat

MOST SUGAR-PACKED FOOD IN AMERICA

1 Baskin-Robbins Made with M&M's Shake

- 287 g sugars
- 2,110 calories
- 73 g fat
  (45 g saturated, 2 g trans)

Sugar equivalent: 19 Little Debbie Marshmallow Pies!

After a year of taking issue with Baskin-Robbins line of so-called "premium" drinks, a funny thing happened: The nutrition information for the shakes vanished from their Web site entirely. At first we celebrated the death of one of the worst lines of drinks ever created, but then we walked into a Baskin-Robbins and saw all of the horrific shakes still on offer, plus a handful of new candy-inspired bombs. If you can't take ownership of your products, then why offer them?

Eat This Instead!

Reese's Peanut Butter Cup Ice Cream (4 ounces) in a Cake Cone
- 29 g sugars • 325 calories

287 grams of sugars
Baskin-Robbins Made with M&M's Shake

Not only does this drink contain dangerous amounts of sugar, but it will also add nearly two-thirds of a pound of fat to your body.

The Best Foods for Yo

SHORT ON THE SWEET STUFF AND LONG ON NUTRIENTS, THESE FOODS

BEST CHICKEN ENTRÉE

Bob Evans Grilled Chicken Breast

- *0 g sugars*
- *232 calories*
- *13 g fat (3 g saturated)*
- *635 mg sodium*

The 29-gram dose of slow-digesting protein in chicken breast is your first guard against escalating blood sugar levels. Your second guard is a powerful B vitamin called niacin. This vitamin has been shown to improve insulin metabolism by helping the body convert proteins, fats, and carbohydrates into usable energy. Chicken's among the best sources, but you also find niacin in mushrooms, tuna, salmon, and asparagus.

BEST DESSERT

Klondike Slim-A-Bear No Sugar Added Ice Cream Sandwich

- *3 g sugars*
- *100 calories*
- *2 g fat (1 g saturated)*

It would be a stretch to call any Klondike bar a health food, but as far as indulgences go, this is as good as you're going to get. The sugars have been replaced with sugar alcohols, drastically cutting down on the insulin response normally needed with ice cream products. Plus each Slim-A-Bear bar comes with 2 grams of fiber, a rarity in a dessert and just enough to give your blood sugar an easy ride.

BEST HOT BREAKFAST

Quaker Cinnamon Swirl High Fiber Instant Oatmeal (1 packet)

- *7 g sugars*
- *160 calories*
- *2 g fat (0.5 g saturated)*
- *10 g fiber*

Ground cinnamon can diminish the severity of your next blood sugar spike. It contains chemicals called methylhydroxychalcone polymers that increase your cells' ability to metabolize sugar by up to 20 times. And according to USDA research, you can see the effect by consuming as little as $\frac{1}{2}$ teaspoon a day. This hot bowl offers the double impact of cinnamon and fiber.

BEST SNACK

Tribe All Natural Hummus (2 Tbsp)

- *0 g sugars*
- *50 calories*
- *3.5 g fat (0 g saturated)*
- *130 mg sodium*

The nutrients needed for a full belly and stable blood sugar are all here: fiber, protein, and healthy fats. But there's another secret weapon at play. Hummus is made from pureed chickpeas, which are one of the world's best sources of manganese. If your body's not getting enough of this essential trace nutrient, it can't produce enough insulin to properly regulate your blood sugar. Carrots and hummus make one of the world's finest snacks.

ur **Blood Sugar**
WILL HELP FEND OFF DIABETES

BEST SIDE DISH
Wendy's Small Chili

- 6 g sugars
- 190 calories
- 5 g fat (2.5 g saturated)
- 14 g protein
- 5 g fiber
- 830 mg sodium

Chili is the ultimate slow-burn food. Thanks to the beans, each bowl is replete with soluble fiber and protein, but here's the best part: The tomatoes in chili are loaded with a hard-to-find mineral called chromium, which helps your body regulate blood sugar. The more refined sugar you eat, the more chromium your body excretes, so if you have a sweet tooth, reach for a bowl of red.

BEST FROZEN ENTRÉE
Kashi Chicken Pasta Pomodoro

- 5 g sugars
- 280 calories
- 6 g fat (1.5 g saturated)
- 6 g fiber

Kashi's Pomodoro contains an all-star list of ingredients that function to regulate blood sugar. Chicken aside, this dish also contains tomatoes and buckwheat, which are loaded with the chemicals chromium and D-chiroinositol, respectively. Together they work to help you create insulin and burn glucose. Plus Kashi's dinners always come loaded with fiber, so you know they'll keep you full longer than the competition.

3 grams of sugars
Klondike Slim-A-Bear Ice Cream Sandwich

No, not a nutritional superstar, but for dessert lovers looking to watch their blood sugar, few treats are better.

313

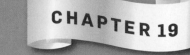

CHAPTER 19

The Best Foods
You've
Never
Heard of

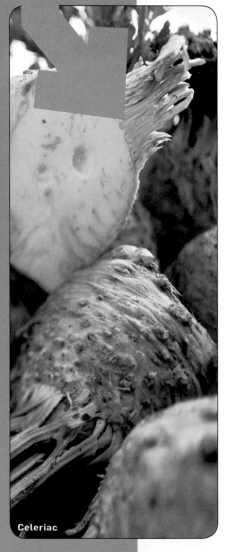

Celeriac

Do you find food shopping boring?

If so, let's do an exercise: Imagine it's breakfast time, your family is hungry, and you're being sent out to go food shopping. But it's not the year 2009 AD. It's the year 2009 BC, and the biggest challenge you face in gathering dinner isn't a shopping cart with a squeaky wheel. It's a little more complicated than that.

You wander through the woods for hours, being stalked by brown bears and mountain lions and packs of hungry wolves. You brave storms and lightning strikes, rival tribes and poisonous plants. And in the end, if you're lucky, maybe all you'll get for your troubles will be a few wild raspberries and a rabbit or two—and then you'll have to go out and do it all again the next day.

Makes the parking lot at Pathmark seem like less of a challenge, doesn't it?

Well, in this chapter, we want to bring back some of the excitement of food shopping. And no, we weren't planning on hiring a roving band of Sumerians to tackle you in the checkout aisle and steal your Cocoa Pebbles at swordpoint. Instead, we'd like you to reassess how you think about your local supermarket. Imagine it not as a sterile, fluorescent migraine of marketing come-ons and disillusioned checkout teens. Imagine it instead as a vast frontier of hidden treasures and untold adventures, a place packed with new sights, flavors, and textures.

See, most big supermarkets are loaded with cool foods that you have never tried—exotic fruits from the Amazon, heirloom vegetables nurtured by family farmers, spices and herbs from Asia, ancient grains loved by civilizations long forgotten. Sure, there are plenty of Frankenfoods concocted by food marketers, but there are even more stalks and roots and vines that have been grown for centuries that deserve more attention.

So, what if your next trip to the supermarket weren't a duty filled with drudgery, but an assignment packed with adventure? Besides breaking up the doldrums and exposing you to a whole new world of tastes, this approach will do one more thing for you: It will improve your health. See, only 20 percent of Americans reach the recommended five to seven servings of fruits and vegetables a day. And what food comprises the largest amount of vegetables eaten most every day by Americans? French fries.

We can do better. The great thing about the foods in this chapter is that they're phenomenally nutrient-dense and nutrient-diverse, meaning they bring potent quantities of the vitamins and minerals we need every day.

Beware of the hype, though. More than a few ambitious entrepreneurs have gotten their hands on great foods and turned them into little more than overpriced marketing gimmicks. Adding a little bit of pomegranate flavor to sugared water or ice cream does not magically turn it into a health food. Your best bet: Go native. Stay as close to the food in its 2009 BC form as possible.

Or we'll have to send the Sumerians after you.

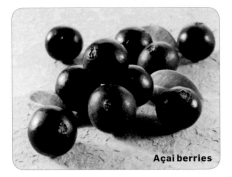

Açai berries

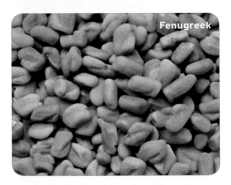

Alligator

Fenugreek

The Ultimate Stealth Health Foods

Açai Berries

Derived from an Amazonian palm tree, açai (ah-SIGH-ee) berries are the size of grapes and taste a bit like chocolate blueberries.

Why they're healthy: A study in the *Journal of Agricultural and Food Chemistry* discovered that the black-purple berries contain higher levels of antioxidants than do pomegranates and blueberries. And a University of Florida study found that an açai extract triggered a self-destruction response in 90 percent of the leukemia cells it came in contact with—a promising finding for scientists working to cure cancer.

How to eat them: You may have to travel to Brazil for the berries themselves, but you can get the benefits by drinking Bossa Nova Açai Juice, available at Whole Foods Market, Wild Oats stores, and bossausa.com.

Aioli

Aioli (eye-OH-lee) is a light, mayonnaise-style sauce made of olive oil, eggs, and garlic. It originated in the south of France and is traditionally served with seafood, hard-boiled eggs, and vegetables.

Why it's healthy: As a replacement for commercial soybean-oil mayonnaise, aioli provides a tasty source of heart-healthy olive oil, protein- and vitamin E—rich eggs, and cholesterol-lowering, cancer-fighting garlic.

How to eat it: Aioli isn't stocked by many regular supermarkets, but it's easy to purchase at online sites, such as savorypantry.com and gourmetfoodstore.com.

Alligator

Popular with chefs and home cooks in the Deep South, alligator has a soft, tender texture similar to veal and a neutral flavor that takes well to big spices and sauces.
Why it's healthy: Alligator fuses the best of surf and turf: It's rich in omega-3 fatty acids and packs more muscle-building protein than beef or chicken. Order at fossilfarms.com.
How to eat it: Rub each pound of gator with 2 tablespoons of blackening seasoning. Cook over high heat on a grill or in a cast-iron skillet.

Amaranth

Like quinoa, this nutrient-packed seed is native to the Americas and was a staple of the Incan diet. The grainlike seeds have a mild, nutty taste.
Why it's healthy: Gram for gram, few grains can compete

with amaranth's nutritional portfolio. It's higher in fiber and protein than wheat and brown rice, it's loaded with vitamins, and it's been shown in studies to help lower blood pressure and harmful LDL cholesterol. Find this super seed at Whole Foods Market or online at bobsredmill.com.
How to eat it: Amaranth cooks up just like rice, but it's even more versatile. Toss it with grilled vegetables as a bed for chicken or steak, or with apples, almonds, and goat cheese for a serious salad.

Aronia Berry

Once revered by Native Americans as a miracle fruit, this tiny, tart berry (also called a chokeberry) has resurfaced as a superfood.
Why it's healthy: No fruit packs more anthocyanins, potent cancer-fighting antioxidants that lend the berry its deep purple color. Because of this, aronia has been shown to fight cardiovascular disease, chronic inflammation, and even liver damage in rats.

How to eat it: Slurp down the benefits of aronia with a bottle of Oki, a juice blend that balances aronia's sharp flavor with the natural sweetness of a mix of other antioxidant powerhouses, including blueberry, black currant, and açaí (orendainternational.com).

Celeriac

What it lacks in aesthetics, this lumpy winter root vegetable makes up for with a pleasant, celerylike flavor.
Why it's healthy: Celeriac is loaded with bone-building vitamin K, and it's a good source of vitamin C and potassium.
How to eat it: It goes well with other root vegetables in soups and stews or shred it raw into coleslaw. You can also swap celeriac for half of your next batch of mashed potatoes. Treat it the same way as the spuds—peel, boil, mash; it'll add a hint of earthy sweetness.

Fenugreek

This tangy, curry-scented herb is used in many tasty Indian dishes.

The Best Foods You've Never Heard Of

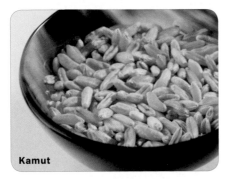

Kamut

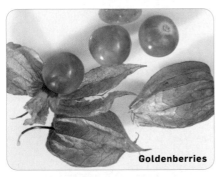

Goldenberries

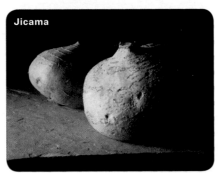

Jicama

Why it's healthy: Several studies show that fenugreek can help regulate blood sugar. Scientists think it may lower your blood-sugar response after a meal by delaying stomach emptying, which slows carbohydrate absorption and enhances insulin sensitivity. Find it in Indian stores or at spicebarn.com.

How to eat it: Fenugreek is a component of most curry powders. You can also mix a teaspoon of pure fenugreek powder into beef stew to kick up the flavor, or add whole seeds to a rice dish to create a Southeast Asian—style pilaf.

Ginger

This fresh, sweet-tasting root is used primarily in Asian cooking.

Why it's healthy: Beyond its role in aiding digestion, ginger may also have cancer-fighting capabilities. That's because it contains 6-gingerol, a nutrient that's been shown to stop the growth of colon-cancer cells, according to researchers at the University of Tennessee.

How to eat it: Grate 1 tablespoon of peeled fresh ginger (discard the skin), and heat it with 1 tablespoon of peanut or canola oil, a chopped garlic clove, and half of a small white onion as the base for your next stir-fry. Or add grated ginger to a marinade of soy and brown sugar for salmon, pork, or chicken.

Goldenberries

These tangy, dark yellow berries are native to South America, where they're sold fresh or made into preserves. In the United States, you're more likely to find the fruit dried and bagged.

Why they're healthy: One serving of dried goldenberries contains 4 grams of protein and 5 grams of fiber. They're also a great source of vitamin A and disease-fighting antioxidants. You can find them at grocers such as Whole Foods Market, or online at elfwholesale.com.

How to eat them: Snack on the dried berries alone like you would raisins, or toss a handful on a salad or your breakfast cereal.

Hemp Seed Nuts

Similar in taste to sunflower seeds, these nuts are derived from hemp seeds, which are also used to grow cannabis. (We know what you're thinking. The answer is no.)

Why they're healthy: By weight, hemp seed nuts provide more high-quality protein—6 grams per tablespoon—than even beef or fish. Each nut is also packed with heart-healthy alpha-linoleic acid. Find them in your local health-food store or in the natural-products section of your grocery store.

How to eat them: Enjoy straight from the bag, or sprinkle a handful on salads or in your morning oatmeal.

Holy Basil

This popular Indian herb, also known as tulsi, is the ideal ingredient for infusing freshness and flavor into almost any meal.

Why it's healthy: Animal studies have shown that natural chemicals in holy basil may help fight diabetes, heart disease, and cancer. You can find it at Asian specialty stores and farmers' markets, but if you're short on time, try fresh sweet basil, available at your local grocery store.

How to eat it: Fresh is best. Chop up a healthy dose of the herb and scatter it on scrambled eggs, soups, or stir-fried dishes.

Jicama

Jicama (HE-kuh-muh) is a Central American root vegetable that looks like a potato or turnip but is juicy and slightly sweet.

Why it's healthy: One cup contains just 49 calories and is loaded with 6 grams of fiber. It also packs a hefty dose of vitamin C. Find it in the produce sections of high-end supermarkets, like Whole Foods and Fresh Market.

How to eat it: You can slice it and eat it raw or boil it like a potato until soft.

Kamut

This cousin of durum wheat was once considered the food of pharaohs. It's now embraced by mere mortals as an alternative to brown rice.

Why it's healthy: Kamut has higher levels of vitamin E and heart-healthy fatty acids than most grains. It also has up to 40 percent more protein than wheat. Pick up kamut products at bobsredmill.com.

How to eat it: Boil it in water for up to an hour, until the grains are tender. Drain and toss with sautéed vegetables, a dash of soy sauce, and a squeeze of lemon.

Kefir

Similar to yogurt, this fermented dairy beverage is made by culturing fresh milk with kefir grains.

Why it's healthy: Because kefir contains gut-friendly bacteria, it's been shown to lower cholesterol, improve lactose digestion, and enhance the immune system. In addition, University of Washington scientists recently demonstrated that kefir was more effective than fruit juice or other dairy beverages at helping people control hunger. Look for kefir in the refrigerated health-food section of your local supermarket, or in the dairy aisle

The Best Foods You've Never Heard Of

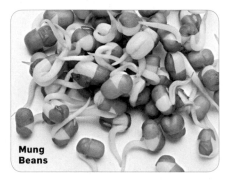

Mung Beans

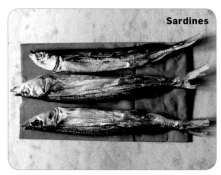

Sardines

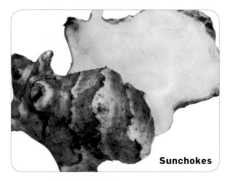

Sunchokes

of health-food stores, such as Whole Foods Market.

How to drink it: Pour a glass for a light breakfast, a sweet snack, or as a milk shake substitute for dessert.

Lemongrass

Grown primarily in warm climates (tropical Asia, for example), this exotic grass exudes a lemon flavor after the stalks are chopped.

Why it's healthy: Lemongrass is loaded with antioxidants, which help protect against oxidative stress, one of the leading causes of heart disease and cancer.

How to eat it: In a stir-fry, start with ½ tablespoon each of minced garlic, grated ginger, and minced lemongrass. Add vegetables, chicken, and soy sauce.

Mung Beans

Commonly eaten in China and India, these beans have a tender texture and a sweet, nutty flavor.

Why they're healthy: Sure, they're high in potassium, iron, and fiber, but they're also 24 percent protein.

What's more, unlike many other legumes, mung beans retain most of their high levels of vitamin C even after they're boiled.

How to eat them: Boil dried mung beans until tender and add them to your next salad. Their natural sweetness will add flavor without piling on extra calories or sodium.

Nori

This algae is popular in Japanese cuisine—you'll recognize it as the dark wrap holding your spicy tuna roll together. It adds a slightly salty, mineral flavor to soups, salads, and sushi.

Why it's healthy: High in fiber and protein, nori also contains a triple dose of cancer fighters, including phytonutrients called lignans, which have been shown to help prevent tumor growth. Look in the international section of your market or online at edenfoods.com.

How to eat it: Roll your own sushi, or for instant use, grind pieces in a coffee grinder and use the powder as a salt substitute to season dishes.

Peppadew Peppers

These sweet-and-spicy fruits look like a cross between a cherry tomato and a red pepper. Native to Africa, they're popular with chefs in the United States.
Why they're healthy: One-third cup of peppadews packs heart-protecting vitamin B_6, cancer-fighting lycopene, and a day's worth of vitamin C. Find this fruit in the salad section of upscale grocers like Wegmans or order the peppers at igourmet.com.
How to eat them: They're great tossed in a salad with avocado and almonds or in a simple pasta with olive oil and garlic. The compact peppers are also perfect for stuffing: For a killer snack or appetizer, try filling them with a hunk of fresh mozzarella or goat cheese.

Rooibos Tea

Rooibos (ROY-bus) is a vibrant red tea made from a South African legume. The tea is caffeine-free and also naturally sweet, so you won't need to add sugar.

Why it's healthy: Rooibos is loaded with disease-fighting antioxidants and has been shown to boost the immune system. In fact, a recent Japanese study on mice and rats suggests that rooibos tea may help prevent both allergies and cancer. Look for Celestial Seasonings rooibos teas (we like Madagascar Vanilla Red) in your local grocery store, or try the Adagio brand, an organic product that features 13 different all-natural flavors (adagio.com).
How to drink it: Make a cup instead of coffee to start your day, or take the chill off a winter's eve before bed.

Sardines

These oily fish are a top source of omega-3 fats, rivaling even salmon. Plus, they're packed with bone-building calcium.
Why they're healthy: Research shows that omega-3s can improve everything from your cholesterol profile to your mood to your ability to ward off Alzheimer's. Look for sardines packed in olive oil. Crown Prince Natu-

ral ($2, thebetterhealthstore.com) brand is inexpensive, but more discerning eaters may want to check Whole Foods or igourmet.com for upscale products.
How to eat them: You can eat them straight from the can, but for a more sophisticated approach, wrap a sardine around an almond-stuffed olive. Or you can chop sardines and stuff them inside a peppadew pepper.

Sunchokes

These vegetables are also called Jerusalem artichokes, but they're neither related to artichokes nor are they from Israel. They look like gnarled potatoes and have a nutty, slightly sweet taste.
Why they're healthy: Sunchokes contain fructooligosaccharides, sweet fibers that promote gut health and may help boost immunity.
How to eat them: Try sunchokes as an alternative to French fries. Slice them into matchstick slivers, toss with olive oil, salt, and pepper, and bake at 350°F for about 15 to 20 minutes.

The Best Foods You've Never Heard Of

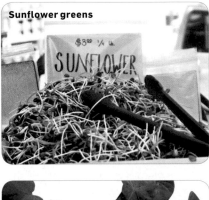

Sunflower greens

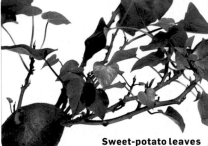

Sweet-potato leaves

Watercress

Sunflower Greens

These crunchy, nutty-tasting sprouts arise when sunflower seeds are grown in soil for about a week.

Why they're healthy: They contain much of the heart-healthy fat, fiber, and plant protein found in sunflower seeds, but with fewer calories. Locate the greens in your local farmers' market or in the produce section of some higher-end grocery stores.

How to eat them: Wash the greens thoroughly, then drizzle olive oil and sprinkle sea salt on them for a simple and crunchy side dish, salad, or bed for grilled chicken. They're also great on sandwiches.

Sweet-Potato Leaves

Typically discarded, sweet-potato leaves are poised to become the next big health-food craze.

Why they're healthy: Sweet-potato leaves are one of the world's richest sources of disease-fighting antioxidants, according to a new report from the University of Arkansas. In all, they're packed with at least 15 different types of healthy compounds that help fight diabetes, heart disease, bacterial infections, and various forms of cancer. You'll have the best shot at finding them in an Asian or specialty grocery store, or you could request them from a vendor at your local farmers' market.

How to eat them: Sauté a handful of the thoroughly washed leaves with onions, garlic, and ginger to create a super-healthy stir-fry base. Then add other vegetables, along with beef, chicken, or shrimp.

Watercress

This leafy green, a member of the cabbage family, has a light, peppery flavor.

Why it's healthy: One cup of watercress has just 4 calories, but it's loaded with vitamins A, C, and K. What's more, it contains lutein and zeaxanthin, antioxidants that are beneficial for eye health.

How to eat it: Swap watercress for the lettuce on your next sandwich, or toss a bowl of the leaves with goat cheese, toasted pistachios, and your favorite vinaigrette.

Yerba Maté

A plant native to Argentina used to make a tealike infusion, maté (MAH-tay) has an herbal taste and half the caffeine of coffee.

Why it's healthy: It's like green tea on steroids, with up to 90 percent more powerful cancer-fighting antioxidants, a cache of B vitamins, and plenty of chromium, which helps stabilize blood-sugar levels. Plus, its bolstering effect on metabolism is so valued that many diet pills list maté as an ingredient.

How to drink it: For the strongest dose of maté's medicine, buy loose-leaf bags at guayaki.com. Bottled maté products are becoming more commonplace in large supermarkets. Look for flavored varieties from Bombilla Gourd at your local Whole Foods Market.

Superfoods in disguise

These common, unsuspecting foods are nutritional Clark Kents—they may look weak and ineffectual, but under their humble facades, they're ready to soar.

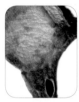 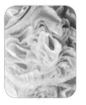   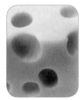

Pork chops
Pork contains almost five times the selenium—a mineral linked to a lower risk of prostate cancer—of beef and twice that of chicken. And Purdue University researchers found that a 6-ounce serving daily helped people preserve muscle while losing weight.

Iceberg lettuce
Conventional wisdom suggests this salad staple is nutritionally bankrupt. But as it turns out, half a head of iceberg lettuce has significantly more alpha-carotene, a powerful disease-fighting antioxidant, than either romaine lettuce or spinach.

Mushrooms
This fungi's metabolites—by-products created when mushrooms are broken down during digestion—have been shown to boost immunity and prevent cancer growth, report researchers in the Netherlands.

Vinegar
Scientists in Sweden discovered that when people consumed 2 tablespoons of vinegar with a high-carb meal, their blood sugar was 23 percent lower than when they skipped the antioxidant-loaded liquid. They also felt fuller.

Red-pepper flakes
A Dutch study found that consuming a gram of red pepper flakes—about half a teaspoon—30 minutes prior to a meal reduced calorie intake by 16 percent. Plus, new research suggests its active ingredient, capsaicin, may help kill cancer cells.

Full-fat cheese
This dairy product is an excellent source of casein protein—one of the best muscle-building nutrients you can eat. Danish researchers found that even when men ate 10 ounces of full-fat cheese daily for 3 weeks, their LDL ("bad") cholesterol didn't budge.

The Best Sources for 14 Vital Vitamins and Minerals

Sure you could just pop a multivitamin pill every day, but research shows that there is no better way to absorb the essential nutrients your body needs than by seeking them out from the fresh food sources that feature them most prominently. Here's a cheat sheet for some of the biggest nutritional players and a bunch of foods that'll deliver them.

VITAMIN A

What it is: A pale yellow crystalline compound also known as retinol.
Why you need it: It preserves and improves your eyesight as well as fights viral infections.

	SERVING SIZE	CALORIES	% DAILY VALUE
Raw carrots	1 cup	53	686
Cooked spinach	1 cup	41	294
Baked sweet potato (with skin)	1	95	262
Cooked turnip greens	1 cup	28	158
Baked winter squash	1 cup	80	145
Cooked collard greens	1 cup	49	118
Cantaloupe	1 cup	56	103
Romaine lettuce	2 cups	16	58
Steamed broccoli	1 cup	43	45
Cooked green peas	1 cup	134	19

VITAMIN B_1

What it is: Also known as thiamin. Helps cells' enzyme systems convert oxygen into usable energy.
Why you need it: Maintains your energy, coordinates nerve and muscle activity, and keeps your heart healthy.

	SERVING SIZE	CALORIES	% DAILY VALUE
Raw sunflower seeds	1/4 cup	205	54
Cooked yellowfin tuna	4 ounces	157	38
Cooked black beans	1 cup	227	28
Cooked corn	1 cup	177	24
Sesame seeds	1/4 cup	206	18
Oatmeal	1 cup	145	17
Cooked asparagus	1 cup	43	14
Brussels sprouts	1 cup	60	11
Cooked spinach	1 cup	41	11
Pineapple	1 cup	76	9

VITAMIN B₆

What it is: Involved in more than 100 enzyme reactions throughout the body.
Why you need it: Helps your nervous system, promotes proper breakdown of starch and sugar, and prevents amino acid buildup in your blood.

	SERVING SIZE	CALORIES	% DAILY VALUE
Banana	1	108	34
Roasted chicken breast	4 ounces	223	32
Roasted turkey	4 ounces	214	27
Cooked cod	4 ounces	119	26
Baked potato	1 medium	133	21
Avocado	1 cup	235	20
Garlic	1 ounce	42	17
Raw red repper	1 cup	24	11
Watermelon	1 cup	48	11
Cooked cauliflower	1 cup	28	10

VITAMIN D

What it is: A vitamin present in just a few foods (but added to some others) that's also produced when UV rays hit the skin.
Why you need it: Essential to calcium absorption—without it, bones don't grow correctly and become thin, brittle, and easily broken. Also helps with the immune system and can reduce inflammation.

	SERVING SIZE	CALORIES	% DAILY VALUE
Halibut	3 ounces	160	130
Mackerel	3.5 ounces	180	90
Salmon	3.5 ounces	185	90
Canned sardines	1.75 ounces	100	70
Oysters	6	60	67
Shrimp	4 ounces	112	40
Vitamin D-fortified milk (reduced fat)	1 cup	125	25
Cod	4 ounces	120	16
Vitamin D-fortified cereal	1 cup	105	10–30
Egg	1	70	6

VITAMIN B₁₂

What it is: An unusual vitamin formed by microorganisms like bacteria and yeast (and found in the various and sundry animals that ingest them).
Why you need it: Plays a key role in developing blood cells and nerve cells and processing protein. Helps protect individuals with anemia and gastrointestinal disorders.

	SERVING SIZE	CALORIES	% DAILY VALUE
Clams	3 ounces	126	1401
Duck liver	3 ounces	114	756
Oysters	6	250	720
Calf liver	4 ounces	187	690
Rainbow trout	3 ounces	130	90
Top sirloin	3 ounces	160	25
Skim yogurt	1 cup	137	25
Milk	1 cup	121	14
Lean cured ham	3 ounces	130	10
Hard-boiled egg	1	80	10
Chicken breast	1	140	6

FOLATE

What it is: Also known as folic acid. A chemically complex vitamin found naturally in foods, folate requires enzymes in the intestine to aid in its absorbtion.
Why you need it: Aids fetal development in pregnancy, helps produce red blood cells, prevents anemia, helps skin cells grow, aids nervous system function, prevents bone fractures, and lowers risk of dementia and Alzheimer's disease.

	SERVING SIZE	CALORIES	% DAILY VALUE
Cooked lentils	1 cup	229	89
Cooked navy beans	1 cup	258	63
Cooked beets	1 cup	74	34
Cooked split peas	1 cup	231	31
Papaya	1	118	28
Mustard greens	1 cup	21	25
Raw peanuts	¼ cup	207	21
Flaxseeds	2 Tbsp	95	13
Orange	1	61	10
Raspberries	1 cup	60	8

The Best Foods You've Never Heard Of

VITAMIN C

What it is: Also known as ascorbic acid. A water-soluble nutrient that acts as an antioxidant to protect us from colds and infections, cardiovascular disease, cancer, joint diseases, and cataracts.

Why you need it: Protects cells from free radical damage, regenerates vitamin E supplies, and improves iron absorption.

	SERVING SIZE	CALORIES	% DAILY VALUE
Steamed broccoli	1 cup	43	205
Cooked brussels sprouts	1 cup	60	161
Strawberries	1 cup	43	136
Orange	1	61	116
Cantaloupe	1 cup	56	112
Kiwi	1	46	95
Grapefruit	1/2 fruit	36	78
Pineapple	1 cup	76	39
Cooked winter squash	1 cup	80	32
Blueberries	1 cup	81	31

VITAMIN E

What it is: A group of fat-soluble vitamins that are found throughout the body.

Why you need it: Protects your skin from ultraviolet rays, promotes communication among your cells, prevents free radical damage, and lowers risk of prostate cancer and Alzheimer's disease.

	SERVING SIZE	CALORIES	% DAILY VALUE
General Mills Total Cereal	3/4 cup cereal, 1/2 cup skim milk	143	100
Raw sunflower seeds	1/4 cup	205	90
Peanut butter	2 Tbsp	189	69
Kashi Heart to Heart Instant Oatmeal, Maple	1 packet	162	68
Roasted almonds	1/4 cup	206	45
Olives	1 cup	154	20
Papaya	1	118	17
Sweet potato chips	1 ounce	139	14
Cooked spinach	1 cup	41	9
Blueberries	1 cup	81	7

CALCIUM

What it is: A mineral that is found in your bones and teeth.

Why you need it: Keeps your bones strong and healthy, promotes efficient function of your nerves and muscles, and helps blood clotting.

	SERVING SIZE	CALORIES	% DAILY VALUE
Sesame seeds	1/4 cup	206	35
2% milk	1 cup	121	30
Plain or vanilla soymilk	1 cup	70	30
Low-fat yogurt	8 ounces	155	25
Cooked spinach	1 cup	40	25
Part-skim mozzarella cheese	1 ounce	72	18
Nature's Path Optimum Slim cereal	1 cup cereal with 1/2 cup skim milk	250	15
Raw tofu	4 ounces	86	10
Cream cheese	1 ounce	29	10

IRON

What it is: A common metal that's essential to nearly all life forms.

Why you need it: Key for oxygen transport, cell growth, and immunity.

	SERVING SIZE	CALORIES	% DAILY VALUE
Chicken liver	3 1/2 ounces	100	70
Soybeans	1 cup	297	50
Spinach	1 cup	40	36
Tofu	4 ounces	86	34
Sesame seeds	1/4 cup	205	30
Kidney beans	1 cup	225	29
Venison	4 ounces	180	28
Lima beans	1 cup	215	25
Beef tenderloin	4 ounces	240	23
Roast turkey	3 1/2 ounces	220	10

MAGNESIUM

What it is: A mineral found mostly in our bones, but also in our muscles. The human body is unable to produce it, so it's vital to seek out foods that contain it.
Why you need it: Helps muscles and nerves relax, strengthens bones, and ensures healthy blood circulation.

	SERVING SIZE	CALORIES	% DAILY VALUE
Cooked salmon	4 ounces	260	35
Raw sunflower seeds	1/4 cup	205	32
Sesame seeds	1/4 cup	206	32
Prickly pear	1 cup	61	32
Cooked black beans	1 cup	227	30
Roasted almonds	1/4 cup	206	25
Cooked pinto beans	1 cup	235	24
Cooked brown rice	1 cup	216	21
Cooked scallops	4 ounces	151	19
Cooked summer squash	1 cup	36	11

SELENIUM

What it is A mineral needed daily, but only in small amounts.
Why you need it: Protects cells from free radical damage, allows thyroid to produce hormones, and protects joints from inflammation.

	SERVING SIZE	CALORIES	% DAILY VALUE
Wild cooked oysters	3 ounces	61	87
Cooked snapper	4 ounces	145	80
Canned white tuna (in water)	3 ounces	109	80
Cooked halibut	4 ounces	158	76
Cooked shrimp	4 ounces	112	65
Roasted turkey breast	4 ounces	215	47
Broiled beef tenderloin	4 ounces	240	40
Grilled portobello mushrooms	1 cup	42	31
Hard-boiled egg	1	68	19
Raw tofu	4 ounces	86	14

POTASSIUM

What it is: Another mineral, stored within cells to regulate muscle contraction and nerve activity.
Why you need it: Keeps your muscles strong, balances electrolytes, and lowers risk of high blood pressure.

	SERVING SIZE	CALORIES	% DAILY VALUE
Baked winter squash	1 cup	80	26
Avocado	1 cup	235	25
Pinto beans	1 cup	243	23
Cooked lentils	1 cup	230	21
Cooked beets	1 cup	75	15
Fresh figs	8 ounces	168	15
Cooked brussels sprouts	1 cup	60	14
Cantaloupe	1 cup	56	14
Banana	1 medium	108	13
Tomato	1 cup	38	11

ZINC

What it is: A mineral that regulates carbohydrate metabolism and blood sugar.
Why you need it: Stabilizes metabolism and blood sugar, helps immune system when you're sick, and heightens your sense of smell and taste. Also plays an important role in male fertility.

	SERVING SIZE	CALORIES	% DAILY VALUE
Broiled beef tenderloin	4 ounces	240	42
Roasted lamb (loin)	4 ounces	230	30
General Mills Cheerios	1 cup cereal with 1/2 cup skim milk	146	30
Wheat germ	1 ounce	101	23
Venison	4 ounces	180	21
Sesame seeds	1/4 cup	206	18
Pastrami	2 slices	82	18
Cooked green peas	1 cup	134	13
Steamed shrimp	4 ounces	112	12
Nonfat shredded mozzarella cheese	1 ounce	42	7

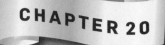

CHAPTER 20

The Best
(&Worst)
Food
Additives

The Incredible Hulk.
The Frankenstein monster.
Major League Baseball.

Don't we have enough evidence already that when scientists fool around with biology, things can go really, really wrong?

Sure, innovations like antibiotics, pain-free dentistry, and that stuff you rub between your toes to stop the itching are pretty great additions to modern life. But when it comes to our food supply, we'd prefer scientists leave well enough alone and put a little more trust in Mother Nature.

See, once upon a time, our food was created by cooks. Some of those cooks were highly paid fancy-pants types, like the great chefs who pioneered French cuisine and, later, fusion foods. But most of them were modest moms and grandmothers, slaving over hot stoves from the Americas to Europe to the Far East, who combined naturally grown grains and bits of meat and vegetables and spices and turned them into everything from spaghetti and meatballs to pad Thai to arroz con pollo. They took what nature handed them and made something miraculous from it.

But today, it's not cooks who are creating our packaged and fast foods anymore—it's teams of scientists. And as they continue to discover emulsifiers to make ice cream taste smoother or strange dyes to make our Popsicles redder, we get further and further away from real food—at least as our ancestors would recognize it. It takes a

Nutrition Facts

Serving Size 1/2 cup (104g)
Servings Per Container 4

Amount Per Serving

Calories 240   Calories from Fat 120

	% Daily Value*
Total Fat 14g	**21%**
Saturated Fat 9g	**47%**
Trans Fat 0g	
Cholesterol 60mg	**20%**
Sodium 50mg	**2%**
Total Carbohydrate 26g	**9%**
Dietary Fiber 1g	**2%**
Sugars 21g	
Protein 4g	

Vit[amin] A 10%	•	Vitamin C 0%
[Calc]ium 15%	•	Iron 4%

[Per]cent Daily Values are based on a 2,000 [c]alorie diet. Your daily values may be higher [o]r lower depending on your calorie needs.

	Calories:	2,000	2,500
Total Fat	Less than	65g	80g
Sat Fat	Less than	20g	25g
Cholesterol	Less than	300mg	300mg
Sodium	Less than	2,400mg	2,400mg
Total Carbohydrate		300g	375g

[IN]GREDIENTS: CREAM, SKIM MILK, LIQUID SUGAR, WATER, CHERRIES, EGG YOLKS, SUGAR, [CO]RN SYRUP, COCONUT OIL, HIGH FRUCTOSE CORN SYRUP, COCOA (PROCESSED WITH [AL]KALI), COCOA, NATURAL FLAVORS, CONCENTRATED LEMON JUICE, CARAMEL & RED [CA]BBAGE EXTRACT (FOR COLOR), GUAR GUM, [MI]LKFAT, SOYA LECITHIN, CARRAGEENAN.

22OA-N2O © Ben & Jerry's Homemade, Inc. 2008 [Cher]ry Garcia is a registered trademark of [th]e Estate of Jerry Garcia and is used under license.

VISIT OUR WEBSITE

TO FIND A SCOOP SHOP NEAREST YOU!

DAIRY K-204

USA
For Approval Numbers, See Bottom

Cherry Garcia

Cows: © Woody Jackson 1987
Your satisfaction guaranteed or your mon[ey]
container bottom, place # date of produ[ct]

Soya lecithin, carrageenan, guar gum: Would your grandma recognize this recipe for ice cream?

The Best (& Worst) Food Additives

degree in chemistry now to fully understand what we're putting into our bodies. And I promise you, my little Ukrainian grandmother never reached into her pantry for xanthan gum, propyl gallate, or phenylacetaldehyde dimethyl acetal to add to her pierogies.

The additives, food substitutes, and unpronounceable chemicals that now infuse our meals like mold through stale bread have two different types of effects on our bodies, which can be summed up thusly: those we understand and those we don't. I'll leave it up to you to decide which is the scarier of the two.

Among those things we do understand: Adding unnatural sweeteners like high-fructose corn syrup to everything from bread to cereal to ketchup has the effect of pushing the calorie counts of even the simplest foods

higher than ever before—meaning you don't have to eat more to weigh more. Adding unnaturally altered fats—called partially hydrogenated or inter-esterified fats—to baked goods and fried foods sharply increases your risk of heart disease and may be linked to everything from diabetes to Alzheimer's. And adding soy where it doesn't belong—everywhere from chocolate bars (you'll often see "soy lecithin" as an ingredient) to canned tuna (look for ingredients like soybean oil or vegetable broth, which can be made from soybeans)—can mess with our hormones, leading to fertility problems and, some research now indicates, eventual memory impairment.

That's what we know. But what about what we don't know? As you'll see from the list at right, a lot of food additives

still come with big black question marks next to their names. (That's why we're hesitant to label anything in this chapter "best.") In this chapter, we've given you what we know about these additives and their effects on your body—and nobody, even the scientists who invented this stuff, knows everything. Some, like ascorbic acid (a form of vitamin C), seem harmless and may even be beneficial. Others should be avoided like the plague. A basic rule of thumb: If you can't pronounce it, don't eat it. Instead, try to cut down on the number of ingredients in your food. There are still brands out there that cling to the last shreds of honesty in the world of packaged foods, products with blissfully few ingredients that represent what food used to be like and could one day be again.

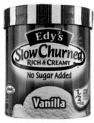

ACESULFAME POTASSIUM (ACESULFAME-K)

A calorie-free artificial sweetener often used with other artificial sweeteners to mask bitterness.

Found in: More than 5,000 food products worldwide, including diet soft drinks and no-sugar-added ice cream

Example: Edy's Slow Churned No Sugar Added Vanilla Light Ice Cream

What You Need to Know: The FDA has approved it for use in most foods, but some health groups claim that the decision was based on flawed tests. Animal studies have linked it to lung and breast tumors.

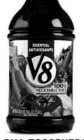

ALPHA-TOCOPHEROL

The form of vitamin E most commonly added to foods and most readily absorbed and stored in the body. An essential nutrient, it helps prevent oxidative damage to the cells and plays a crucial role in skin health and disease prevention.

Found in: Meats, foods with added fats, and foods that boast vitamin E health claims; also occurs naturally in seeds, nuts, leafy vegetables, and vegetable oils

Example: Campbell's Essential Antioxidants V8

What You Need to Know: In the amount added to foods, tocopherols pose no apparent health risks, but concentrated supplements might bring on toxicity symptoms such as cramps, weakness, and double vision.

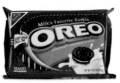

ARTIFICIAL FLAVORING

Denotes any of hundreds of allowable chemicals such as butyl alcohol and phenylacetaldehyde dimethyl acetal. The exact chemicals used in flavoring are the proprietary information of food processors, used to imitate specific fruits, butter, spices, and so on.

Found in: Thousands of highly processed foods such as cereals, beverages, and cookies

Example: Oreo cookies

What You Need to Know: The FDA has approved every item on the list of allowable chemicals, but because flavorings can hide behind a blanket term, there is no way for consumers to pinpoint the cause of a reaction they might have had.

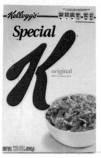

ASCORBIC ACID

The chemical name for the water-soluble vitamin C.

Found in: Juices and fruit products, meat, cereals, and other foods with vitamin C health claims

Example: Kellogg's Special K

What You Need to Know: Although vitamin C is associated with no known risks, it is often added to junk foods to make them appear healthy.

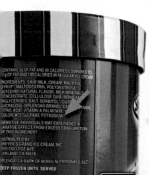

CONTAINS 3g OF FAT AND 90 CALORIES COMPARED TO 11g OF FAT AND 199 CALORIES IN REGULAR ICE CREAM

INGREDIENTS: SKIM MILK, CREAM, MALTITOL SYRUP, MALTODEXTRIN, POLYDEXTROSE, GLYCERIN, NATURAL FLAVOR, MILK MINERALS CONCENTRATE, CELLULOSE GUM, MONO- AND DIGLYCERIDES, SALT, SORBITOL, GUAR, SUCRALOSE (SPLENDA® BRAND), CARRAGEENAN, CITRIC ACID, VITAMIN A PALMITATE, COLOR, ACESULFAME POTASSIUM.

SENSITIVE INDIVIDUALS MAY EXPERIENCE A LAXATIVE EFFECT FROM EXCESS CONSUMPTION OF THIS INGREDIENT.

DISTRIBUTED BY DREYER'S GRAND ICE CREAM, INC. 5929 COLLEGE AVE OAKLAND, CA 94618

SPLENDA IS A MARK OF McNEIL NUTRITIONALS, LLC

KEEP FROZEN UNTIL SERVED

100% VEGETABLE JUICE
INGREDIENTS: TOMATO JUICE FROM CONCENTRATE (WATER, TOMATO CONCENTRATE), RECONSTITUTED VEGETABLE JUICE BLEND (WATER AND CONCENTRATED JUICES OF CARROTS, CELERY, BEETS, PARSLEY, LETTUCE, WATERCRESS, SPINACH), CONTAINS LESS THAN 2% OF THE FOLLOWING: SALT, VITAMIN C (ASCORBIC ACID), BETA CAROTENE, FLAVORING, VITAMIN E (ALPHA TOCOPHERYL ACETATE), ZINC GLUCONATE, CITRIC ACID.

INGREDIENTS: SUGAR, ENRICHED FLOUR (WHEAT FLOUR, NIACIN, REDUCED IRON, THIAMINE MONONITRATE (VITAMIN B1), RIBOFLAVIN (VITAMIN B2), FOLIC ACID), HIGH OLEIC CANOLA OIL AND/OR PALM OIL AND/OR CANOLA OIL AND/OR SOYBEAN OIL, COCOA (PROCESSED WITH ALKALI), HIGH FRUCTOSE CORN SYRUP, CORNSTARCH, LEAVENING (BAKING SODA AND/OR CALCIUM PHOSPHATE), SALT, SOY LECITHIN (EMULSIFIER), VANILLIN - AN ARTIFICIAL FLAVOR, CHOCOLATE.
CONTAINS: WHEAT, SOY.

CONTAINS WHEAT AND MILK INGREDIENTS.

Distributed by Kellogg Sales Co.
Battle Creek, MI 49016 USA
®, TM, © 2008 Kellogg NA Co.

Consumers: Visit Kelloggs.com
or call 1-800-962-1413

ASCORBIC ACID (VITAMIN C), ALPHA TOCOPHEROL ACETATE (VITAMIN E), REDUCED IRON, NIACINAMIDE, PYRIDOXINE HYDROCHLORIDE (VITAMIN B6), RIBOFLAVIN (VITAMIN B2), THIAMIN HYDROCHLORIDE (VITAMIN B1), VITAMIN A PALMITATE, FOLIC ACID AND VITAMIN B12.

No percentage for sugar is given since no Daily Value (DV) for sugars has not been established. The Institute of Medicine suggests that less than 25% of daily calories come from added sugars to help minimize the consumption of foods with empty calories (IOM, 2002/2005). For a 2,000 calorie diet, this would equal 12.5g of added sugar per day.

Exchange: 1½ Carbohydrates
The dietary exchanges are based on the Exchange Lists for Meal Planning. ©2003 by The American Diabetes Association, Inc. and The American Dietetic Association.

Consumers: Visit www.kelloggnutrition.com to learn how to use **Nutrition at a Glance™** for you and your family.

The Best (& Worst) Food Additives

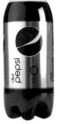

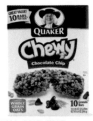

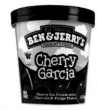

ASPARTAME

A near-zero-calorie artificial sweetener made by combining two amino acids with methanol. Most commonly used in diet soda, aspartame is 180 times sweeter than sugar.

Found in: More than 6,000 grocery items, including diet sodas, yogurts, and the tabletop sweeteners NutraSweet and Equal
Example: Diet Pepsi
What You Need to Know:
Over the past 30 years, the FDA has received thousands of consumer complaints due mostly to neurological symptoms such as headaches, dizziness, memory loss, and, in rare cases, epileptic seizures. Many studies have shown aspartame to be completely harmless, while others indicate that the additive might be responsible for a range of cancers.

BHA AND BHT (BUTYLATED HYDROXYANISOLE AND BUTYLATED HYDROXYTOLUENE)

Petroleum-derived antioxidants used to preserve fats and oils.

Found in: Beer, crackers, cereals, butter, and foods with added fats
Example: Quaker Chewy Granola Bar Chocolate Chip
What You Need to Know:
Of the two, BHA is considered the more dangerous. Studies have shown it to cause cancer in the forestomachs of rats, mice, and hamsters. The Department of Health and Human Services classifies the preservative as "reasonably anticipated to be a human carcinogen."

BLUE #1 (BRILLIANT BLUE) AND BLUE #2 (INDIGOTINE)

Synthetic dyes that can be used alone or combined with other dyes to make different colors.

Found in: Blue, purple, and green foods such as beverages, cereals, candy, and icing
Example: Skittles Original
What You Need to Know:
Both dyes have been loosely linked to cancers in animal studies, and the Center for Science in the Public Interest recommends that they be avoided.

CARRAGEENAN

A thickener, stabilizer, and emulsifier extracted from red seaweed.

Found in: Jellies and jams, ice cream, yogurt, and whipped topping
Example: Ben & Jerry's Cherry Garcia Ice Cream
What You Need to Know:
In animal studies, carrageenan has been shown to cause ulcers, colon inflammation, and digestive cancers. While these results seem limited to degraded carrageenan—a class that has been treated with heat and chemicals—a University of Iowa study concluded that even undegraded carrageenan could become degraded in the human digestive system.

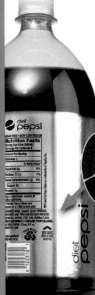

act], whole grain rolled wheat, partially with natural tocopherol added to prese veet chocolate chips (sugar, chocolate r, corn syrup solids, glycerin, partially artificial flavors, BHT (a preservative),

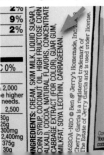

2%
9%
2%

0%

2,000
e higher
needs.
2,500

30g
25g
300mg
2,400mg
375g
30g

INGREDIENTS: CREAM, SKIM MILK, LIQUID SUGAR, CORN SYRUP, COCONUT OIL, HIGH FRUCTOSE CORN ALKALI), COCOA, NATURAL FLAVORS, CONCENTRATE CABBAGE EXTRACT FOR COLOR), GUAR GUM, MILKFAT, SOYA LECITHIN, CARRAGEENAN.

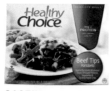

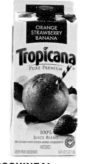

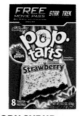

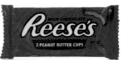

CASEIN

A milk protein used to thicken and whiten foods and appearing often by the name sodium caseinate. It is a good source of amino acids.

Found in: Protein bars, shakes, ice cream, and other frozen desserts
Example: Healthy Choice Beef Tips Portobello with Gravy
What You Need to Know: Although casein is a by-product of milk, the FDA allows it and its derivatives—sodium and calcium caseinates—to be used in "nondairy" and "dairy-free" creamers. Most lactose intolerants can handle casein, but those with broader milk allergies might experience reactions.

MALTODEXTRIN, DRIED WHEY, DRIED CAULIFLOWER, SESAME OIL), JVIGNON WINE, MODIFIED FOOD STARCH, BEEF EXTRACT, ROASTED RROT EXTRACT, MALTODEXTRIN, SOYBEAN OIL, AUTOLYZED YEAST, TE, CITRIC ACID, SODIUM BISULFITE AND BHT (TO PROMOTE COLOR RED CREAM (CREAM, NON-FAT MILK, CULTURE ENZYMES), SALI GAR, HIGH FRUCTOSE CORN SYRUP SUGAR, SOYBEAN OIL, HONEY, FAT MILK SOLIDS, SODIUM CASEINATE, (TOCOPHEROL), CARAMEL FLAVOR

ConAgra Foods Inc.
ConAgra Foods® P.O. Box 3768, Dept. H
Omaha, NE 68103-0768 U.S.A.

COCHINEAL EXTRACT OR CARMINE

A pigment extracted from the dried eggs and bodies of the female Dactylopius coccus, a beetlelike insect that preys on cactus plants. It is added to food for its dark-crimson color.

Found in: Artificial crabmeat, fruit juices, frozen-fruit snacks, candy, and yogurt
Example: Tropicana Orange Strawberry Banana
What You Need to Know: Cochineal extract is comprised of about 90 percent insect-body fragments. Although the FDA receives very few complaints, some organizations are asking for a mandatory warning label to accompany cochineal-colored foods.

• Percent Daily Values are based on a 2,000 calorie diet.

Ingredients: 100% Pure orange juice, banana puree concentrate, grape juice concentrate, strawberry juice concentrate, cochineal extract (color) and natural flavors.

Tropicana Manufacturing Company, Inc.

CORN SYRUP

A liquid sweetener and food thickener made by allowing enzymes to break corn starches into smaller sugars. USDA subsidies to the corn industry make it cheap and abundant, placing it among the most ubiquitous ingredients in grocery food products.

Found in: Every imaginable food category, including bread, soup, sauces, frozen dinners, and frozen treats
Example: Kellogg's Pop-Tarts Frosted Strawberry
What You Need to Know: Corn syrup provides no nutritional value other than calories. In moderation, it poses no specific threat—other than an expanded waistline.

Calories per gram: Fat 9 • Carbohydrate 4

INGREDIENTS: ENRICHED FLOUR (WHEAT FLOUR, NIACINA IRON, THIAMIN MONONITRATE [VITAMIN B₁], RIBOFLAVIN [VI ACID), CORN SYRUP, HIGH FRUCTOSE CORN SYRUP, DEXTR OIL (SOYBEAN, PALM, COTTONSEED AND/OR HYDROGENAT OIL) WITH TBHQ AND CITRIC ACID FOR FRESHNESS), SUGAR, CONTAINS TWO PERCENT OR LESS OF WHEAT STARCH, SALT BERRIES, DRIED APPLES, DRIED PEARS, CORNSTARCH, LEA SODA, SODIUM ACID PYROPHOSPHATE, MONOCALCIUM PHO ACID, MILLED CORN, MODIFIED WHEAT STARCH, GELATIN, C MONO- AND DIGLYCERIDES, SODIUM STEAROYL LACTYLAT TIALLY HYDROGENATED SOYBEAN AND/OR COTTONSEED CORN STARCH, XANTHAN GUM, SOY LECITHIN, COLOR ADDE

DEXTROSE

A corn-derived caloric sweetener. Like corn syrup, dextrose contributes to the American habit of more than 200 calories of corn sweeteners per day.

Found in: Bread, cookies, and crackers
Example: Reese's Peanut Butter Cups
What You Need to Know: As with other sugars, dextrose is safe in moderate amounts.

Nutrition Facts   Amount/serving %DV² Amount/servin
Total Fat 12 g   00%   Total Carb 24

INGREDIENTS: MILK CHOCOLATE (SUGAR, COCOA BUTTER, CHOCO EMULSIFIER); PEANUTS; SUGAR; DEXTROSE; SALT; TBHQ (PRESER
Mfd. by **H.B. Reese Candy Co.**
Hershey, PA 17033-0815, U.S.A.
A Division of **The Hershey Company**

337

The Best (& Worst) Food Additives

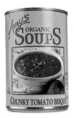

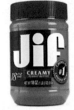

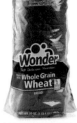

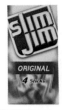

EVAPORATED CANE JUICE

A sweetener derived from sugarcane, the same plant used to make refined table sugar. It's also known as crystallized cane juice, cane juice, or cane sugar. Because it's subject to less processing than table sugar, evaporated cane juice retains slightly more nutrients from the grassy cane sugar.

Found in: Yogurt, soy milk, protein bars, granola, cereal, chicken sausages, and other natural or organic foods

Example: Amy's Organic Chunky Tomato Bisque Soup

What You Need to Know: Although pristine sugars are often used to replace ordinary sugars in "healthier" foods, the actual nutritional difference between the sugars is miniscule. Both should be consumed in moderation.

FULLY HYDROGENATED VEGETABLE OIL

Extremely hard, wax-like fat made by forcing as much hydrogen as possible onto the carbon backbone of fat molecules. To obtain a manageable consistency, food manufacturers often blend the hard fat with unhydrogenated liquid fats.

Found in: Baked goods, frozen meals, and tub margarine

Example: Jif Creamy Peanut Butter

What You Need to Know: In theory, fully hydrogenated oils, as opposed to partially hydrogenated oils, should contain zero trans fat. But the process of hydrogenation isn't completely perfect, which means that trans fat will inevitably occur in small amounts.

HIGH-FRUCTOSE CORN SYRUP (HFCS)

A corn-derived sweetener representing more than 40 percent of all caloric sweeteners in the supermarket. In 2005, there were 59 pounds produced per person.

Found in: Nearly everything: ice cream, chips, cereal, bread, ketchup, canned fruits, yogurt, and two-thirds of all sweetened beverages

Example: Wonder Bread Whole Grain Wheat

What You Need to Know: Since 1980, the US obesity rate has risen proportionately to the increase in HFCS, and Americans are now consuming at least 200 calories of the sweetener each day. Still, research shows that the body metabolizes HFCS no differently than sugar.

HYDROLYZED VEGETABLE PROTEIN (HVP)

A flavor enhancer created when heat and chemicals are used to break down vegetables—most often soy—into their component amino acids. HVP allows food processors to achieve stronger flavors from fewer ingredients.

Found in: Canned soups and chili, frozen dinners, beef- and chicken-flavored products

Example: Slim Jim Meat Sticks

What You Need to Know: One effect of hydrolyzing proteins is the creation of MSG, or monosodium glutamate. When MSG in food is the result of hydrolyzed protein, the FDA does not require it to be listed on the packaging.

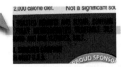

INTERESTERIFIED FAT

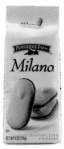

Developed in response to demand for trans-fat alternatives, this semisoft fat is created by chemically blending fully hydrogenated and nonhydrogenated oils.

Found in: Pastries, margarine, frozen dinners, and canned soups
Example: Pepperidge Farm Milano Cookies
What You Need to Know: Testing on these fats has not been extensive, but the early evidence doesn't look promising. A study by Malaysian researchers showed a 4-week diet of 12 percent interesterified fats increased the ratio of LDL to HDL cholesterol, not a good thing. This study also showed an increase in blood glucose levels and a decrease in insulin response.

MADE FROM: UNBLEACHED ENRICHED WHEAT FLOUR (FLOUR, NIACIN, REDUCED IRON, THIAMIN MONONITRATE [VITAMIN B1], RIBOFLAVIN [VITAMIN B2], FOLIC ACID), SEMI-SWEET CHOCOLATE (SUGAR, CHOCOLATE LIQUOR, COCOA BUTTER, CHOCOLATE LIQUOR PROCESSED WITH ALKALI (DUTCHED), MILK FAT, SOY LECITHIN ADDED AS AN EMULSIFIER, VANILLA EXTRACT), SUGAR, VEGETABLE OILS (PALM AND/OR INTERESTERIFIED AND HYDROGENATED SOYBEAN AND/OR HYDROGENATED COTTONSEED), NONFAT MILK, WHOLE EGGS, CONTAINS 2 PERCENT OR LESS OF: CORNSTARCH, EGG WHITES, SALT, NATURAL FLAVOR, BAKING SODA AND SOY LECITHIN.

LECITHIN

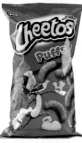

A naturally occurring emulsifier and antioxidant that retards the rancidity of fats. The two major sources of lecithin as an additive are egg yolks and soybeans.

Found in: Pastries, ice cream, and margarine
Example: Nutella
What You Need to Know: Lecithin is an excellent source of choline and inositol, compounds that help cells and nerves communicate and play a role in breaking down fats and cholesterol. There is some concern, however, that the naturally occurring estrogens in soy lecithin can cause hormonal problems in men who consume excessive amounts of it.

MALTODEXTRIN

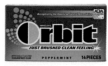

A caloric sweetener and flavor enhancer made from rice, potatoes, or, more commonly, cornstarch. Through treatment with enzymes and acids, it can be converted into a fiber and thickening agent.

Found in: Canned fruit, instant pudding, sauces, dressings, chips, and chocolates
Example: Cheetos Cheese Snacks
What You Need to Know: Like other sugars, maltodextrin has the potential to raise blood glucose and insulin levels.

Dietary Fiber	
Calories per gram:	
Fat 9	• Carbohydrate 4

Ingredients: Enriched Corn Meal Sulfate, Niacin, Thiamin Mononitrat Acid), Vegetable Oil (Contains Following: Corn, Soybean, or Su Seasoning (Whey, Cheddar Ch Cultures, Salt, Enzymes], and L Following: Partially Hydrogenate Maltodextrin, Disodium Phosphate, Cream, Nonfat Milk], Artificial Glutamate, Lactic Acid, Artificial C 6], Citric Acid), and Salt.
CONTAINS MILK INGREDIENTS.

MANNITOL

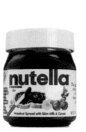

A sugar alcohol that's 70 percent as sweet as sugar. It provides fewer calories and has a less drastic effect on blood sugar.

Found in: Sugar-free candy, low-calorie and diet foods, and chewing gum
Example: Orbit Peppermint Sugar-Free Gum
What You Need to Know: Because sugar alcohols are not fully digested, they can cause intestinal discomfort, gas, bloating, flatulence, and diarrhea. But in small quantities, you should be safe from any ill effects.

MADE OF: SORBITOL, GUM BASE, GLYCEROL, MANNITOL, NATURAL AND ARTIFICIAL FLAVORS, LESS THAN 2% OF: XYLITOL, ACESULFAME K, ASPARTAME, SOY LECITHIN, BHT (TO MAINTAIN FRESHNESS), SUFAME K, ASPARTAME, SOY LECITHIN. PHENYLKETONURICS: CONTAINS PHENYLALANINE.

The Best (& Worst) Food Additives

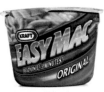

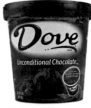

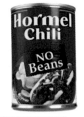

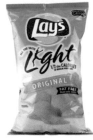

MODIFIED FOOD STARCH

A catch-all term describing starches (derived from corn, wheat, potato, or rice) that are modified to change their response to heat or cold, improve their texture, and create efficient emulsifiers, among other reasons.

Found in: Most highly processed foods, low-calorie and diet foods, cookies, frozen meals

Example: Kraft Easy Mac

What You Need to Know: The starches themselves appear safe, but the nondisclosure of the chemicals used in processing causes some nutritionists to question their effects on health.

MONO- AND DIGLYCERIDES

Fats added to foods to bind liquids with fats. They occur naturally in foods and constitute about 1 percent of normal fats.

Found in: Peanut butter, ice cream, margarine, baked goods, and whipped topping

Example: Dove Unconditional Chocolate Ice Cream

What You Need to Know: Aside from being a source of fat, the glycerides themselves pose no serious health threats.

MONOSODIUM GLUTAMATE (MSG)

The salt of the amino acid glutamic acid, used to enhance the savory quality of foods. MSG alone has little flavor, and exactly how it enhances other foods is unknown.

Found in: Chili, soup, and foods with chicken or beef flavoring

Example: Hormel Chili No Beans

What You Need to Know: Studies have shown that MSG injected into mice causes brain-cell damage, but the FDA believes these results are not typical for humans. The FDA receives dozens of reaction complaints each year for nausea, headaches, chest pains, and weakness.

OLESTRA

A synthetic fat created by pharmaceutical company Procter & Gamble and sold under the name Olean. It has zero-calorie impact and is not absorbed as it passes through the digestive system.

Found in: Light chips and crackers

Example: Lay's Light Original Potato Chips

What You Need to Know: Olestra can cause diarrhea, intestinal cramps, and flatulence. Studies show that it impairs the body's ability to absorb fat-soluble vitamins and vital carotenoids such as beta-carotene, lycopene, lutein, and zeaxanthin.

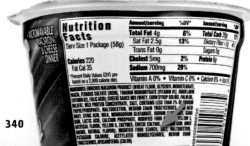

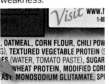

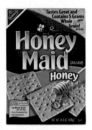

PARTIALLY HYDROGENATED VEGETABLE OIL

A manufactured fat created by forcing hydrogen gas into vegetable fats under extremely high pressure, an unintended effect of which is the creation of trans-fatty acids. Food processors like this fat because of its low cost and long shelf life.

Found in: Margarine, pastries, frozen foods, cakes, cookies, crackers, soups, and nondairy creamers

Example: Honey Maid Graham Crackers

What You Need to Know: Trans fat has been shown to contribute to heart disease more so than saturated fat. While most health organizations recommend keeping trans-fat consumption as low as possible, a loophole in the FDA's labeling requirements allows processors to add as much as 0.49 gram per serving and still claim zero in their nutrition facts. Progressive jurisdictions such as New York City, California, and Boston have approved legislation to phase trans fat out of restaurants, and pressure from watchdog groups might eventually lead to a full ban on the dangerous oil.

REDIENTS: ENRICHED FLOUR (WHEAT FLOUR, NIAC
DUCED IRON, THIAMINE MONONITRATE (VITAMIN B
OFLAVIN (VITAMIN B2), FOLIC ACID), SUGAR, GRAH
UR (WHOLE GRAIN WHEAT FLOUR), SOYBEAN
D/OR PARTIALLY HYDROGENATED COTTONSEED OIL, H
UCTOSE CORN SYRUP, HONEY, LEAVENING (BAKING SO
D/OR CALCIUM PHOSPHATE), SALT, ARTIFICIAL FLAVC
Y LECITHIN - AN EMULSIFIER, CORNSTARCH.

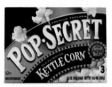

PROPYL GALLATE

An antioxidant used often in conjunction with BHA and BHT to retard the rancidity of fats.

Found in: Mayonnaise, margarine, oils, dried meats, pork sausage, and other fatty foods

Example: Pop-Secret Kettle Corn

What You Need to Know: Rat studies in the early '80s linked propyl gallate to brain cancer. Although these studies don't provide sound evidence, it is advisable to avoid this chemical when possible.

NTS: WHOLE GRAIN POPC(
LY HYDROGENATED SOYBEA
CRALOSE, NONFAT MILK.
ED BY PROPYL GALLATE.
S MILK INGREDIENTS.

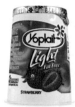

RED #3 (ERYTHROSINE) AND RED #40 (ALLURA RED)

Food dyes that are cherry red and orange red, respectively. Red #40 is the most widely used food dye in America.

Found in: Fruit cocktail, candy, chocolate cake, cereal, beverages, pastries, maraschino cherries, and fruit snacks

Example: Yoplait Light Fat Free Strawberry

What You Need to Know: The FDA has proposed a ban on Red #3 in the past, but so far the agency has been unsuccessful in implementing it. After the dye was inextricably linked to thyroid tumors in rat studies, the FDA managed to have the liquid form of the dye removed from external drugs and cosmetics.

HIGH IN CALCIUM
WITH ACTIVE YOGURT CULTURES
INCLUDING L. ACIDOPHILUS
INGREDIENTS: CULTURED PASTEUR-
IZED GRADE A NONFAT MILK, HIGH
FRUCTOSE CORN SYRUP, STRAWBER-
RIES, MODIFIED CORN STARCH,
NONFAT MILK, KOSHER GELATIN,
CITRIC ACID, TRICALCIUM PHOS-
PHATE, *ASPARTAME, POTASSIUM
SORBATE ADDED TO MAINTAIN
FRESHNESS, NATURAL FLAVOR, RED
#40, VITAMIN A ACETATE, VITAMIN D₃

DISTRIBUTED BY YOPLAIT USA, INC.
BOX 200 YC, MPLS, MN 55440 USA

tion Facts
1 container
Calories from Fat 0
% Daily Value*
0%
Fat 0g
0%
0g
erol less than 5mg
1%
0mg
4%

The Best (& Worst) Food Additives

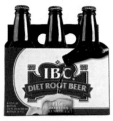

SACCHARIN

An artificial sweetener 300 to 500 times sweeter than sugar. Discovered in 1879, it's the oldest of the 5 FDA-approved artificial sweeteners.

Found in: Diet foods, chewing gum, toothpaste, beverages, sugar-free candy, and Sweet 'N Low

Example: IBC Diet Root Beer

What You Need to Know: Rat studies in the early '70s showed saccharin to cause bladder cancer, and the FDA, reacting to these studies, enacted a mandatory warning label to be printed on every saccharin-containing product on the market. The mandate was removed after 20 years, but the question over saccharin's safety was never resolved. More recent studies show that rats on saccharin-rich diets gain more weight than those on high-sugar diets.

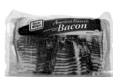

SODIUM NITRITE AND SODIUM NITRATE

Preservatives used to prevent bacterial growth and maintain the pinkish color of meats and fish.

Found in: Bacon, sausage, hot dogs, and cured, canned, and packaged meats

Example: Oscar Mayer Bacon

What You Need to Know: Under certain conditions, sodium nitrite and nitrate react with amino acids to form cancer-causing chemicals called nitrosamines. This reaction can be hindered by the addition of ascorbic acid, erythorbic acid, or alpha-tocopherol.

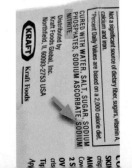

SORBITOL

A sugar alcohol that occurs naturally in some fruits. It's about 60 percent as sweet as sugar and used to both sweeten and thicken.

Found in: Dried fruit, chewing gum, and reduced-sugar candy

Example: Fudgsicle No Sugar Added

What You Need to Know: Sorbitol is digested slower than sugars, which makes it a better choice for diabetics. But like other sugar alcohols, it can cause intestinal discomfort, gas, bloating, flatulence, and diarrhea.

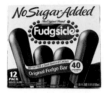

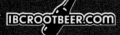

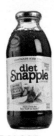

SUCRALOSE

A zero-calorie artificial sweetener made by joining chlorine particles and sugar molecules. It's 600 times sweeter than sugar and largely celebrated as the least damaging of the artificial sweeteners.

Found in: Sugar-free foods, pudding, beverages, some diet sodas, and Splenda

Example: Snapple Diet Lemonade Tea

What You Need to Know: After reviewing more than 110 human and animal studies, the FDA concluded that use of sucralose does not cause cancer. The sweetener is one of only 3 artificial sweeteners deemed safe by the Center for Science in the Public Interest.

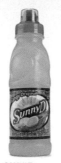

YELLOW #5 (TARTRAZINE) AND YELLOW #6 (SUNSET YELLOW)

The second and third most common food colorings, respectively.

Found in: Cereal, pudding, bread mix, beverages, chips, cookies, and condiments

Example: SunnyD Original

What You Need to Know: Several studies have linked both dyes to learning and concentration disorders in children, and there are piles of animal studies demonstrating potential risks such as kidney and intestinal tumors. One study found that mice fed high doses of sunset yellow had trouble righting themselves in water. The FDA does not view these as serious risks to humans.

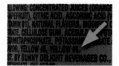

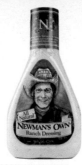

XANTHAN GUM

An extremely common emulsifier and thickener made from glucose in a reaction requiring a slimy bacteria called Xanthomonas campestris—*the same bacterial strain that appears as black rot on cruciferous vegetables like broccoli.*

Found in: Whipped topping, dressings, marinades, custard, and pie filling

Example: Newman's Own Ranch Dressing

What You Need to Know: Xanthan gum is associated with no adverse effects.

CANOLA OIL), WATER, BUTTERMILK (MILK),
VINEGAR, SUGAR, EGG YOLK, GARLI
LT, CONTAINS 2% OR LESS OF: BUTTERM
(MILK), ONION*, GARLIC*, NA
R, LACTIC ACID, XANTHAN GUM, LEMO
CE CONCENTRATE. CHIVES. SPICE *DRIED

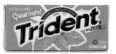

XYLITOL

A sugar alcohol that occurs naturally in strawberries, mushrooms, and other fruits and vegetables. It is most commonly extracted from the pulp of the birch tree.

Found in: Sugar-free candy, yogurt, and beverages

Example: Trident Spearmint Sugarless Gum with Xylitol

What You Need to Know: Unlike real sugar, sugar alcohols don't encourage cavity-causing bacteria. They do have a laxative effect, though, so heavy ingestion might cause intestinal discomfort or gas.

ent Daily Values (DV) are
d on a 2,000 calorie diet.

EAL TEA STARTS WITH THE FINEST TE
AND IS MADE FROM: FILTERED WATER
JUICE CONCENTRATE, NATURAL FLAVO
A, POTASSIUM CITRATE, SUCRALOSE, ACESULFAME
UM.   Ⓚ KOSHER PAREVE
tains 41 mg per 1 cup serving/81 mg per
f natural antioxidants (as tea polyphenols).

LOWING: CONCENTRATED JUICES (ORAN
PEFRUIT), CITRIC ACID, ASCORBIC ACID (
AMIN C), NATURAL FLAVORS, MODIFIE
TATE, CELLULOSE GUM, ACESULFA
METAPHOSPHATE, POTASSIU
TOR, YELLOW #5, YELLOW #6
ST. BY SUNNY DELIGHT BEVERAGES CO.

INGREDIENTS: SORBITOL, GUM BASE, XYLITOL, GLYCERIN, NATURAL AND ARTIFICIAL FLAVORING, MANNITOL, ASPART
ACESULFAME POTASSIUM, SOY LECITHIN, YELLOW 5 LAKE, BLUE 1 LAKE AND BHT (TO MAINTAIN FRESHNESS).
© 2006   **PHENYLKETONURICS: CONTAINS PHENYLALANINE**   Comments?
CADBURY ADAMS USA LLC DIST: CADBURY ADAMS USA LLC, PARSIPPANY, NJ 07054 Call 1-800-524-2

The Purest Packaged

LESS IS ALWAYS MORE IN THE SUPERMARKET, WHICH IS WHAT MAKES

Packaged foods typically come teeming with unpronounceable food additives. The good news is that not all pre-made products are so overprocessed. It's rare, but certain boxed and bagged items lining your grocery aisles contain natural ingredients and—prepare yourself for this—actual food. Here are a few of the best-of-the-best packaged foods almost completely un-tainted by suspicious additives.

BEST PLAIN YOGURT

Stonyfield Farm Oikos Organic Greek Yogurt (Plain)

Cultured pasteurized organic nonfat milk. Contains five live and active cultures, including L. acidophilus, L. bifidus, and L. casei.

- 80 calories (per 5.3 ounces)
- 0 g fat
- 15 g protein
- 6 g sugars

Fruit-flavored yogurts contain as much high-fructose corn syrup as they do actual fruit. This cup trades in the sugar for a double shot of protein.

BEST INSTANT RICE

Uncle Ben's Ready Rice Whole Grain Brown

Whole grain par-boiled brown rice, canola oil, and/or sunflower oil

- 220 calories (per 1 cup cooked)
- 4 g fat (0.5 g saturated)
- 5 g protein
- 2 g fiber
- 41 g carbo-hydrates

It takes just 90 seconds to pre-pare this perfect side to your lunch-time salad. There may be better whole grains, but in terms of convenience, Uncle Ben is hard to top.

BEST READY-TO-EAT TUNA

Ortiz Bonito del Norte in Olive Oil

White tuna, olive oil, sea salt

- 160 calories (per ¼ cup)
- 11 g fat
- 14 g protein

Sure, it's more expensive than the standard canned kind. But it tastes so delicious you can skip the mayo. Try it flaked on anything: salads, pasta, sandwiches, or a pile of Triscuits.

BEST COTTAGE CHEESE

Friendship 4% California Style

Cultured pasteurized grade A skim milk, milk, cream, salt

- 110 calories (per ½ cup)
- 5 g fat (3 g saturated)
- 15 g protein
- 0 g fiber
- 2 g sugars
- 380 mg sodium
- 3 g carbo-hydrates

Cottage cheese makes a low-calorie afternoon snack. And the protein is great for postworkout fuel.

Foods in America

THESE UNADULTERATED EATS SO GREAT

BEST
FRUIT JUICE
Lakewood Organic Pure Cranberry

Fresh pressed juice from certified organic cranberries

- 70 calories (per 8 ounces)
- 0 g fat
- 10 g sugars

Most juices—even 100 percent juices—are made mostly from apple and white grape juices, since they're inexpensive and high in natural sugars. Juice should have one ingredient: the fruit that's on the label. Lakewood offers exactly that.

BEST CEREAL
Post Shredded Wheat

Whole grain wheat

- 160 calories (per 1 cup)
- 1 g fat
- 6 g fiber
- 0 g sugars
- 0 mg sodium
- 40 g carbo-hydrates

You won't find another cereal as pure as Post. The more fiber you consume in the morning, the fewer calories you'll consume later in the day.

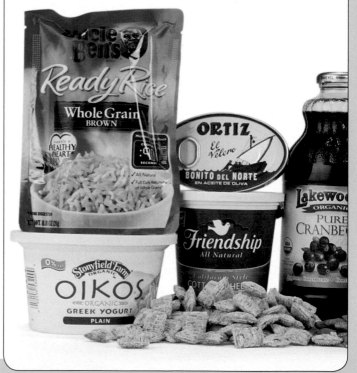

Tuna, olive oil, salt
Ortiz Bonito del Norte

345

The Purest Packaged Foods in America—*Continued*

Dates, pecans, almonds
Lärabar Pecan Pie

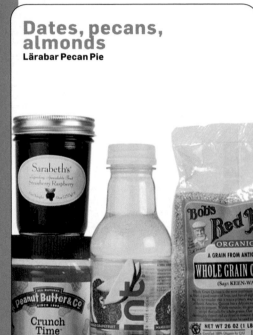

BEST ALMONDS

Blue Diamond Natural Oven-Roasted Almonds

Almonds

- 170 calories (per 24 nuts)
- 15 g fat (1 g saturated)
- 6 g protein
- 3 g fiber
- 0 mg sodium
- 5 g carbohydrates

Almonds are an excellent source of protein and heart-healthy fats. Enjoy them in their purest state.

BEST SNACK BAR

Lärabar Pecan Pie

Dates, pecans, almonds

- 200 calories (per bar)
- 14 g fat (1 g saturated)
- 3 g protein
- 4 g fiber
- 16 g sugars

Lärabar bucks the trend of bogus bars spiked with added sugars and hidden fats by making tasty treats with just dried fruit and nuts.

BEST JELLY

Sarabeth's Strawberry Raspberry Preserves

Strawberries, raspberries, sugar, lemon juice

- 40 calories (per 1 Tbsp)
- 0 g fat
- 9 g sugars

Most jams and jellies come packed with a candy bar's worth of sugar. Sarabeth's is almost all fruit (with just a little sugar added)—so it's both delicious and safe for your blood sugar levels.

BEST PEANUT BUTTER

Peanut Butter & Co. Crunch Time

Peanuts, salt

- 190 calories (per 2 Tbsp)
- 16 g fat (2 g saturated)
- 8 g protein
- 2 g fiber
- 40 mg sodium

Too many major peanut butter brands rely on partially hydrogenated oils in their products—meaning they come packed with hidden artery-clogging trans fat. Peanut butter should never have more than 2 ingredients. You may have to stir a bit before using, but it's worth it in the name of a healthier heart.

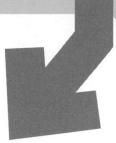

BEST FLAVORED WATER
Hint Mango Grapefruit

Purified water with mango, grapefruit, and other natural flavors

- *0 calories*
- *0 g fat*
- *0 g sugars*

The cooler section is overcrowded with so-called functional beverages, each one claiming to offer a robust package of vitamins and nutrients. What they really offer, though, is a glut of excess sugar and unpronounceable ingredients. This refreshing beverage contains no calories, sugar, or artificial sweeteners—just H$_2$0 and a touch of fruit.

BEST GRAIN
Bob's Red Mill Organic Quinoa

Organic whole grain quinoa

- *170 calories (per $1/4$ cup, uncooked)*
- *2.5 g fat*
- *7 g protein*
- *3 g fiber*

The Incas, lovers of this oft-overlooked seed, knew a thing or two about nutrition. Quinoa is rich in protein, packs twice the fiber of brown rice, and contains all of the essential amino acids your body needs for peak performance. Use it as a substitute for rice or toss it with roasted asparagus and goat cheese for an amazing salad.

BEST SOUP
Lucini Italia Rustic Italian Minestrone Soup

Filtered water, San Marzano plum tomatoes, Lucini premium select extra virgin olive oil, celery, carrots, potatoes, borlotti beans, string beans, penne rigate pasta, chick peas, peas, spinach, onion, sea salt, parsley, garlic, basil, chili pepper, oregano

- *160 calories (per 1 cup)*
- *7 g fat (1.5 g saturated)*
- *6 g protein*
- *9 g fiber*
- *760 mg sodium*

Plenty of ingredients, but they're almost exclusively A-list, fiber-rich vegetables.

BEST FROZEN VEGETABLE
Birds Eye Garden Peas

Peas

- *70 calories (per $2/3$ cup)*
- *4 g fiber*
- *12 g carbohydrates*

Frozen meals tend to come with ingredient lists dozens of items long. Stick to simpler frozen items, like these versatile peas, and you reap the same cost benefits and make huge gains in nutrition.

BEST SLICED DELI MEAT
Hormel Natural Choice Oven-Roasted Deli Turkey

Turkey breast meat, water, natural salt, natural turbinado sugar, carrageenan (from seaweed), baking soda

- *60 calories (per 4 slices)*
- *1 g fat*
- *10 g protein*
- *440 mg sodium*

The Hormel Natural Choice line of sliced meats is one of the only lines of deli cuts that avoid nitrates and nitrites. While there are one or two more ingredients in here than we'd like, when it comes to simplicity, it still trounces the competition.

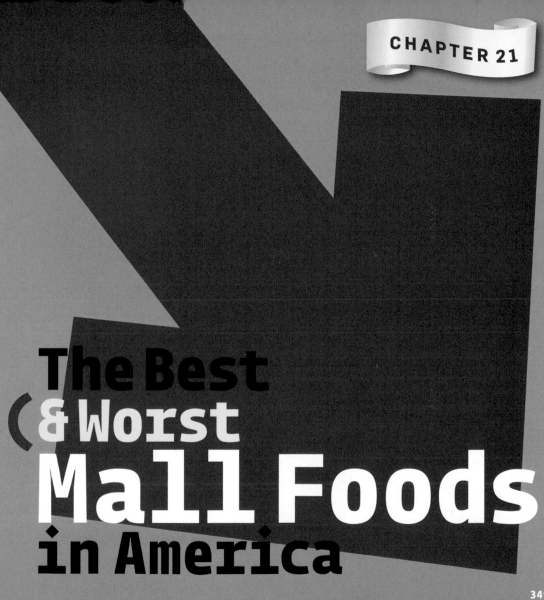

CHAPTER 21

The Best (& Worst Mall Foods in America

Eat This

Auntie Anne's Cinnamon Sugar Pretzel

No butter

380 calories
1 g fat
(0 g saturated)
29 g sugars
84 g carbohydrates

Save 55 g fat!
Plus, cut 10 bacon strips' worth of saturated fat from your diet.

Save 730 calories!
And those calories are the worst kind—almost pure added fat and refined carbs.

Trans fat free!
A rare feat in the world of mall sweets.

Not That!

Cinnabon Regular Caramel Pecanbun

1,110 calories
56 g fat
(10 g saturated, 5 g trans)
47 g sugars
141 g carbohydrates

The only speck of nutrition to be found in the bun comes from the nuts. Too bad they're coated in a river of sugar.

This isn't breakfast, this is dessert. And an atrocious one at that. There are dozens of ways to curb a sweets craving at the mall, but your sugar fix should never climb above 400 calories.

If the food court at your local mall had a slogan, it would say: Resistance Is Futile.

Because no matter how dedicated you are to eating well, the mall is the perfect machine for dashing your discipline and sending you careening over the edge of the carbohydrate canyon.

In the airtight electric ecosystem of the mall, all signs point to consumption. See, studies have shown that the more temptation people resist, the harder it becomes to continue resisting. That means after hours of being surrounded by last-minute offers and cloying salespeople, your ability to stave off the enticing edibles of the mall food court may be severely compromised. And when you've already dropped a few hundred bucks at Radio Shack or Gap, what's another 5 bucks on that warm, gooey little snack with an aroma that's wafting in the air like a sugarplum dream? Problem is, that "little snack" could translate into half a day's worth of calories, and that $5 is likely your worst investment of the day.

The same seven or eight places are found in nearly every mall in America—the greasy Chinese buffet line, the oversize-pizza-slice purveyor, the pretzel lady. It's up to you to have enough nutritional wherewithal to avoid being handed a weighty sentence in the food court. What follows is a list of the worst foods we discovered in our scramble to save shoppers serious calories. Proceed with caution.

1,025 calories

Panda Express Orange Chicken with Fried Rice

Orange chicken, General Tso's, and sweet and sour chicken make up a troubling trinity of calamitous chicken dishes found at Chinese places. All are floured, fried, and sauced with nondescript sugar-based sauces. And all are lousy for you.

The Worst Mall Foods in America

WORST HOT DOG
12 Hot Dog on a Stick's Hot Dog on a Bun

- *470 calories*
- *26 g fat (12 g saturated)*
- *1,220 mg sodium*

The name of the store is Hot Dog on a Stick—and when you venture from that concept, choosing the traditional bun-swaddled dog, you add 200 calories to your lunch, not to mention tripling your intake of saturated fat. Want a meal that you can carry while you shop? Pick the stick over the bun every time (and make sure to pass on the 700-calorie side of fries!).

Eat This Instead!
Hot Dog on a Stick
- *250 calories • 14 g fat (4 g saturated)*
- *780 mg sodium*

WORST SNACK
11 Auntie Anne's Sesame Pretzel
with Hot Salsa Cheese Dip

- *510 calories*
- *18 g fat (7 g saturated)*
- *1,440 mg sodium*

Auntie Anne can be like the old calorie-pushing hag from Hansel and Gretel if

you're not careful. The secret to success (or failure) at her pretzel lair is choosing your condiments wisely. Skip the butter and salt and be sure to find a solid dip. The Hot Cheese Salsa is the worst dip, and marinara's the best (by a healthy margin); start there and work backward.

Eat This Instead!
Jalapeño Pretzel with Marinara, no butter, no salt
- *320 calories • 1 g fat*
- *810 mg sodium*

WORST SLICE OF PIZZA
10 Sbarro Stuffed Pepperoni Pizza (1 slice)

- *890 calories*
- *42 g fat*
- *3,200 mg sodium*

The architecture of this thing makes it less like a slice of pizza and more like a pizza-inspired Chipotle Burrito. It relies on an oversize shell of oily bread to hold together a gooey wad of cheese and pepperoni. The net result is a pizza pocket with two-thirds of your day's fat and more than a day's worth of sodium. And the traditional

pizza slices aren't much better; few fall below 600 calories. If you want to do well at Sbarro, think thin crust with nothing but produce on top.

Eat This Instead!
New York Style Fresh Tomato Pizza (1 slice)
- *450 calories • 14 g fat*
- *1,040 mg sodium*

WORST BURGER
9 Five Guys Bacon Cheeseburger

- *920 calories*
- *62 g fat (29.5 g saturated)*
- *1,310 mg sodium*

We applaud Five Guys, first for their delicious burgers and second because said burgers don't come coated with trans-fatty oils (unlike too many of their competitors). But their regular-size burgers are still way too big, and the fact that they call their substantial single-patty option a "small" burger encourages overconsumption. The bacon cheeseburger is the most caloric, but none of the other options are less than 700 calories either. Instead, consider a "little" burger, which will

1,070 calories
Panera Bread Full Chipotle Chicken

There are 2 sides to the chicken sandwich genre: the lean grilled chicken breast, produce-topped and weighing in around 400 calories, and this, the bacon-veiled, condiment catastrophe with dizzying amounts of calories. Know the difference.

fill your stomach without requiring you to plug a new hole at the end of your belt. Plus, you can load it up with all the produce you want.

Eat This Instead!
Little Hamburger
· 480 calories · 26 g fat
(11.5 g saturated) · 380 mg sodium
· 39 g carbohydrates

WORST FROZEN TREAT

8 Dairy Queen Georgia Mud Fudge Blizzard (medium)

· 1,010 calories
· 54 g fat
(16 g saturated, 4 g trans)
· 97 g sugars

Somehow the Blizzard and its ilk have become so commonplace that they seem to slip unnoticed beneath the radar of normal nutritional pru-

dence. It's just an innocent cup of ice cream, right? Eh, not exactly. Dairy Queen blends its Blizzards with copious amounts of fat and sugar, and not a single one of any size has less than 1 gram of trans fat. Until DQ agrees to use a lighter cream, we can't endorse a Blizzard of any size or flavor. Nor can we endorse any of their malts,

Conquer the Food Court

5 SAVVY STRATEGIES FOR ENLIGHTENED MALL MUNCHING

Be a Bargain Shopper
You spend countless hours comparing prices and hunting for bargains, so why drop that wall of prudence when you hit the food court? Instead, look around and see what calorie bargains you can find. Maybe the chicken noodle bread bowl isn't the best option when you can get the same soup from a real bowl somewhere else. And maybe you'll feel better about passing on the fried chicken drumstick when there's a grilled chicken breast just 200 feet away. Sure the food court is teeming

with waistline-expanding temptations, but every temptation has a healthy substitution. You just have to shop smart.

Shop It Off
It seems a little cruel how they insist on placing the sweet-tooth kiosk right in the middle of the mall, seducing shoppers with the enticing aromas of freshly made fudge, warm gooey brownies, and soft-baked cookies. How are you supposed to resist an allure like that? One battle at a time, that's how. Sail straight past the cookie counter with-

out stopping and promise yourself that if the cravings persist, you'll double back and have your treat. Believe it or not, there's a good chance you'll forget all about it. A UK study found that chocolate cravings diminished by 12 percent for regular chocolate eaters after they walked for 15 minutes. That means so long as you keep moving, you'll keep your cravings at bay.

Carry a Water Bottle
This is a rule that can save you calories anytime, anywhere. That's because thirst

is far too often confused with hunger. Your brain just does a lousy job differentiating between the two. Keep yourself hydrated and you'll be much better prepared to spend your time in the stores instead of the grub lines. And here's the really good part: Guzzling just 1 bottle of cold water will help you burn more calories while you shop. That's because, as German researchers discovered, 16 ounces of cold water can boost metabolism by 24 percent for a full 90 minutes. Swing by the beverage vending shakes, cakes, or waffle treats. Thankfully, the DQ Sandwich and the extensive line of small sundaes should be enough to stave off even the sweetest tooth.

Eat This Instead!
DQ Sandwich
• *190 calories* • *5 g fat (3 g saturated)*
• *18 g sugars*

WORST CHINESE MEAL
7 Panda Express Orange Chicken with Fried Rice

• *1,025 calories*
• *44 g fat (9 g saturated)*
• *1,640 mg sodium*

It's unfortunate that this dish happens to be one of the most popular on Panda's menu. Consider the recipe: battered and fried, then coated in a sugary syrup. It's like Colonel Sanders meets Willy Wonka. Pair with a scoop of fried rice and you've got a dish with serious flab-enhancing potential. Here's a better survival strategy: Skip the rice altogether and choose steamed veggies instead. Then pick any entrée besides orange chicken.

Eat This Instead!
Broccoli Beef and Mixed Veggies
• *260 calories* • *15 g fat (3 g saturated)*
• *680 mg sodium*

machine as you enter the mall and then sip away as you shop.

Pack a Snack
The mall's selection of snacks is lackluster at best; think French fries, pretzels, muffins, and other quick-fix carbs. The irony is you'll probably need a small snack to help you make it through the day without racing to the nearest deep fryer. A study at Florida State University found that men with low blood sugar (i.e., men who went too long without a snack) performed the worst on tests that evaluate self-control, which means they're liable to make bad decisions in the food court. So what's the key to a good snack? Protein. French researchers found that a high-protein snack eaten 4 hours after lunch delayed the desire to eat dinner by 60 minutes. That will put off your hunger long enough for you to make your final purchases and head home for a real meal. Try stuffing into your purse or pocket a bag of nuts, jerky, or a protein bar. We like Odwalla's Super Protein.

Plan for a Small Dinner
Sometimes your defenses flop and you find yourself bellied up to an oversize plate of noodles and fried chicken covered in a murky brown sauce of dubious oriental origin. It's okay; don't panic. You might have one more chance to salvage your day. When Boston researchers tried to pin down the cause of weight gain, they looked at the eating habits of adolescents. As it turns out, both "lean" and "overweight" subjects overate in the food court. What set the two groups apart was the amount of food consumed the rest of the day; the lean students cut back on other meals, while the overweight students continued to eat full-size portions. Why does this matter? Because it's not the number of calories consumed in one meal that makes or breaks your diet: It's total calories consumed over the course of the day. Compensate for your food-court blunder by cutting your normal dinner in half and you can fall asleep no bigger than when you woke up.

The Worst Mall Foods in America

6 Steak Escape Ranch and Bacon Fries

- *1,044 calories*
- *71 g fat*
- *1,398 mg sodium*

Consuming half your day's allowance of calories in one meal is bad enough—but in one side dish? Claiming innocence will never hold up in a food court of law, though—not when a flood of ranch, a flurry of bacon, and a mountain of fried potatoes are involved. Add on the namesake cheesesteak and you may need a wheelbarrow to make it back to your car.

Until some nutritionally savvy company starts baking their fries in the oven, you'll need to seek out alternative treatments to get your spud fix. The Smashed Potatoes are about as good as a potato gets anywhere in the world of chain restaurants.

Eat This Instead!

Smashed Potatoes

- *246 calories • 0 g fat • 43 mg sodium*
- *53 g carbohydrates*

5 Panera Bread New England Clam Chowder

in a Sourdough Bread Bowl

- *1,070 calories*
- *44.5 g fat*
  (28 g saturated, 1 g trans)
- *2,320 mg sodium*

Soup in an edible bowl? The only more egregious nutritional pairing we've seen lately is Domino's audacious idea of serving pasta in a similarly hulking bread vessel. Next thing you know you'll be ordering your cheeseburger on a plate of pizza. Okay, maybe not, but here's the deal: This sourdough bowl contributes an

Crime & Punishment

The sentences handed down in the food court of law can be cruel and unusual. That's because the caloric content of so many of our favorite foods there can be alarmingly high. Next time you're feeling like a little pick-me-up when you're out shopping, consider the consequences.

Crime:
Panera Bread Cinnamon Crunch Bagel with 2 ounces plain cream cheese
- *610 calories*
- *26 g fat (16 g saturated)*
- *31 g sugars*

Punishment:
153 minutes vacuuming the house

Crime:
Au Bon Pain Pecan Roll
- *630 calories*
- *32 g fat (11 g saturated)*
- *38 g sugars*

Punishment:
55 minutes vigorously treading water

Crime:
Cold Stone Creamery Peanut Butter Ice Cream (large)
- *890 calories*
- *58 g fat.*
  (30 g saturated, 1 g trans)
- *66 g sugars*

Punishment:
182 minutes raking the lawn

extra 590 calories to an already dubious bowl of chowder. Switch to a better soup and nix the soggy vessel or you might drop before you shop.

Eat This Instead!
Forest Mushroom Soup (bowl)
· *250 calories* · *18 g fat (8 g saturated)*
· *1,150 mg sodium*

WORST SANDWICH
4 Panera Bread Full Chipotle Chicken
on Artisan French

· *1,070 calories*
· *55 g fat*
  (15 g saturated, 1 g trans)
· *2,570 mg sodium*

Panera, home to soups, salads, and a general feeling of well-being (not to mention free Wi-Fi!), benefits from a beaming health halo— a perceived virtuousness that doesn't necessarily play out in the hard realities of their nutritional stats. Yes, you can carefully construct a well-balanced 500-calorie meal, but you can also unknowingly consume 1,500 calories without breaking a sweat. Take this sandwich: It begins innocently enough (chicken and white bread), but is supported by a scurrilous cast of bacon strips, high-fat chipotle sauce, and a tarp of Cheddar cheese, the most fattening of the cheese choices. The result is a lunch with more calories than 11 Rice Krispies Treats and a serious crack in the health halo.

Eat This Instead!
Full Smoked Turkey on Sourdough
· *470 calories* · *17 g fat (2.5 g saturated)*
· *1,680 mg sodium*

Crime:
Taco Bell Chipotle Steak Fully Loaded Taco Salad
· *950 calories*
· *59 g fat*
  (11 g saturated, 1 g trans)
· *1,760 mg sodium*

Punishment:
116 minutes on the elliptical trainer

Crime:
Dairy Queen Chocolate Chip Cookie Dough Blizzard (medium)
· *1,010 calories*
· *40 g fat*
  (20 g saturated, 4.5 g trans)
· *109 g sugars*

Punishment:
2,220 sit-ups
(3 seconds apiece)

Crime:
Charley's Grilled Subs Cheddar Bacon Fries
· *1,089 calories*
· *87 g fat*
  (18 g saturated, 2.5 g trans)
· *1,762 mg sodium*

Punishment:
152 minutes speed walking through the mall

Crime:
Regular Quiznos Tuna Melt
· *1,230 calories*
· *92 g fat*
  (18 g saturated, 1 g trans)
· *1,510 mg sodium*

Punishment:
72 minutes running up stairs

The Worst Mall Foods in America

WORST SMOOTHIE
3 Smoothie King Grape Expectations II (40 ounces)

- *1,096 calories*
- *0 g fat*
- *250 g sugars*

Smoothie King calls this a way to "snack right," but we call it one of the quickest ways to fill out the midsection. The bulk of the juice in this smoothie is grape, which is the sweetest, most fructose-packed of all common juices. Then, to make a mediocre smoothie worse, Smoothie King adds the usual heap of turbinado sugar and honey, leaving this barrel-size cup with as much sugar as 13 Dunkin' Donuts Chocolate Frosted Cake Donuts! Eliminate the added sugars by asking for a slim smoothie; eliminate the excess calories by ditching the bathtub-size 40-ouncer for a more restrained 20.

Drink This Instead!
Slim-N-Trim Orange, Vanilla (20 ounces)
- *215 calories • 1 g fat • 38 g sugars*

WORST MALL DRINK
2 Jamba Juice Peanut Butter Moo'd (Power)

- *1,170 calories*
- *30 g fat (7 g saturated)*
- *169 g sugars*

The scary thing about this 30-ounce shake is that you can consume more than half a day's worth of calories in 3 minutes of spirited sipping, all under the pseudohealthy banner of the sacred smoothie. What's even scarier is you'll be slurping up the sugar equivalent of 8 packs of peanut M&M's, all while thinking you're doing your body a favor. Though no mall food packs more calories, the Moo'd at least offers a touch of nutrition (unlike the dreaded Pecanbun) in the form of peanut butter's protein and healthy fat. Still, don't mistake it for anything other than a serious threat to your waistline. When at Jamba, stick to their impressive list of smoothies in the All Fruit and Light categories.

Drink This Instead!
Mango Mantra (16 ounces)
- *170 calories • 0.5 g fat • 33 g sugars*

WORST MALL FOOD IN AMERICA
1 Cinnabon Regular Caramel Pecanbun

- *1,100 calories*
- *56 g fat*
  (10 g saturated, 5 g trans)
- *47 g sugars*
- *141 g carbohydrates*

Cinnabon and malls are inseparable. Consider it a symbiotic relationship: Researchers have found that men are turned on by the smell of cinnamon rolls, and further studies have shown that men are more likely to spend money when they're thinking about sex. But just because Cinnabon might be good for Gap doesn't mean it's at all good for you. This dangerously bloated bun contains nearly an entire day's worth of fat and more than half of your daily allotment of calories. (For those keeping score, that's as much as you'll find in 8 White Castle hamburgers).

Eat This Instead!
Cinnabon Stix
- *379 calories*
- *21 g fat (6 g saturated, 4 g trans)*
- *14 g sugars • 41 g carbohydrates*

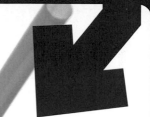

1,170 calories
Jamba Juice Peanut Butter Moo'd

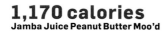

This milk shake in disguise is what Hollywood superstars drink when they need to bulk up for a role. There are just too many solid options on the Jamba menu to ever settle for something this bad.

The Best Mall Foods in

THESE SIX STANDOUTS WOULD BE CONSIDERED ROYALTY IN ANY FOOD

BEST CHINESE MEAL
Panda Express Mushroom Chicken
with Mixed Vegetables

- *240 calories*
- *14 g fat (3 g saturated)*
- *710 mg sodium*

You'd be hard pressed to find anything better in the food court. Panda's all-star entrée, coupled with mixed veggies, prepares you for some serious bargain hunting by filling your belly with zucchini, carrots, broccoli, mushrooms, and chicken. Taken together, these ingredients create a trifecta of protein, fiber, and B vitamins, which will ensure that your energy sustains you until you can get home and loot your purchases.

BEST BREAKFAST SANDWICH
Panera Bread Egg and Cheese Breakfast Sandwich

- *380 calories*
- *14 g fat (6 g saturated)*
- *620 mg sodium*

Researchers in Connecticut determined that, compared with people who ate bagels for breakfast, people who ate eggs consumed fewer calories throughout the rest of the day. The primary reason is protein, which digests slower than carbohydrates. This sandwich has 18 grams of the muscle-building, stomach-filling nutrient, so you can browse easier knowing your morning shopping spree won't turn into an afternoon eating binge.

BEST ICE CREAM
Cold Stone Creamery Sinless Sans Fat Sweet Cream with Raspberries (Like It)

- *165 calories*
- *0 g fat*
- *11 g sugars*

Bet you didn't think anything at Cold Stone could be good for you. Now you know. Order Sinless Cream with fruit on top and you'll be doing your body a favor. All the sugar in this cup comes from real fruit and naturally occurring lactose, and 1 small serving has 20 percent of your day's calcium.

BEST TREAT
Auntie Anne's Cinnamon Sugar Pretzel, no butter

- *380 calories*
- *1 g fat*
- *29 g sugars*
- *400 mg sodium*

Let's be clear: This is no health food. But by the standard set by the food court's oversize and oversweetened pastries (we're looking at you, Cinnabon), this bread knot's actually not so bad. The pretzel twisters will gladly bake you one without butter, which eliminates a quick 90 calories of pure fat, and if you can manage to bring along a partner in crime, you can enjoy your treat for only 190 calories.

America

COURT

BEST COOKIE
Jamba Juice Omega-3 Oatmeal Cookie

- 150 calories
- 6 g fat (1.5 g saturated)
- 15 g sugars

It's a misconception with dire health consequences that every cookie we eat has to be made from white flour and loaded with fat and sugar. The truth is, even cookies can have a place in a healthy diet, and none makes that more clear than Jamba's. It's made from fiber-rich rolled oats and sweetened with a blend of dried cranberries and raisins. Then, to work in the healthy fats, it's filled out with pumpkin seeds and ground flax. It's a cookie that eats like a meal.

BEST SOUP
Au Bon Pain Jamaican Black Bean Soup (medium)

- 250 calories
- 1 g fat
- 440 mg sodium

If you ever doubted the nutritional heft of black beans, here's your proof: This bowl packs in an astounding 23 grams of fiber, not to mention a motley array of antioxidants. But here's where Au Bon Pain scores major points: It keeps the sodium in this soup at a manageable level. The Low-Fat Black Bean Soup at Panera, for comparison, has 1,490 milligrams of sodium. Just be sure to order the *Jamaican* version; Pain's regular Black Bean soup is swimming in sodium.

240 calories
Panda Express Mushroom Chicken with Mixed Vegetables

Whether it's Panda, Manchu Wok, or any generic Chinese food court purveyor, the key to success is replacing the rice and lo mein with a base of vegetables. Here, it saves you 340 calories and 84 g carbs over steamed rice.

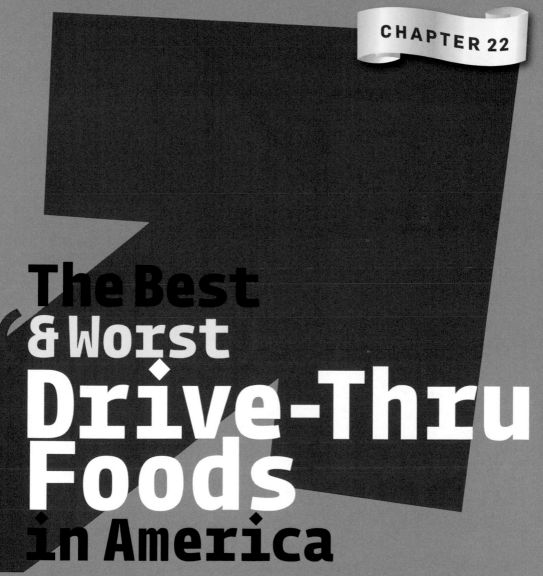

CHAPTER 22

The Best
& Worst
Drive-Thru
Foods
in America

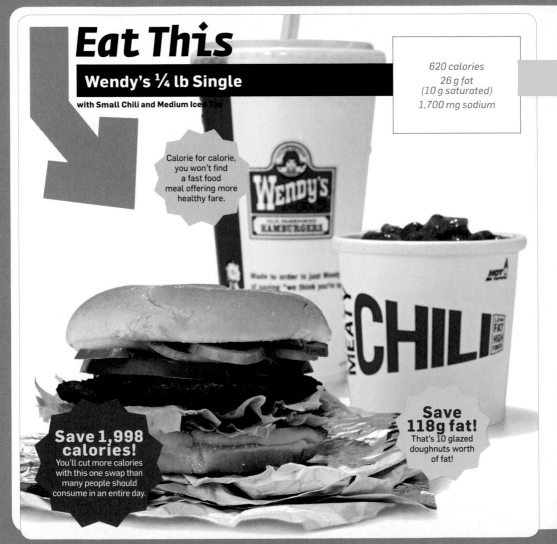

Eat This

Wendy's ¼ lb Single

with Small Chili and Medium Iced Tea

620 calories
26 g fat
(10 g saturated)
1,700 mg sodium

Calorie for calorie, you won't find a fast food meal offering more healthy fare.

Save 1,998 calories! You'll cut more calories with this one swap than many people should consume in an entire day.

Save 118g fat! That's 10 glazed doughnuts worth of fat!

2,618 calories
144 g fat
(51.5 g saturated)
2,892 mg sodium

Not That!

Carl's Jr. Double Six Dollar Burger

with Medium Natural Cut Fries and 32-Ounce Coke

Carl's seems to take a certain sadistic pleasure in dispensing the country's most consistently atrocious fast food. (Don't believe us? Just watch their commercials.) Unless you're a marathoner or Michael Phelps, stay away at all costs.

You're better off dusting 29 Rice Krispies Treats than tussling with this combo meal.

One day in the far-distant future,

archaeologists will be digging through the ruins of a once-great civilization and will suddenly become very confused.

They will discover a large metal object that appears to be a vehicle for transportation: It will have bucket seats, a combustion engine, and a posterior space that seems designed to carry one's belongings over long distances. But inside, they'll find remnants that suggest this metal object wasn't, in fact, a vehicle for transportation at all. They'll find petrified food, plastic eating utensils, and lots of stained napkins. And those far-off future scientists will think, "Aha! This isn't a transportation vehicle! It's an eating pod!"

Well, to a certain extent, they'll be right. We use today's cars as much for "eating pods" as we do for getting around. A recent study by the Culinary Institute of America found that almost one in five of our meals are eaten not in restaurants, or at the dining room table, or in front of the TV. They're eaten in our cars.

There are two big reasons for that: time and money. They're our two most precious resources, and what's better, when it comes to saving both time and money, than drive-thru food? The average American eats 32 restaurant meals in his or her car every month—up more than 50 percent in the last 25 years. That's a lot of Tater Tots rolling around under the seats.

Unfortunately, it's also a lot of flab rolling around on top of the seats. Drive-thru foods may be convenient and easy on the wallet, but they're loaded with unhealthy fats, added sugars, and excess sodium. Translation: They're no bargain at all when it comes to your health. But jam-packed schedules and a dismal economy make the occasional drive-thru meal a part of life. That's why

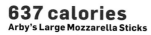

637 calories
Arby's Large Mozzarella Sticks

Fried cheese is never a good idea, but as a sandwich sidekick, it spells certain disaster. Eat these with a Market Fresh Pecan Chicken Salad sandwich and you've got 1,507 calories and 89 grams of fat on your hands.

we studied the open-air menu boards and compiled a list of the worst items out there, plus better alternatives. Avoid these dietary land mines and save more than a few minutes and a couple of bucks—how does up to 20 pounds in a year sound? Next time you're barking orders into a speakerphone, make sure you know what to say—and what not to.

WORST BEVERAGE

17 Sonic Route 44 Cherry Limeade (44 ounces)

- *460 calories*
- *0 g fat*
- *120 g sugars*

"Ade" is the suffix attached to "juices" with more sugar water than fruit. Don't fall for the health head-fake; this is the worst way to round out a drive-thru meal. For as many dubious drinks taking up space on Sonic's menu, they do have an impressive line of low-sugar flavored iced teas. Take advantage.

Drink This Instead!
Route 44 Peach Ice Tea
- *10 calories • 0 g fat • 0 g sugars*

WORST SIDE

16 Arby's Large Mozzarella Sticks

- *637 calories*
- *42 g fat (19 g saturated fat)*
- *2,047 mg sodium*

Anything with as much saturated fat as a Double Whopper should not be called a side. Arby's menu presents a sides conundrum, given that their entire roster of "Sides and Sidekickers" receives the deep-fried treatment. Best to skip over this section entirely. If it's cheese you crave, order the French Dip 'N Swiss or Ham and Swiss Melt instead to save more than 300 calories.

Eat This Instead!
Martha's Vineyard Salad with Light Buttermilk Ranch Dressing
- *389 calories*
- *14 g fat (5 g saturated)*
- *923 mg sodium*

WORST FISH ENTRÉE

15 Burger King Big Fish Sandwich

- *640 calories*
- *32 g fat (5 saturated)*
- *1,540 mg sodium*

The Big Fish is a whale of a sandwich. Seriously, when BK first released the sandwich, it was under the unfortunate name of the Whaler. Even though the marketing team has corrected the flaws in its original moniker, it still outpaces every other fish sandwich around by a few hundred calories. Part of that is due to its substantial size, the rest due to the thick application of calorie-dense tartar sauce. If you have a soft spot for fried fish sandwiches, you can't do much better than the Filet-O-Fish, so pull across the street to the Golden Arches if you really need a fix and save a quick 260 calories. If not, switch to chicken and stick with the King.

Eat This Instead!
Tendergrill Chicken Sandwich without Mayo
- *380 calories • 9 g fat (2 g saturated)*
- *1,130 mg sodium*

640 calories
Burger King Big Fish

Looks almost identical to a McDonald's Filet-O-Fish, right? It is, except for the fact that it packs an extra 260 calories and 14 grams of fat. We subscribe to a strict catch-and-release policy on this fried fish.

Does this really look like a breakfast for *one person*? Of course not. That's why this is the worst fast-food breakfast in America by an unhealthy margin.

1,370 calories
McDonald's Deluxe Breakfast

WORST MEXICAN ENTRÉE

14 Taco Bell Grilled Stuft Beef Burrito

- *680 calories*
- *30 g fat (10 g saturated)*
- *2,120 mg sodium*

One of the Bell's biggest hits of the past decade is also a serious hit to your dreams of slimming down. Beyond the caloric heft, there's also the sodium equivalent of 20 cups of buttered popcorn wrapped up in that toasted tortilla. Ditch this and order two grilled steak soft tacos (or any menu item) "fresco" style, and the Bell boys will replace cheese and sauces with a chunky tomato salsa, helping to cut calories in half and trim the fat by at least 25 percent. Oh, and no need to favor chicken over steak for nutritional reasons here; Taco Bell's protein options all have nearly identical nutritional stats.

Eat This Instead!
Grilled Steak Soft Tacos, Fresco Style (2)

- *320 calories • 9 g fat (3 g saturated)*
- *1,100 mg sodium*

WORST GRILLED CHICKEN

13 Jack in the Box Chipotle Chicken Ciabatta

- *690 calories*
- *28 g fat (9 g saturated)*
- *1,850 mg sodium*

Chicken sandwiches—even grilled chicken sandwiches —are one of America's most misunderstood foods. They're uniformly accepted as healthier than burgers, but it's more about the supporting cast than the headliner. Case in point: Jack's Chicken Ciabatta. We'll give it points for being one of the few items on their menu free of trans fat, but the oversize ciabatta roll should be the first warning sign; the application of bacon and cheese should be the others. Thankfully, Jack in the Box has one of the best chicken entrées in the drive-thru world in the Fajita Pita.

Eat This Instead!
Chicken Fajita Pita

- *300 calories • 9 g fat (3.5 g saturated)*
- *1,090 mg sodium*

WORST POTATO SIDE

12 Jack in the Box Bacon Cheddar Potato Wedges

- *720 calories*
- *48 g fat*
  (15 g saturated, 12 g trans)
- *1,360 mg sodium*
- *52 g carbohydrates*

You probably don't need us to tell you that bacon, cheese, and fried potatoes don't make for healthy eating. What you do need to know, though, is that Jack in the Box cooks in trans-fatty vegetable shortening, which has been linked to heart disease. It's no secret that French fries can ruin an otherwise sensible meal, but these things take destruction to another level entirely. Cheese sticks, surprisingly enough, mitigate the damage of the oil bath substantially, but if you want to skip the trans fat totally, turn to the side salad standby.

Eat This Instead!
Mozzarella Cheese Sticks (3)

- *240 calories*
- *12 g fat (5 g saturated, 2 g trans)*
- *420 mg sodium*

WORST HOT SANDWICH
11 Sonic Chicken Club Toaster Sandwich

- 740 calories
- 46 g fat (11 g saturated)
- 1,740 mg sodium

How can a chicken sandwich pack so much fat? Start with a chicken breast, bread it, deep-fry it, then add bacon, cheese, and mayo. Tack on nearly an entire day's worth of sodium and you're looking at a serious dietary disaster.

Eat This Instead!
Sonic Burger with Mustard
- 560 calories • 25 g fat (9 g saturated)
- 750 mg sodium

WORST DRIVE-THRU BREAKFAST SANDWICH
10 Jack in the Box Sausage, Egg & Cheese Biscuit

- 740 calories
- 55 g fat
  (17 g saturated, 6 g trans)
- 1,430 mg sodium

Skip biscuits at all costs. Even when you're not at Jack's, biscuits are bound to be loaded with partially hydrogenated oils, since bakers rely so heavily on shortening to make them flaky. The simple solution is to keep your breakfast sandwich habit focused on English muffins, rolls, or (if you're lucky) wheat toast. The Bacon Breakfast Jack packs 16 grams of protein into a low-impact roll.

Eat This Instead!
Bacon Breakfast Jack
- 300 calories • 14 g fat (5 g saturated, 0.5 g trans) • 730 mg sodium

WORST "HEALTHY" FOOD
9 Arby's Pecan Chicken Salad Market Fresh Sandwich

- 769 calories
- 39 g fat (10 g saturated)
- 1,240 mg sodium

Best and Worst Cheap Eats in America

Things didn't look so bright for the Golden Arches in the early moments of the new millennium. Customer lawsuits, declining yearly profits, and the one-two critical punch of the films *Fast Food Nation* and *Super Size Me* had McDonald's reeling and stocks plummeting. But in 2003, execs for the fast-food titan decided to fight back, launching the groundbreaking Dollar Menu, which used cheap double cheeseburgers and chicken sandwiches to help fuel McDonald's 6-year run of record-breaking profits.

Where McDonald's goes, so goes the rest of the fast-food world, and the big players have all adopted the value menu approach in recent years. And with tough economic times tightening the collective American budget, don't expect the dollar deals to go away anytime soon. To help you better negotiate this new era of cheap eats, we went through the value menus of the major fast-food joints in the country, picking out the best and worst options on each, all in an attempt to help you spend your money—and your calories—wisely.

Arby's Market Fresh line of sandwiches sounds particularly virtuous, especially when you throw in the fact that most are served on honey wheat bread. But it's the bread that proves to be the sandwiches' undoing, made from a dizzying number of food additives—including partially hydrogenated oil and high-fructose corn syrup—which combined pack a 361-calorie wallop. Request the sandwich on a sesame bun and cut the bread calories in half or opt for the decadent-sounding Super Roast Beef and save even more.

Eat This Instead!
Super Roast Beef
- *398 calories • 19 g fat (6 g saturated)*
- *1,061 mg sodium*

WORST CRISPY CHICKEN SANDWICH

8 Hardee's Big Chicken Fillet Sandwich

- *800 calories*
- *37 g fat (6 g saturated)*
- *1,890 mg sodium*

Forget about the embarrassment of ordering something called "the big chicken."

Making this nutritional gaffe just once a month will add more than a pound of flab to your frame, compared to the charbroiled chicken, which, to Hardee's credit, is one of the best sandwiches you'll ever find at a drive-thru.

Eat This Instead!
Charbroiled BBQ Chicken Sandwich
- *340 calories • 4 g fat (1 g saturated)*
- *1,070 mg sodium*

*Cheap calories are the sign of foods heavy on inexpensive ingredients like fat, salt, and sugar and lacking in true nutrition.

WENDY'S

Eat This!
5-Piece Crispy Nuggets ($1.29)
- *230 calories*
- *15 g fat (3 g saturated)*
- *520 mg sodium*

Cost per 100 calories: $0.56*
Calories from fat: 144

Free your chicken from bun and tortilla and you'll cut down on carbohydrates, plus the unencumbered chicken doesn't have an opportunity to get greased over with oily sauces.

Not That!
Crispy Chicken Sandwich ($1.29)
- *360 calories*
- *18 g fat (3.5 g saturated)*
- *710 mg sodium*

Cost per 100 calories: $0.36*
Calories from fat: 160

Nearly every value menu has a fried chicken sandwich, and in nearly every case, it's the worst possible investment you could make.

KFC

Eat This!
Hot Wings Snack Box ($1.99)
- *470 calories*
- *27 g fat (6 g saturated)*
- *1,190 mg sodium*

Cost per 100 calories: $0.42
Calories from fat: 240

This is the leanest snack box KFC has to offer. Just don't ask for any biscuits with it; each one will set you back an extra 180 calories.

Not That!
Popcorn Chicken Snack Box ($1.99)
- *660 calories*
- *38 g fat*
  (7 g saturated, 0.5 g trans)
- *1,900 mg sodium*

Cost per 100 calories: $0.30
Calories from fat: 340

It's simple math: The smaller the chicken pieces, the more surface there is to bread. More breading = more oil soakage = more calories.

The Worst Drive-Thru Foods in America

WORST DESSERT
7 Dairy Queen Large Strawberry CheeseQuake Blizzard

- 930 calories
- 37 g fat (24 g saturated)
- 97 g sugars

This creation combines ice cream, strawberry syrup, and hunks of cheesecake for a high-fat dairy dessert. If you're set on a Blizzard, go bananas. A small Banana Split Blizzard has 7 grams less than the small Oreo, Cookie Dough, Peanut Butter Cup, or Strawberry Cheese-Quake. Or stray from the Blizzard and satisfy your sweet tooth with a small chocolate sundae instead to save major calories and fat.

Eat This Instead!
Small Chocolate Sundae
- 280 calories • 7 g fat (4.5 g saturated)
- 42 g sugars

WORST DRIVE-THRU KIDS MEAL
6 Burger King Kids Double Cheeseburger and Kids Fries with Small Coke

- 960 calories
- 46 g fat
  (17.5 g saturated, 1.5 g trans)
- 1,640 mg sodium

BK's dubious double burger earns the distinction of being the fattiest meal for an on-the-go kid, with nearly a day's worth of saturated fat for the average 8-year-old. It's going to have to come with one heck of an action toy to help your child burn off all of these calories!

Eat This Instead!
4-Piece Chicken Tenders with Fresh Apple Fries and unlimited H$_2$0
- 205 calories
- 11 g fat (2 g saturated)
- 490 mg sodium

Best and Worst Cheap Eats in America—*Continued*

BURGER KING

Eat This!
Whopper Jr. without Mayo ($1.00)
- 290 calories
- 12 g fat (4.5 g saturated)
- 500 mg sodium

Cost per 100 calories: $0.34
Calories from fat: 108

The key here is to ask for "no mayo." Otherwise, you can expect an extra 9 grams of fat.

Not That!
Spicy Chick'n Crisp Sandwich ($1.00)
- 450 calories
- 30 g fat (5 g saturated)
- 810 mg sodium

Cost per 100 calories: $0.22
Calories from fat: 270

The word "crisp" should tip you off that this chicken has been breaded and fried.

TACO BELL

Eat This!
Crunchy Taco ($0.89)
- 170 calories
- 10 g fat (3.5 g saturated)
- 350 mg sodium

Cost per 100 calories: $0.52
Calories from fat: 90

You're better off eating 2 crunchy tacos over 1 bean burrito. You'll earn a few extra grams of protein and save yourself the sodium overload.

Not That!
Triple Layer Nachos ($0.79)
- 340 calories
- 18 g fat
  (2.5 g saturated, 1.5 g trans)
- 720 mg sodium

Cost per 100 calories: $0.23
Calories from fat: 162

As a general rule, the less it costs your wallet, the more it costs your health. What you want is a nutritional bargain, not free calories.

5 McDonald's Large Triple Thick Chocolate Milkshake

- *1,160 calories*
- *27 g fat (16 g saturated)*
- *168 g sugars*
- *510 mg sodium*

You'd be better off eating 2 Quarter Pounders than sucking down 1 of these belt-breaking shakes. Most of McDonald's entrée offerings are relatively restrained (except for the Chicken Selects and that Double Quarter Pounder, of course), but their milk shakes are treacherous. If you must have a frozen dessert, order a vanilla ice cream cone to save more than 1,000 calories. Make three swaps like that a week and you'll melt 44 pounds in a year.

Eat This Instead!
Vanilla Reduced-Fat Ice Cream Cone

- *150 calories*
- *3.5 g fat (2 g saturated)*
- *18 g sugars • 60 mg sodium*

4 McDonald's Deluxe Breakfast with margarine and syrup

- *1,370 calories*
- *64.5 g fat (21.5 g saturated)*
- *2,335 mg sodium*
- *161 g carbohydrates*

The fact that this breakfast is 210 calories worse than McDonald's Large Triple Thick Chocolate Milkshake tells you everything you need to know. Carbohydrate-based breakfasts are the scourge of healthy eating habits and a hard-working metabolism,

---

McDONALD'S

Eat This!
Fruit 'n Yogurt Parfait ($1.00)

- *160 calories*
- *2 g fat (1 g saturated)*
- *21 g sugars*

Cost per 100 calories: $0.62
Calories from fat: 20

McDonald's calls it a dessert, but we say it's a perfect treat anytime. Each cup of low-fat yogurt is loaded with calcium and vitamin A and gut-friendly bacteria.

Not That!
2 Baked Hot Apple Pies ($1.00)

- *500 calories*
- *25 g fat (14 g saturated)*
- *26 g sugars*

Cost per 100 calories: $0.20
Calories from fat: 225

McDonald's charges $0.89 for 1 apple pie or $1.00 for 2, which makes it incredibly inexpensive to get 25 percent of your day's calories with hardly a shred of redeeming nutrition.

JACK IN THE BOX

Eat This!
Hamburger Deluxe ($1.00)

- *344 calories • 18 g fat*
  (5 g saturated, 1 g trans)
- *548 mg sodium*

Cost per 100 calories: $0.29
Calories from fat: 162

Unfortunately, Jack's value menu is riddled with trans fat, so with the exception of a side salad, this is the best you can do. But at least there are 14 grams of protein.

Not That!
Jumbo Jack ($1.39)

- *578 calories*
- *33 g fat*
  (12 g saturated, 1 g trans)
- *916 mg sodium*

Cost per 100 calories: $0.24
Calories from fat: 297

In one handheld meal, Jack's super-size value burger sucks up more than half your day's saturated fat. It's not worth saving a buck.

and this one platter packs more cheap carbs than you'd get from 11 slices of Wonder Bread. Unless you're ordering yogurt, breakfast at McDonald's shouldn't require utensils.

Eat This Instead!
Egg McMuffin and Large Coffee
• *300 calories* • *12 g fat (5 g saturated)*
• *820 mg sodium* • *30 g carbohydrates*

WORST CHEESEBURGER
3 Hardee's Monster Thickburger

• *1,420 calories*
• *108 g fat (43 g saturated)*
• *2,770 mg sodium*

Ever since Carl's Jr. purchased Hardee's back in 1997, the two have been teaming up to wreak havoc on the American waistline. This burger is the Double Six Dollar Burger's evil East Coast twin, packing two-thirds of a pound of ground beef, 3 slices of cheese, and 4 slices of bacon. Opt for the significantly less monstrous Low Carb Thickburger instead, which subtracts a patty and swaps in lettuce leaves for a bun, all in the

name of saving you 1,000 calories in a single sitting.

Eat This Instead!
Low Carb Thickburger
• *420 calories* • *32 g fat (12 g saturated)*
• *1,010 mg sodium*

WORST CHICKEN STRIPS
2 Dairy Queen 6-Piece Chicken Strip Basket with Country Gravy

• *1,640 calories*
• *74 g fat*
  (12 g saturated, 1 g trans)
• *3,690 mg sodium*

Kudos to DQ for aggressively cutting trans-fat content across their menu (these strips used to carry 11 grams of the stuff), but as they've cut back on the nasty fat, they've also increased overall portion size. The result is a basket packing more calories than 10 ice cream sand-wiches. Take the chicken out of the fryer, stuff it into a bun, and save 1,240 calories. It's that simple.

Eat This Instead!
Grilled Chicken Sandwich
• *400 calories* • *16 g fat (2.5 g saturated)*
• *790 mg sodium*

THE WORST DRIVE-THRU MEAL IN AMERICA
1 Carl's Jr. Double Six Dollar Burger
with Medium Natural Cut Fries and 32-Ounce Coke

• *2,618 calories*
• *144 g fat (51.5 g saturated)*
• *2,892 mg sodium*

Of all the gut-growing, heart-threatening, life-shortening burgers in the drive-thru world, there is none whose damage to your general well-being is as potentially catastrophic as this. A bit of perspective is in order: This meal has the caloric equivalent of 13 Krispy Kreme Original Glazed doughnuts, the saturated fat equivalent of 52 strips of bacon, and the salt equiva-lent of 7½ large orders of McDonald's French fries!

Eat This Instead!
Famous Star with Side Salad with Low-Fat Balsamic Dressing and 32-Ounce Iced Tea
• *685 calories* • *38 g fat*
  (10.5 g saturated) • *1,520 mg sodium*

Do you really want to eat this bloated burrito in your car? Let's hope not, because the Combo Meal—with a hard taco and a soft drink—will eat up 1,100 calories.

680 calories
Taco Bell Grilled Stuft Beef Burrito

The Best Drive-Thru Me

ROLL DOWN YOUR WINDOW FOR THESE GRAB-AND-GO BITES

BEST DRIVE-THRU MEAL

Chick-fil-A Chargrilled Chicken Sandwich
with Large Fruit Cup and Unsweetened Iced Tea

- *360 calories*
- *3 g fat
  (0.5 g saturated)*
- *1,310 mg sodium*

One of the features we love most about Chick-fil-A's menu is that they allow you to swap in healthy sides for the standard fried fare. That sets the stage for a perfectly balanced meal, not just low in calories but high in protein (28 grams) and fiber (10 grams) and soaked in the metabolism-spiking antioxidants of a simple glass of zero-calorie iced tea.

BEST DRIVE-THRU MEXICAN

Taco Bell Grilled Steak Soft Tacos,
Fresco Style (2)

- *320 calories*
- *9 g fat (3 g saturated)*
- *1,100 mg sodium*

Taco Bell's smart addition of the Fresco Style option to their menu saves diners hundreds of calories by replacing cheese and fatty sauces with a chunky tomato salsa. This two-taco combo, paired with H_2O or iced tea, makes for a good lunch in a pinch. (But go easy on the hot sauce; this baby already packs enough sodium as it is.)

BEST DRIVE-THRU SANDWICH

Arby's Melt

- *298 calories*
- *12 g fat (4 g saturated)*
- *922 mg sodium*

Perhaps one of the most surprising things about the Arby's menu is that this cheese-smothered beef sandwich trounces most of their turkey and chicken options. In fact, Arby's signature roast beef is surprisingly lean in all of its iterations, making it one of the most reliable options on their menu.

BEST DRIVE-THRU BURGER

Whopper Jr.
without Mayo

- *290 calories*
- *12 g fat
  (4.5 g saturated)*
- *500 mg sodium*

It's rare enough to find a burger in the drive-thru world that weighs in at less than 300 calories, but what makes this one so great is that it comes with a pile of vegetation, too (lettuce, tomatoes, onions, pickles). Miss the mayo? Request ketchup and mustard or even a packet of 10-calorie barbecue sauce on the side.

als in America

Wendy's Jr. Original Chocolate Frosty

- *160 calories*
- *4 g fat (2.5 g saturated)*
- *21 g sugars*

Fast food milk shakes are usually something to avoid at all costs, but what makes this one different is that Wendy's was smart enough to make it available in such a perfect portion—that is, just large enough to satisfy your sweet tooth without doing any real damage.

Real Mexican tacos never come with Cheddar or sour cream, and neither does anything on Taco Bell's Fresco Menu. Not a single item—each strewn with tomato salsa instead of fatty condiments—tops the 350-calorie mark.

320 calories
Taco Bell Grilled Steak Soft Tacos

CHAPTER 23

The Best & Worst Foods for Kids

Eat This

McDonald's Chicken McNuggets

with Apple Dippers, Caramel Dip, and 1% Low-Fat Milk

395 calories
15 g fat
(3.5 g saturated)
560 mg sodium

Save 64g fat!
Kids also get a serving of fruit and a big dose of calcium.

Save 875 calories!
8-year-olds should take in about 1,600 calories a day. They'll win back more than half of that with this one swap.

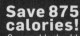

Rich, ready-to-eat apple slices with low fat caramel dip*

Rich in Vitamin C

Net Wt. 2.4 oz (68g)

Keep refrigerated

TEAR HERE

Not all kids' meals at Mickey Ds are so happy. Swap in fries and a soft drink and this meal swells to 635 calories.

1,270 calories
79 g fat
(11.5 g saturated)
2,850 mg sodium

Not That!

Uno Chicago Grill Kid's Kombo

with French Fries

By swapping fried chicken for grilled and fries for fruit, your kid will save 1,085 calories and 75 grams of fat at Uno's.

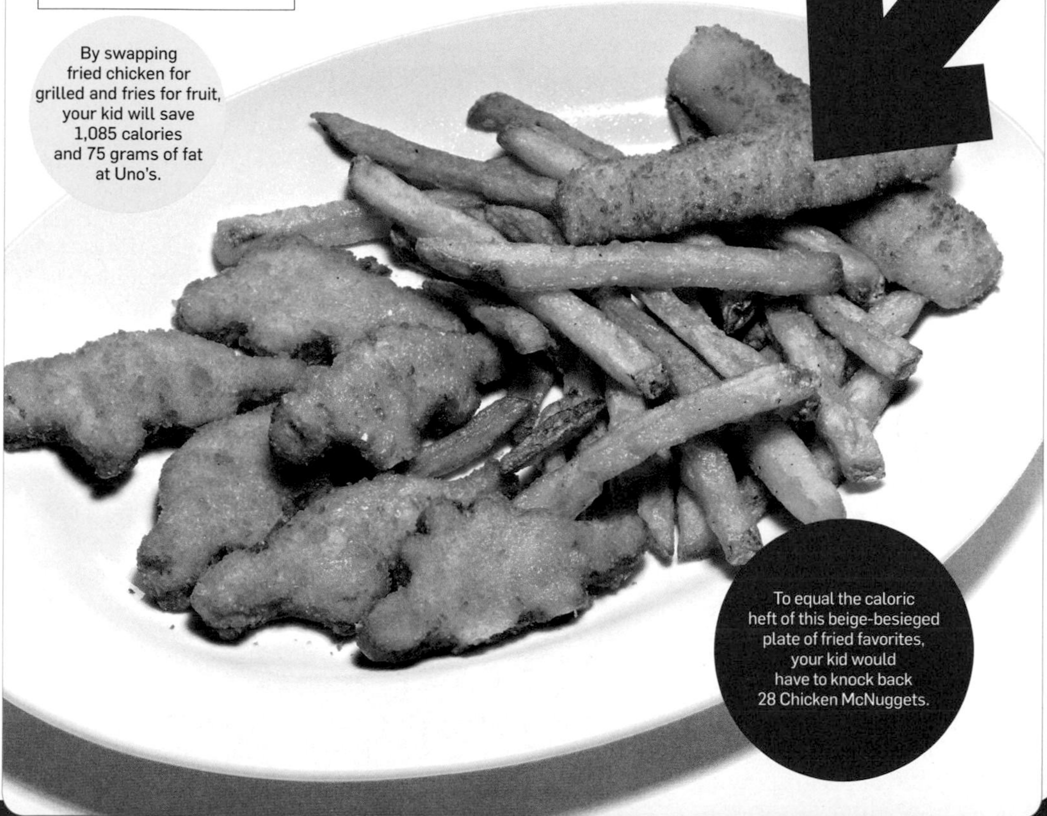

To equal the caloric heft of this beige-besieged plate of fried favorites, your kid would have to knock back 28 Chicken McNuggets.

Here's a pop quiz:

If you have young children at home, which of the following is likely to eat up the larger percentage of your household income?

A. Books and other educational materials
B. DVDs, CDs, music downloads, and trips to the movies
C. Video games
D. Fast food

You're probably not surprised to discover that the right answer is D. But you might be surprised to discover that, if you're a parent, you will most likely spend more on fast food this year than on A, B, and C combined.

Restaurants are no more kind to our children's health and well-being than they are to our own: The typical burger, soda, and fries that you and I ate as kids contains an average of 214 more calories today than that same meal did in the 1970s—enough to add at least 3 pounds of weight a year to your child's body, even if he or she ate that fast-food meal just once a week.

Indeed, some of the nutritional stats in the foods restaurants are selling as "kids' meals" are terrifying. A grilled cheese with as much fat as 25 strips of bacon? A child-size dessert with more than half a day's worth of calories? And the supermarket aisles offer little salvation.

As a result, childhood obesity rates in America have tripled since 1980— today, 16 percent of children between the ages of 6 and 19 are overweight or obese. An additional 15 percent of kids are "at risk of becoming overweight or obese."

Seventy percent of overweight adolescents end up overweight or obese in adulthood. And since obesity increases your odds of heart attack, stroke, and early death, consider the impact of an entire generation of overweight children on our country's health care system—and families. It's a chilling thought, especially if one of those children is your own. That's why we've created this list, to help your family make smarter choices today for a healthier tomorrow.

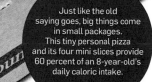

980 calories
**Uno Chicago Grill's Deep Dish
Pepperoni Pizza** for kids

Just like the old
saying goes, big things come
in small packages.
This tiny personal pizza
and its four mini slices provide
60 percent of an 8-year-old's
daily caloric intake.

The Worst Foods for Kids in America

WORST SWEETENED CEREAL
20 Cap'n Crunch (1 cup)

- *146 calories*
- *2 g fat (1 g saturated)*
- *16 g sugars*
- *1 g fiber*

The Cap'n's cereal is the archetypal hypersweetened breakfast. It didn't make our list by its abundance of fat or calories; it made the list by being among the dominant sources of empty calories in a child's diet. Aside from the small amount of added vitamins, which are mandated by the government, this cereal is a food scientist's concoction of worthless foodlike particles and chemicals. Corn flour makes the bulk of each crunch, and sugar, brown sugar, and coconut oil hold it together. This cereal is also coated with loads of the food colorings yellow 6 and 5, which have been linked to irritability and poor behavior in children.

Eat This Instead!
Cascadian Farm Clifford Crunch (1 cup)
- *100 calories • 1 g fat (0 g saturated)*
- *25 g carbohydrates • 6 g sugars*

WORST PACKAGED SNACK
19 Austin Cheese Crackers with Cheddar Jack Cheese (1 package)

- *210 calories*
- *10 g fat*
  (2 g saturated, 4 g trans)
- *370 mg sodium*

The calorie count is the least of your concerns with these ubiquitous orange cracker snacks. They made the list because each package contains 2 days' worth of trans fats. Most of the food industry has figured out how to make foods free of these nasty lipids (which have been proven to raise bad cholesterol); we suggest Austin do the same.

Eat This Instead!
Laughing Cow Mini Babybel
- *70 calories • 6 g fat (4 g saturated)*
- *170 mg sodium*

WORST BEVERAGE
18 SunnyD Smooth Style (16 ounces)

- *260 calories*
- *60 g sugars*

Remember those commercials where the kid with SunnyD in the fridge always had the coolest mom? What they didn't tell you was that Mom's love of the orange stuff was quietly undermining her kid's well-being. Don't mistake SunnyD for OJ; there's just 5 percent real juice in this bottle, which means the other 95 percent is well-marketed sugar water. Do you really want your child slurping down the sugar equivalent of a dozen Chips Ahoy cookies?

Drink This Instead!
Capri Sun Tropical Fruit Roarin' Water (6.8 ounces)
- *35 calories • 0 g fat • 9 g sugars*

WORST SIDE
17 Bob Evans Smiley Face Potatoes

- *524 calories*
- *31 g fat (6 g saturated)*
- *646 mg sodium*

These incessantly smiling potatoes are more than just creepy; they're more fat- and calorie-packed than Bob's Sirloin Steak. Let this be a lesson to you youngsters: Just because they're smiling doesn't make them nice.

Eat This Instead!
Home Fries
- *159 calories • 3 g fat (1 g saturated)*
- *533 mg sodium*

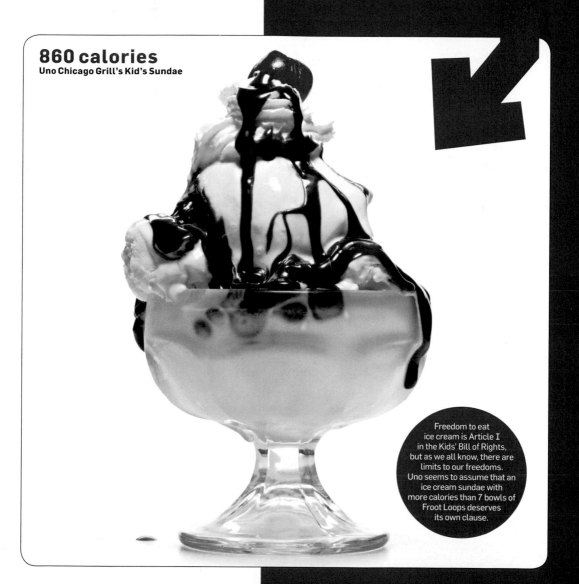

860 calories
Uno Chicago Grill's Kid's Sundae

Freedom to eat
ice cream is Article I
in the Kids' Bill of Rights,
but as we all know, there are
limits to our freedoms.
Uno seems to assume that an
ice cream sundae with
more calories than 7 bowls of
Froot Loops deserves
its own clause.

The Worst Foods for Kids in America

WORST PB&J

16 Atlanta Bread Company Peanut Butter & Jelly

- 550 calories
- 15 g fat (3.5 g saturated)
- 690 mg sodium
- 34 g sugars

Apparently it's a bad idea to stick an American classic on French bread. How else could we explain a 550-calorie peanut butter and jelly sandwich? Toss some chips onto that plate and you've got a meal that can quickly make a small child big. Make this meal at home instead and you not only save a ton of money, but you can also cut the caloric load by half.

Eat This Instead!
Kids Cheese Pizza
· 300 calories · 7 g fat (3.5 g saturated)
· 660 mg sodium

WORST MALL SNACK

15 Auntie Anne's Pepperoni Pretzel Pocket

- 650 calories
- 27 g fat (12 g saturated)
- 1,120 mg sodium
- 11 g sugars

Oversize pretzels are already precarious, because they pack a ton of empty carbohydrates. So stuffing a pretzel with sausage is wrapping barbed wire around a fire ax. It will take more than a day of walking around the mall for your kid to burn off all the fat in this greasy fat sponge. (Better warm up that credit card!)

Eat This Instead!
Pretzel Dog
· 360 calories · 20 g fat (9 g saturated)
· 740 mg sodium

WORST SANDWICH

14 Au Bon Pain Kids' Grilled Cheese

- 670 calories
- 41 g fat (25 g saturated)
- 1,060 mg sodium

You wouldn't even consider feeding your child this if they called it by its real name: an oil sandwich with cheese. So soaked is this sandwich that you'd need to eat 25 strips of cooked bacon to equal the amount of saturated fat found between the two slices. Wait until you get home—in about 5 minutes you can make a pretty mean 300-calorie grilled cheese sandwich.

Eat This Instead!
Kids' Macaroni and Cheese
· 250 calories · 14 g fat (9 g saturated)
· 690 mg sodium

WORST PREPARED LUNCH

13 Oscar Mayer Maxed Out Turkey & Cheddar Cracker Combo Lunchables

- 680 calories
- 22 g fat (9 g saturated)
- 61 g sugars
- 1,440 mg sodium

Lunchables has established itself as the prepackaged lunch choice for kids, but just because your kids love Lunchables doesn't mean Lunchables loves your kids. The Maxed Out line is the worst of the lot; Oscar Mayer packs this one with nearly half of an 8-year-old's daily calorie allotment and sweetens it with more than twice the sugar and fat of most candy bars.

Eat This Instead!
Hillshire Farm Deli Wrap Smokehouse Ham & Swiss Wrap Kit
· 260 calories · 11 g fat (4 g saturated)
· 960 mg sodium

12 Uno Chicago Grill Kid's Sundae

- *860 calories*
- *38 g fat (20 g saturated)*
- *94 g sugars*

Consider the repercussions of slapping three Baby Ruth bars' worth of fat and sugar onto the end of your child's meal. Weighing in at an astounding ¾ pound, this abominable sundae is twice as big as the Kid's Pasta, and twice as caloric as his entire meal should be.

Eat This Instead!
Kid's Slush

- *70 calories • 0 g fat • 17 g sugars*

11 Ruby Tuesday Kids Turkey Minis & Fries

- *873 calories*
- *46 g fat*
- *88 g carbohydrates*

When we first pointed out how bad this restaurant kids' meal was, Ruby Tuesday sprang into action, shrinking the meal down to save . . . a total of 20 calories. That's not going to help your child fight obesity and all the health problems that can

873 calories
Ruby Tuesday Kids Turkey Minis & Fries

In a perfect world, ground turkey is leaner than ground beef and a turkey burger is a decent thing to feed your kid. But Ruby Tuesday finds a way to confound all expectations by cramming more calories than you'd find in Wendy's Baconator into this kid's plate.

come with it, not when these mini burgers still have more calories than a Wendy's formidable Baconator. The best solution? Avoid Ruby's burgers entirely. Chicken and broccoli, at just 201 calories, is best, but the chop steak plate is like eating a burger without the bun (not to mention all those excess calories).

Eat This Instead!
Chop Steak & Mashed Potatoes
· 403 calories · 30 g fat
· 15 g carbohydrates

WORST HOMESTYLE MEAL
10 **Boston Market's Kids' Meat Loaf** with Sweet Potato Casserole and Cornbread
· 890 calories
· 46.5 g fat (17.5 g saturated)
· 131 g carbohydrates
· 1,500 mg sodium

This is not your mother's meat loaf—and that's too bad. This slab-o-meat begins as beef and ends as a science project with 55 ingredients that include the understandable (cheese cultures), the detestable (partially hydrogenated cottonseed oil), and the unpronounceable (azodicarbonamide). Stack the amalgamation next to a sugar- and cream-injected sweet potato and a starchy piece of cornbread and you're asking your kid to be the lab rat. We can tell you right now, the results will be big. Roast turkey provides a safe haven for discerning eaters.

Eat This Instead!
Kids' Roasted Turkey with Green Bean Casserole and Cornbread
· 390 calories · 9 g fat (3 g saturated)
· 36 g carbohydrates
· 1,045 mg sodium

How to Pack the Perfect School Lunch

Concerned that the sludge they're slopping at the cafeteria is ruining your kid's appetite and maybe even his waistline? Then it's time to take control of the midday meal by packing a heroic lunch for your loved ones each morning. Not only will you ensure optimum nutrition, you'll also be able to cater to his likes and dislikes, which means there's a darn good shot he'll actually eat this lunch, rather than leaving it behind in the rush to get to the playground.

A good lunch is formed around a dependable main course and punctuated with a solid supporting cast of nutrient-packed sides, a low- or no-calorie drink, and even a little treat. Mix and match like you would when ordering Chinese takeout—though, unlike sweet-and-sour goop, this stuff is actually good for your kid. Master the mix and your kid will be the envy of every mystery-meat-eating student in the second grade.

Dependable Drink
This is a high-stakes decision that few parents really think about. Considering that many kids' beverages have nearly as much sugar per ounce as soft drinks, tossing the wrong drink in the lunchbox could translate into 3 to 5 extra pounds by the end of the school year. Drinks should be either zero- or low-cal (water, diet drinks), high in nutrition (milk, 100 percent juice), or both (tea). Here are the best picks, in descending order.

· Water
· Lightly sweetened iced tea, like Honest Tea
· Low-fat milk
· 100 percent juice drinks
· Low-calorie kids' drinks, like Minute Maid Fruit Falls and Tropicana Fruit Squeeze

Sturdy Anchor
Avoid a lunch built on refined carbohydrates, as the intake of quick-burning carbs will leave your kid with an energy and attention deficit for the rest of the day. Focus instead on

9 Romano's Macaroni Grill Fettuccine Alfredo

- *890 calories*
- *67 g fat (38 g saturated)*
- *1,480 mg sodium*

This plate of noodles has 2 days' worth of saturated fat—for a full-grown adult! For a kid, this could serve as a precursor for obesity. And to make matters worse, Macaroni Grill likes to throw in a free ice cream with every kid's meal. They sure don't make it easy to be a responsible parent.

Eat This Instead!

Cheeseoli

- *440 calories • 20 g fat (12 g saturated)*
- *1,280 mg sodium*

WORST MEXICAN MEAL

8 On the Border Kids' Bean and Cheese Nachos

- *980 calories*
- *57 g fat (29 g saturated)*
- *1,850 mg sodium*

On the Border's Beef Soft Taco meal has been downsized just enough to keep it from topping our list this year. But we've spotted several other troubling dishes in the kids' domain, especially this plate of nachos. It's hard to imagine how chips, cheese, and beans are transformed into a day and a half worth of saturated fat, but once you see the train wrecks on the adult side of the menu, you begin to understand.

Eat This Instead!

Kids' Grilled Chicken with black beans

- *310 calories • 9 g fat (3 g saturated)*
- *1,230 mg sodium*

---

protein, fiber, and healthy fats that will help keep your kid satisfied, keep his metabolism running high, and provide some important nutrients, too.
- Turkey or roast beef and Swiss on wheat bread (sans mayo, but loaded with produce, if you can get away with it)
- Sliced ham, cheese, and Triscuits
- PB&J (made on whole wheat bread with a pure-fruit jelly like Smucker's Simply Fruit)
- Thermos of hot soup

- Grilled chicken breast
- Hard-boiled eggs
- Tuna or cubed chicken tossed with light mayo, mustard, celery, and carrot

Sides with Substance

Only 1 in 4 kids consumes the recommended 5 servings of fruits and vegetables daily, so pack a lunch sans produce and you're missing a golden opportunity to slip some much-needed nutrients back into their diets. As long as you have at least 1 piece of fruit or

a serving of vegetables, adding a second crunchy snack is fine.
- Carrot sticks
- Celery sticks
- Apple slices with peanut butter
- Fruit salad
- Banana, pear, peach, or any other whole fruit
- Olives
- Almonds and raisins (mixed 50–50)
- Triscuits
- Small bag of pretzel sticks or Goldfish pretzels
- Baked! Lay's

Low-Impact Treat

You've gotta give them something they can brag to their friends about, right? A treat should have no trans fats, less than 12 grams of sugar, and no more than 100 calories. If you can eke some extra nutrition out of it, all the better.
- Fruit leather
- Squeezable yogurt
- Low-fat, low-sugar chocolate pudding
- Sugar-free Jell-O
- Rice Krispies Treats
- A square of chocolate

The Worst Foods for Kids in America

WORST PIZZA
7 Uno Chicago Grill Kid's Deep Dish Pepperoni Pizza

- *980 calories*
- *70 g fat (20 g saturated)*
- *1,860 mg sodium*

We analyzed every kids' pizza in every chain restaurant in America, and these sloppy slices beat out the next closest competitor by 27 grams of fat. Calorie-wise, it's like eating more than two whole boxes of Bagel Bites.

Eat This Instead!
Macaroni and Cheese
- *480 calories • 16 g fat (5 g saturated)*
- *1,200 mg sodium*

WORST CHICKEN MEAL
6 Chili's Pepper Pals Little Chicken Crispers with Ranch and Homestyle Fries

- *1,010 calories*
- *75 g fat (13 g saturated)*
- *1,780 mg sodium*

A moderately active 8-year-old kid should eat around 1,600 calories a day. This single meal plows through about 65 percent of that allotment. Unless he plans on munching on nothing but celery the rest of the day, he ought to plan on skipping the country-fried crispers.

Eat This Instead!
Pepper Pals Grilled Chicken Platter with Cinnamon Apples
- *340 calories • 8 g fat (2.5 g saturated)*
- *755 mg sodium*

WORST FINGER FOOD
5 Denny's Little Dipper Sampler with Honey Mustard Dressing Dipping Sauce and Deep Space French Fries

- *1,030 calories*
- *61 g fat (15 g saturated)*
- *1,590 mg sodium*

Nuggets, mozzarella sticks, and fries make an unholy trinity of sodium and saturated fat. Parents can choose the convenience of giving their tots something that doesn't require a fork to eat, but not if it delivers two-thirds of the kid's daily calories.

Eat This Instead!
Moons & Stars Chicken Nuggets with BBQ Sauce and Moon Crater Mashed Potatoes and Gravy
- *430 calories • 17 g fat (3.5 g saturated)*
- *1,480 mg sodium*

WORST DRINK
4 Baskin-Robbins Small Snickers Shake

- *1,040 calories*
- *50 g fat (26 g saturated, 1 g trans)*
- *112 g sugars*

Baskin-Robbins has a whole line of these candy-themed shakes to help nudge your child toward a lifetime of elevated blood sugar. How they manage to fit so much fat and sugar into a 16-ounce cup is a mystery of modern food science. This one's the equivalent of nearly 4 whole Snickers bars. You're better off giving your kid the real candy.

Drink This Instead!
Small Strawberry Citrus Fruit Blast
- *350 calories • 1 g fat (0 g saturated)*
- *85 g sugars*

WORST DRIVE-THRU MEAL
3 Burger King Kids Double Cheeseburger with Small Fries and Coke

- *1,100 calories, • 52 g fat (17.5 g saturated, 1.5 g trans)*
- *1,870 mg sodium*

BK's double beef earns the distinction of being the

As America's worst side dish for kids, these creepy Smiley Face Potatoes are no laughing matter.

524 calories
Bob Evans Smiley Face Potatoes

Best and Worst Cafeteria Breakfasts

BEST CAFETERIA BREAKFASTS
Scrambled eggs and bacon

· 250 calories
· 10 g fat (4 g saturated)
· 550 mg sodium

A study from St. Louis University found that people starting their day with eggs consumed 264 fewer calories than people eating bagels for breakfast. The reason? Protein and good fat are important elements of satiety, working diligently to keep your kid's belly full and prevent those midmorning cravings that lead to empty-calorie consumption.

Apple-cinnamon oatmeal

· 280 calories
· 3 g fat (0 g saturated)
· 5 g carbohydrates

True, the calories from oatmeal come mostly from carbohydrates, but with each bowl comes a dose of soluble fiber, which helps slow the absorption of the carbs, keeping kids' blood sugar levels—and thus their energy and concentration levels—more stable.

Ham and egg on an English muffin

· 240 calories
· 8 g fat (3 g saturated)
· 610 mg sodium

Not even the most malicious cafeteria cook could mess this one up: low-calorie bread, an egg, and a few slices of lean ham. Protein and healthy fat are two great ways to wake up; the only thing that's missing is fiber, and that can be corrected easily enough by using a whole-grain English muffin.

WORST CAFETERIA BREAKFASTS
Sausage biscuit

· 400 calories
· 22 g fat
  (12 g saturated, 3 g trans)
· 1,100 mg sodium

Here's the standard biscuit recipe: flour, lard, buttermilk. So it's not hard to imagine how this greasy, sausage-stuffed breakfast sandwich packs such a wallop. The fact that biscuits are one of the biggest transporters of trans fat only makes the need to avoid this breakfast bomb all the more vital.

French toast with syrup and margarine

· 450 calories
· 18 g fat (5 g saturated)
· 67 g carbohydrates

The only thing vaguely nutritious about French toast is the egg in which the bread is battered, but even that is drowned out by a flood of melted margarine and sugary syrup.

Bagel with jelly

· 390 calories
· 12 g fat (1 g saturated)
· 385 mg sodium

Bagels may look harmless, but behind each bite is a mouthful of refined carbohydrates. When a flood of quick-burning carbs enters the bloodstream, blood sugars rise rapidly and your body panics and begins to store fat. Jelly only makes matters worse, since most jellies found in school cafeterias have more sugar in them than fruit.

fattest meal for an on-the-go kid. It has 18 more grams of fat than the same meal at McDonald's. The meal might be quick, but it takes a long time for a 90-pound child to burn all those calories.

Eat This Instead!
Kraft Macaroni and Cheese with Apple Fries, Caramel Dipping Sauce, and Low-Fat Milk

· 340 calories · 8 g fat (3 g saturated)
· 505 mg sodium

WORST CHINESE ENTREE
2 P.F. Chang's Crispy Honey Chicken on Brown Rice

· 1,210 calories
· 51 g fat (9 g saturated)
· 610 mg sodium

Although P.F. Chang's doesn't offer a proper kids' menu, this is the item it identifies on its menu as the "Kids' #1 Favorite." As a single entrée, this dish will saddle your child with two-thirds of her day's calories and nearly an entire day's worth of fat. They put the lazy Susan on the tables at Chang's for a reason; these dishes need to be shared.

Eat This Instead!
Almond and Cashew Chicken on Brown Rice

· *294 calories* · *10 g fat (2 g saturated)*
· *1,694 mg sodium*

THE WORST KIDS' MEAL IN AMERICA

1 Uno Chicago Grill Kid's Kombo with French Fries

· *1,270 calories*
· *79 g fat (11.5 g saturated)*
· *2,850 mg sodium*

For food marketers, the color of money isn't green—it's beige. Any parent knows that most foods kids clamor for, from fries to white bread to chicken nuggets, come in beige. It's also a marker of cheap, calorie-rich, nutritionally bankrupt foodstuffs. So when you see this monochromatic cluster of cheese sticks, dinosaur-shaped chicken, and fried potatoes, you know your kid's in trouble. Make it a rule when eating out: All dishes must come with at least two colors (and ketchup doesn't count).

Eat This Instead!
Kid's Pasta

· *300 calories* · *3 g fat (0 g saturated)*
· *270 mg sodium*

Best and Worst Cafeteria Lunches

BEST CAFETERIA LUNCHES

Roast beef and gravy

· *240 calories*
· *11 g fat (4 g saturated)*
· *625 mg sodium*

Made from a lean cut of beef, a few slices of roast beef prove to be a relatively low-fat, low-calorie source of protein. And since cafeteria gravies are invariably of the "instant" variety, the only minor threat they pose is of adding a bit of extra sodium to the meal.

Chili with shredded cheese

· *300 calories*
· *12 g fat (4 g saturated)*
· *570 mg sodium*

This cheesy, gooey mess is actually good for your kid? Hard to believe, but beyond being packed with enough protein to keep her full and focused the rest of the school day, a bean-laced bowl of red gives your kid plenty of fiber and disease-fighting antioxidants. Tastes great, is more filling, fights against cancer. What more could you want?

Grilled chicken sandwich

· *280 calories*
· *10 g fat (2 g saturated)*
· *550 mg sodium*

The nonfried corollary to one of the cafeteria's most ubiquitous items is about as good as it gets. Skip the mayo in favor of ketchup, mustard, or barbecue sauce and, with any luck, your kid will welcome the addition of a bit of produce.

Tater Tots

· *150 calories*
· *7 g fat (1 g saturated)*
· *200 mg sodium*

Cafeteria Tots usually avoid the harsh fry treatment in favor of a simple bake, which keeps the calorie count down.

WORST CAFETERIA LUNCHES

Turkey wrap

· *375 calories*
· *14 g fat (5 g saturated)*
· *575 mg sodium*

Wraps start with the dreaded tortilla, to which the lunch ladies add fatty dressing (usually ranch or Italian), cheese (usually processed), and produce (usually token shreds of lettuce).

French bread cheese pizza

· *440 calories*
· *19 g fat (8 g saturated)*
· *930 mg sodium*

The thick, doughy crust used by most school cafeterias packs on a heavy carb and sodium load, plus it provides the structural integrity for a haphazard application of cheese, doubling down on the calorie count.

Crispy chicken sandwich

· *400 calories*
· *19 g fat (7 g saturated)*
· *735 mg sodium*

If they're going to take an innocent chicken breast, bread it, deep-fry it, and cover it in mayo, your kid may as well opt for the hamburger.

French fries

· *310 calories*
· *18 g fat (7 g saturated)*
· *400 mg sodium*

French fries probably won't be lucky enough to avoid the boiling oil, where they soak up most of their saturated fat. More often than not, they contain as many calories as the entrée sharing the plate with them.

The Best Kids' Meals

WIN THE WAR ON THEIR WAISTLINES WITH THESE TASTY STANDBYS

BEST KIDS' MEAL

Uno Chicago Grill Kid's Grilled Chicken with Apples and Mandarin Oranges

- *185 calories*
- *4 g fat (0 g saturated)*
- *600 mg sodium*
- *31 g protein*

Oddly enough, the restaurant that serves the Worst Kids' Meal in America also serves one of the best. This meal is just about perfect. It offers a massive dose of protein to help your child grow, it keeps the sodium to an acceptable level, and it does it all in under 200 calories. If only all their meals were so reliable.

BEST PASTA

Fazoli's Spaghetti with Marinara and Broccoli

- *295 calories*
- *1.5 g fat (0 g saturated)*
- *930 mg sodium*
- *7 g fiber*

Here's what's great about Fazoli's kids' menu: It offers proper portion sizes, all around 8 ounces or less of food. And if you ask, you can get vegetables added on top. Once the greens are covered in antioxidant-loaded marinara, your child won't even know he's eating right. That's what we call health food in disguise.

BEST DRIVE-THRU MEAL

McDonald's Chicken McNuggets with Apple Dippers, Caramel Dip, and 1% Low-Fat Milk

- *395 calories*
- *15 g fat (3.5 g saturated)*
- *560 mg sodium*
- *18 g protein*

McDonald's may be synonymous with cheap, often-bad-for-you food, but to be fair, the fast-food purveyor has spent a lot of time trying to clean up its act, and it might have finally succeeded. This meal cuts out the trans fat completely, and by subbing apple dippers for fries, it offers your child a nice dose of vitamins and fiber.

BEST PIZZA

Domino's Crunchy Thin Crust Cheese Pizza (2 slices)

- *278 calories*
- *14 g fat (5 g saturated)*
- *480 mg sodium*

There's an important lesson to be learned here: Kids' menus are often less healthy than adult fare, especially when it comes to pizza. Places like Così and Uno offer kids their own personal pie, but that translates into adult-like serving sizes and big caloric costs. More often than not, a few slices of Mom and Dad's pizza will serve them better—especially when that pizza is as restrained as Domino's thin crust standby.

in America

BEST SNACK
Au Bon Pain Cheddar, Fruit, and Crackers

- 200 calories
- 12 g fat (6 g saturated)
- 280 mg sodium

You won't find this meal on the kids' menu. Instead it's located on our all-time favorite menu category: Au Bon Pain's Portions menu. It's loaded with small-appetite selections like this, and it's the perfect spot to find a meal proportioned to your little one's little appetite. You might even find a little something for yourself.

BEST TREAT
Rice Krispies Treat

- 90 calories
- 2.5 g fat (1 g saturated)
- 7 g sugars

No, it's not loaded with nutrients, but what treats are? Instead, what you get is a kid-favorite sweet with 200 fewer calories than most candy bars, which makes it ideal for a little reward or impromptu dessert.

278 calories
Two slices of Domino's Thin Crust Cheese Pizza

Domino's is home to the lowest calorie slice we've found from any national pizza peddler. Keep it thin, and if you can persuade the little ones to add a few vegetables to the pie, all the better.

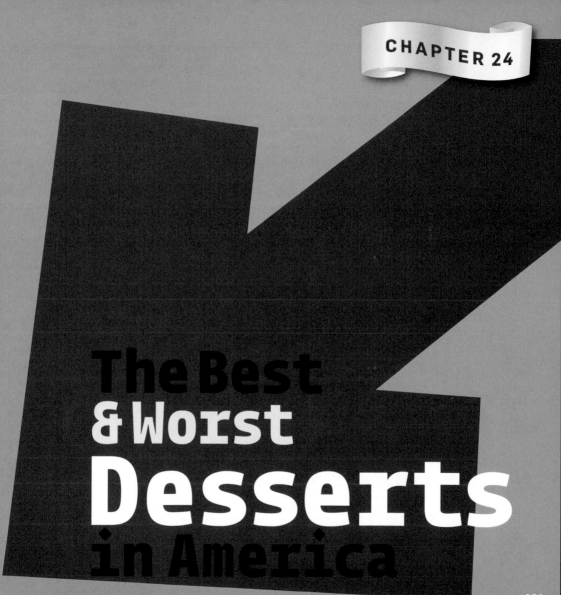

CHAPTER 24

The Best
& Worst
Desserts
in America

Eat This

Chili's Sweet Shot Key Lime Pie

*240 calories
12 g fat (8 g saturated)
30 g carbohydrates*

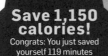

Save 1,150 calories!
Congrats: You just saved yourself 119 minutes on the treadmill.

Save 57 g fat!
You could knock back 5 shots of key lime pie and still cut calories and fat.

1,390 calories
69 g fat
205 g carbohydrates

Not That!

Red Robin Mountain High Mudd Pie

You'd be better off eating 9 scoops of Breyers All Natural Rocky Road ice cream.

Red Robin's Jackson Pollock imitation suffers from the disease afflicting all too many restaurant desserts in this country: gigantism. Split among 4 forks, it would still ruin even the healthiest meal eaten before it.

Indulgence.

It's part of what makes life worth living—giving in to temptation, letting go of one's inhibitions.

We all need an occasional crazy blowout, but in today's society, it's hard to find a reasonable, happy medium. We're bombarded constantly with competing messages about food and the nature of indulgence. One message says, "You must diet, exercise, feel the burn, stay hungry, and keep your body-fat percentage in the non-existent range or else you're a failure." The other message says, "Sugar-coated, cream-filled, chocolaty goodness three for a dollar—you gotta have it or you're missing out!"

So, like anyone who is constantly sold two wildly different value systems, we get pretty darn confused. After all, how are we supposed to supersize our food and downsize our bodies at the same time? No wonder we find ourselves in an ongoing cycle of splurge-guilt-purge.

It doesn't need to be this way. See, people have been happily indulging in cakes and cookies and ice cream for thousands of years. Yet the obesity crisis—and the accompanying rise in diabetes and heart disease rates—has only come into being in the past 30 years or so.

Why? Because the simple, delicious, indulgent desserts of previous generations have been replaced with monstrosity versions of themselves. Like Bruce Banner getting hit with a dose of gamma rays, today's desserts have become giant Hulk-like incarnations of once-innocent delights, thanks to all the added fats, sugars, and chemicals. And if you make the wrong choice, indulging once can be the caloric equivalent of indulging two, three, or four times.

Here, you'll learn how to indulge more often but with less damage. You could literally have dessert after most dinners and still stay slim or have dessert once a week and grow fat. How? Simply by knowing the truth about America's Best and Worst Desserts!

360 calories
Häagen-Dazs Chocolate Peanut Butter (½ cup)

Ever have one of those days when you can't wait to drown your sorrow in a pint of chocolaty ice cream? Make it this pint and you'll have gained nearly half a pound of body fat by the time you take the last spoonful.

The Worst Desserts in America

13 Tofutti Vanilla (½ cup)

- *210 calories*
- *13 g fat (2 g saturated)*
- *15 g sugars*

The label touts the fact that Tofutti has no butterfat and no cholesterol. While these claims are technically true (Tofutti is not made from dairy, so by definition it can't have butterfat or cholesterol), they might as well advertise "no razor blades inside!" Because touting what's not in this product simply obscures the truth about what is: Tofutti is as loaded with fat and sugar as most full-fledged ice creams. (It also has about 10 ingredients too many, including a big helping of corn oil.) If you're looking for an honest, low-calorie nondairy ice cream, stick with It's Soy Delicious; their whole line of products is great, and you'll cut your calorie intake nearly in half.

Eat This Instead!
It's Soy Delicious Vanilla (½ cup)

- *110 calories · 1.5 g fat (0 g saturated)*
- *9 g sugars*

12 Häagen-Dazs Chocolate Peanut Butter (½ cup)

- *360 calories*
- *24 g fat (11 g saturated)*
- *24 g sugars*

Häagen-Dazs produces their ice creams using only a few simple ingredients; problem is, those ingredients are heavy cream, egg yolks, and sugar, making their ice creams consistently the most calorie-dense in the freezer section. This peanut-butter blast to your gut takes the cake—literally—packing an astounding 1,440 calories into every pint-size carton. Compare it with what Breyers has to offer, for a third of the calories. Wouldn't you rather have dessert three times, instead of just once? You can, if you make the right choice.

Eat This Instead!
Breyers All Natural Vanilla and Chocolate

- *130 calories · 7 g fat (4.5 g saturated)*
- *15 g sugars*

11 Einstein Bros. Iced Sugar Cookie

- *480 calories*
- *15 g fat (6 g saturated)*
- *46 g sugars*

This iced sugar cookie has as much sugar as 2½ Twinkies and more calories than a McDonald's Quarter Pounder. Indulging too often in a fearsome flood of sugar like this can set you up for insulin resistance later on, the first step in a long, sad march toward diabetes. Much better to snack when you want but to keep the portion size down so you don't wallop your body all at once with a giant caloric hit. That's why the decadent, but mini, chocolate mudslide is a solid choice.

Eat This Instead!
Mini Chocolate Mudslide Cookie

- *160 calories · 8 g fat (4.5 g saturated)*
- *19 g sugars*

1,610 calories

Baskin-Robbins York Peppermint Pattie Brownie Sundae

It's bad enough to build an entire dessert around a candy bar, but then you throw in a brownie, too? The only safe strategy at Baskin-Robbins is to stick to the straight ice cream. Single scoop.

The Worst Desserts in America

WORST PACKAGED DESSERT
10 Toll House Chocolate Chip Ice Cream Sandwich

- *520 calories*
- *23 g fat (9 g saturated)*
- *44 g sugars*

Do you really want more than a quarter of your day's calories to come from an ice-cream novelty? If you're going to take in this much fat and calories in a single sitting, it had better be dinner. There are too many solid indulgences in the freezer section to fall back on this bad habit.

Eat This Instead!
Breyers Oreo Ice Cream Sandwich
- *170 calories • 6 g fat (2.5 g saturated)*
- *13 g sugars*

WORST ICE CREAM
9 Cold Stone Creamery Nutter Butter Ice Cream, Gotta Have It size (large)

- *940 calories*
- *59 g fat*
  (30 g saturated, 1 g trans)
- *84 g sugars*

Wow. If you strapped a hand grenade to a stick of dynamite and put it in a nitroglycerin bath, you'd have a good idea of the kind of caloric energy that this ice cream is packing. That's great if you're planning to run a marathon the next day, but not if you're waking up and going to work. This monstrous serving delivers a payload of nearly half your daily calories and has the saturated fat equivalent of 30 strips of bacon. The sugar shock is equally terrifying— as much as you'd find in 4 packs of peanut M&Ms. The good news is that Cold Stone offers a number of reasonable choices on its menu. Choose any of the "sinless" options and you'll consume only a tenth of the sugars and a sixth of the calories.

Eat This Instead!
Sinless Sans Fat Sweet Cream Ice Cream, Like It size (small)
- *140 calories • 0 g fat • 9 g sugars*

3 Steps to Dessert Nirvana

The best way to cut calories from your dessert tab is to replace the slices of store-bought pies, cakes, and brownies with simple, honest sweets that can be made at home in minutes. Consider any of these three unconventional desserts blueprints for a delicious, relatively healthy end to a meal.

1 Combine a pint of sliced strawberries with $\frac{1}{4}$ cup of good-quality balsamic vinegar. Let the fruit macerate for at least 15 minutes, then serve over a scoop of vanilla ice cream or hunk of angel food cake for an enlightened strawberry shortcake.

2 Place a scoop of ice cream in a chilled bowl and drizzle $\frac{1}{2}$ tablespoon of fruity olive oil over the top. Sprinkle with a few coarse crystals of sea salt. Trust us; the salty-sweet-savory combination is amazing.

3 Place peaches halves directly on a hot grill. At the same time, grill wedges of angel food cake until lightly charred and crispy. Serve half a grilled peach with each piece of hot cake and top with a small dollop of whipped cream.

8 Ruby Tuesday Strawberries and Ice Cream

- *1,009 calories*
- *62 g fat*
- *99 g carbohydrates*

What could be so wrong about a bowl of strawberries and a scoop of ice cream? Turns out plenty, when placed in the reckless hands of the line cooks over at Ruby Tuesday. First off, the serving size is predictably and unreasonably massive. Then, they encapsulate the whole concoction in a buttery, fat-strewn shell of puff pastry, ratcheting up the calorie and fat counts into the stratospheric levels. If you must have something sweet before signing the bill, stick to the good old-fashioned chocolate chip cookies.

Eat This Instead!
Chocolate Chip Cookies

- *320 calories · 15 g fat*
- *40 g carbohydrates*

WORST DRIVE-THRU DESSERT
7 Dairy Queen Raspberry Truffle Blizzard (large)

- *1,140 calories*
- *44 g fat*
  (31 g saturated, 1 g trans)
- *141 g sugars*

The decadent offerings at DQ span the nutritional spectrum, ranging from smart indulgences to caloric catastrophes and everything in between. So choose wisely or you'll end up wolfing down two-thirds of your daily caloric allotment without ever leaving the driver's seat. Being smart at DQ means skipping over the malts and Blizzards entirely and opting instead for a relatively restrained sundae. Stick to a small and you can have any flavor your hungry heart desires.

Eat This Instead!
Small Strawberry Sundae

- *260 calories*
- *7 g fat (4.5 g saturated, 0 g trans)*
- *36 g sugars*

The Ultimate At-Home, Make-It-Yourself Indulgence

Even the most carefully prepared restaurant dessert could never contend with a true homemade masterpiece. This one combines our favorite store-bought ice cream (at just 130 calories a scoop) with a one-two punch of delicious fruit and the heart-healthy fats and antioxidants of walnuts. Oh, and did we mention it's totally delicious? That's the best part!

½ cup Breyers All Natural Vanilla Ice Cream

½ banana, sliced

6 strawberries, sliced

1 Tbsp hot fudge

1 Tbsp chopped walnuts

1 maraschino cherry

- *300 calories · 11 g fat (3.5 g saturated fat) · 23 g sugars*

Place the ice cream in a chilled bowl and scatter the fruit around it. Drizzle the hot fudge, scatter the walnuts, and top it all with a cherry.

The Worst Desserts in America

6 Red Robin Mountain High Mudd Pie

- *1,390 calories*
- *69 g fat*
  (unknown saturated and trans)
- *205 g carbohydrates*

You're surprised that a "mountain high" dessert packs in the caloric equivalent of 7 Crunchy Taco Supremes from Taco Bell? Red Robin doesn't list sugar content in its nutrition information, but based on the 205 grams of carbohydrates, you can bet that it's well over 100 grams of the sweet stuff (not to mention, oddly enough, nearly 1,000 milligrams of sodium—half as much salt as you should eat in a whole day!). Unfortunately, Red Robin doesn't offer any reasonable pie alternatives. The good news is that you can enjoy a (slightly modified) sundae without completely destroying your diet.

Eat This Instead!
Birthday Sundae with Peanuts and Whipped Cream
- *312 calories • 17 g fat*
- *49 g carbohydrates*

WORST CAKE
5 Red Lobster Chocolate Wave

- *1,490 calories*
- *81 g fat (25 g saturated)*
- *172 g carbohydrates*

Chocolate Tidal Wave is more like it: This fat-packed mega-cake accounts for three-quarters of your daily calories and as many carbohydrates as you'll find in 14 slices of white bread. (Just sit and digest that statistic for a second.) The dessert menu at Red Lobster isn't great—2 out of 5 options break the 1,000-calorie mark, and the "lightest" choice is a little over half that—but if you split the cheesecake with a friend, you could eat a delicious dessert without bursting from your pants when you're done.

Eat This Instead!
New York–Style Cheesecake with Strawberries
- *520 calories • 36 g fat (21 g saturated)*
- *270 mg sodium • 39 g carbohydrates*

WORST CHOCOLATE DESSERT
4 Chili's Chocolate Chip Paradise Pie

- *1,590 calories*
- *76 g fat (37 g saturated)*
- *220 g carbohydrates*

Here is empirical evidence that food marketers are making our food worse and worse: In 2008, we listed this chocolate pie as the Worst Dessert in America. In 2009, it doesn't even take the bronze! Yet this hulking slice still packs as many calories as 3 Big Macs. That's right: Nobody would ever consider capping a meal with 3 Macs, so why would they order a slice of this stuff? When choosing dessert at Chili's, the only safe options are the Sweet Shots, drinkable treats with built-in portion control. Avoid the chocolate one, which rings in at 420 calories; any of the others should be fine.

Eat This Instead!
Sweet Shot Red Velvet Cake
- *250 calories • 9 g fat (4.5 g saturated)*
- *39 g carbohydrates*

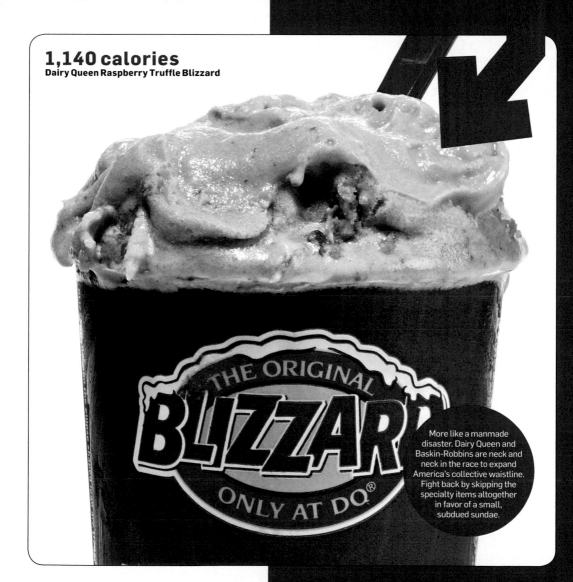

1,140 calories
Dairy Queen Raspberry Truffle Blizzard

More like a manmade disaster. Dairy Queen and Baskin-Robbins are neck and neck in the race to expand America's collective waistline. Fight back by skipping the specialty items altogether in favor of a small, subdued sundae.

The Worst Desserts in America

3 Uno Chicago Grill Chocolate Peanut Butter Cup

- *1,600 calories*
- *104 g fat*
  (42 g saturated)
- *110 g sugars*
- *142 g carbohydrates*

You'd have to eat a dozen Reese's Peanut Butter Cups to take in as many calories as you do with this one peanut butter bomb. Uno's entrée options are terrifying enough, so to avoid further calamity, learn to do dessert the right way. You really have only 2 options that you won't need to split with a hungry crew, and both are labeled "mini." But just because they're labeled mini doesn't mean you shouldn't share with your hungry comrades.

Eat This Instead!
Mini Hot Chocolate Brownie Sundae
- *370 calories • 16 g fat (8 g saturated)*
- *38 g sugars • 54 g carbohydrates*

2 Baskin-Robbins York Peppermint Pattie Brownie Sundae

- *1,610 calories*
- *80 g fat*
  (32 g saturated, 1 g trans)
- *183 g sugars*
- *222 g carbohydrates*

Warning: Not a single sundae from Baskin-Robbins contains less than 500 calories. Furthermore, anything with chocolate that can be sucked through a straw should be avoided at all costs. That means the only real viable route at the popular dessert parlor is to stick with a single scoop of ice cream. (At least you'll have 31 flavors to choose from.)

Eat This Instead!
Made with Snickers Ice Cream (4 ounces)
- *290 calories*
- *15 g fat (8 g saturated, 0 g trans)*
- *31 g sugars • 36 g carbohydrates*

1 Romano's Macaroni Grill New York Cheesecake with Caramel Fudge Sauce

- *1,660 calories*
- *97 g fat (57 g saturated)*
- *950 mg sodium*
- *165 g carbohydrates*

Considering the fact that Macaroni Grill's savory menu is already cluttered with one of the country's most potent arrays of calorie, fat, and sodium bombs, its lineup of destructive desserts only adds insult to injury. There's the Dessert Ravioli (1,630 calories), the Lemon Passion (1,360 calories), and the always classic and catastrophic caramel-smothered cheesecake, which, with more calories than 3 Big Macs and as much saturated fat as 57 strips of bacon, is the worst dessert in America. Seek solace in a scoop of sorbetto—one of the country's best sit-down sweets.

Eat This Instead!
Italian Sorbetto with Biscotti
- *240 calories • 1 g fat (0.5 g saturated)*
- *58 g carbohydrates*

1,660 calories
Romano's Macaroni Grill New York Cheesecake

What makes cheesecake such a guaranteed calamity? Start with two of the planet's most calorie-dense ingredients—cream cheese and sugar—then whisk in egg yolks and sour cream. Finish with a butter-soaked crust and a chocolate drizzle.

The Best Desserts in

THERE'S NOTHING GUILTY ABOUT THESE WELL-PROPORTIONED PLEA

BEST SUPERMARKET ICE CREAM

Breyers All Natural Vanilla and Chocolate

(½ cup)

- 130 calories
- 7 g fat
  (4.5 g saturated)
- 15 g sugars

Many light ice cream lines cram their ingredient list full of strange emulsifiers, stabilizers, and artificial sweeteners, turning a simple indulgence into a science experiment. We love the Breyers All Natural line because it delivers great-tasting, low-calorie scoops with a pretty honest list of ingredients. Choose your favorite flavor and have at it; you really can't go wrong.

BEST LIGHT DESSERT

Romano's Macaroni Grill Sorbetto with Biscotti

- 240 calories
- 1 g fat
  (0.5 g saturated)
- 58 g carbohydrates

Macaroni Grill shows a dose of atypical restraint with this Italian take on cookies and ice cream. Sorbets in general are usually a safe call for dessert; since they're dairy free, they're also nearly fat free and lower in calories than most ice creams. Enjoy: It's the only dessert on the menu that you don't have to divide among a legion of eaters.

BEST SUNDAE

Uno Chicago Grill Mini Hot Chocolate Brownie Sundae

- 370 calories
- 16 g fat
  (8 g saturated)
- 54 g carbohydrates

BEST FROZEN BAR

Natural Choice Full of Fruit Organic Strawberry

- 60 calories
- 0 g fat
- 13 g sugars

The organic strawberries and strawberry puree in this bar contain a heaping load of disease-fighting antioxidants.

BEST MINI DESSERT

Chili's Sweet Shot Key Lime Pie

- 240 calories
- 12 g fat
  (8 g saturated)
- 30 g carbohydrates

Most restaurant desserts creep into the 4-digit calorie range for one reason: portion distortion. But Chili's has smartly addressed the problem by inventing this line of miniature sweets based around classic dessert flavors. Perhaps it's their penance for providing a menu otherwise awash in sugary sins. Either way, a shot of this stuff is a fairly safe bet, as far as nightcaps go.

America

SURES. FIND OUT FOR YOURSELF

BEST DRINKABLE DESSERT

Starbucks Grande Cinnamon Dolce Frappuccino Light Blended Coffee

- 140 calories
- 5 g fat
  (0.5 g saturated)
- 21 g sugars

Not all frappuccinos were created equal. Exhibit A: The 750-calorie Strawberries and Cream, which is one of the worst drinks in America. But this cinnamon-flavored sippable is sweet enough to qualify as dessert but restrained enough to not do any real damage to a day of careful eating. If you like blended coffee drinks, make this your go-to.

BEST DESSERT SPLURGE

Dairy Queen Banana Split

- 520 calories
- 13 g fat
  (10 g saturated)
- 73 g sugars

You'll be lucky to find another banana split in this country with fewer than 800 calories, so consider this DQ creation a sweet deal when it comes time to do some serious splurging. But seriously, the banana split thing can develop into a nasty habit, so limit yourself to one a month.

370 calories
**Uno Chicago Grill
Mini Hot Chocolate
Brownie Sundae**

In restaurant dessert vernacular, "mini" usually means just right. The rest of Uno's menu is weighed down by industrial-strength dessert bombs, but this sundae makes for a smart indulgence.

Index

Boldface page references indicate photographs.
<u>Underscored</u> references indicate boxed text and tables.

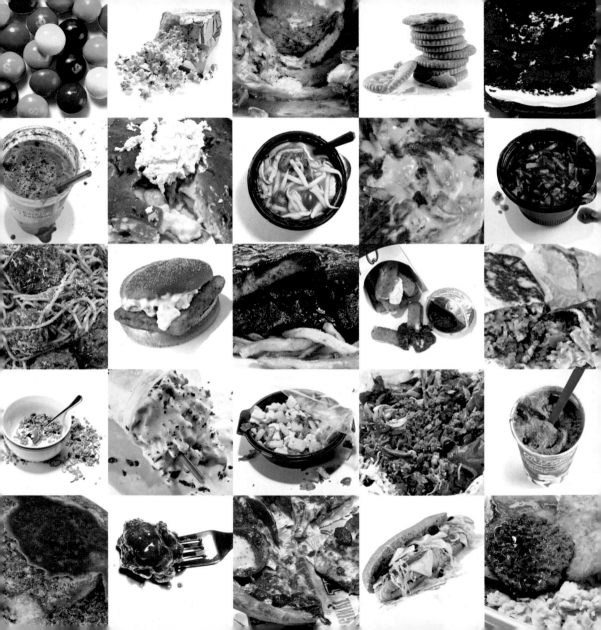